VOICE
TRADITION
AND
TECHNOLOGY

A State-of-the-Art Studio

VOICE
TRADITION
AND
TECHNOLOGY
A State-of-the-Art Studio

Garyth Nair

Associate Professor of Music
Drew University
Madison, New Jersey

SINGULAR PUBLISHING GROUP, INC.
SAN DIEGO

Singular Publishing Group, Inc.
401 West "A" Street, Suite 325
San Diego, California 92101-7904

Singular Publishing Group, Inc., publishes textbooks, clinical manuals, clinical reference books, journals, videos, and multimedia materials on speech-language pathology, audiology, otorhinolaryngology, special education, early childhood, aging, occupational therapy, physical therapy, rehabilitation, counseling, mental health, and voice. For your convenience, our entire catalog can be accessed on our website at **http://www.singpub.com**. Our mission to provide you with materials to meet the daily challenges of the ever-changing health care/educational environment will remain on course if we are in touch with you. In that spirit, we welcome your feedback on our products. Please telephone (**1-800-521-8545**), fax (**1-800-774-8398**), or e-mail (**singpub@singpub.com**) your comments and requests to us.

© 1999 by Garyth Nair

Typeset in 10/12 Stone Informal by So Cal Graphics
Printed in Canada by Transcontinental

Library of Congress Cataloging-in-Publication Data

Nair, Garyth
  Voice tradition and technology: a state-of-the-art studio/by Garyth Nair
      p.   cm.
    Includes bibliographical references and index.
    ISBN 0–7693–0028–6
    1. Singing—Instruction and study.   2. Voice culture.   3. User
interfaces (Computer systems)   I. Title
MT820.N292   1999
783'.00285—dc21
                                                          99–16180
                                                                CIP

CONTENTS

CHAPTER 10 THE NONPITCH CONSONANTS   153

CHAPTER 11 A SPECTROGRAPHIC MISCELLANY   169

CHAPTER 12 THE USE OF SPECTRUM ANALYSIS IN THE
VOICE STUDIO   189

CHAPTER 13 THE USE OF THE ELECTROGLOTTOGRAPH
IN THE VOICE STUDIO   211

Donald Miller and Harm K. Schutte

CHAPTER 14 SOME CONSIDERATIONS ON THE
SCIENCE OF SPECIAL CHALLENGES IN
VOICE TRAINING   227

Katherine Verdolini and David E. Krebs

FOREWORD

Garyth Nair's new book, *Voice Tradition and Technology: A State-of-the-Art Studio,* stands out as a milestone in the interdisciplinary evolution of vocal art and science. Throughout history, a few enlightened teachers have tried to make sense out of voice pedagogy. Unfortunately, little credible scientific and medical information has been available until the last two decades. During the 1980s and 1990s, however, dramatic advances have occurred in our knowledge of the anatomy and physiology of the voice, our ability to analyze and quantify voice function and dysfunction, the ability of physicians to diagnose and treat voice disorders (in collaboration with speech-language pathologists, singing voice specialists and others), and the evolution of interdisciplinary guidelines for healthy voice use to prevent the development of vocal pathology.

Although the recent developments have been based on interdisciplinary research in which voice teachers have collaborated in invaluable ways, most new publications have been driven by scientists and clinicians and published primarily for them. Garyth Nair is not a scientist, but rather a voice teacher, singer, and conductor. A few, farsighted voice teachers before him have attempted to integrate new knowledge and technology into the studio, including the pioneer in this field William Vennard at the University of Southern California, and more recently Richard Miller at Oberlin. Nair's new book represents the next logical (but giant) step in the practical integration of new knowledge into musical training. As such, it also holds an important place in the evolution of voice pedagogy literature.

Through the eyes of an enlightened, experienced voice pedagogue, this book synthesizes in simple terms many of the latest findings of voice science and medical research and teaches the reader how to apply them in a practical, accessible in the studio, way in order to enhance (not replace) traditional voice training. In the process, he provides a window for teachers and singers into the world of voice science and its language and a "how-to" guide for the teacher who wishes to advance his or her studio capabilities.

Perhaps more important, Nair also makes clear not merely the "how," but also the "why." He explains how techniques such as computer-assisted, real-time analysis can provide feedback to the teacher and student that expedites and enhances the training process in a natural way, serving as an important, additional tool in the armamentarium of a modern voice teacher.

Several special features enhance Nair's text. The book is accompanied by a CD-ROM package. In keeping with the message of the book, Nair has provided the first multimedia contribution toward understanding the relationship between voice, science, and voice pedagogy. The CD-ROM package is particularly helpful in elucidating and simplifying the practical uses of computer programs to augment traditional voice training. The interactive CD-ROM also contains a functional spectrogram/power spectrum, and spectrograms for all of the illustrations included in the book, substantially advancing the value of the text. In addition, Nair has included in the book contributions by Donald Miller and Harm K. Schutte on the use of spectrum analysis in the voice studio, Katherine Verdolini and David E. Krebs on the science of special challenges in voice training, and Robert A. Volin on the applications of computerized feedback systems to voice therapy and to the learning process. These invited contributions add information and scope that expand the value of the book for professionals in all disciplines.

Voice Tradition and Technology: A State-of-the-Art Studio is concise and engaging. It will enhance the library of anyone interested in voice, including not only teachers and singers, but also physicians, therapists, scientists, and others. It seems likely that it will be followed by future editions that update information in this rapidly changing field, and by books by other authors. Nevertheless, this initial offering will continue to hold a special place in the history of the evolution of voice pedagogy.

Robert Thayer Sataloff, M.D., D.M.A.
Chairman, Department of Otolaryngology—Head and Neck Surgery,
Graduate Hospital, Philadelphia, Pennsylvania
Professor of Otolaryngology—Head and Neck Surgery,
Department of Otolaryngology—Head and Neck Surgery,
Thomas Jefferson University, Philadelphia, Pennsylvania
Chairman, Board of Directors, The Voice Foundation

PREFACE

How wonderful life's path can be! As a youth, my two principle passions were music and biology. At the end of my high school education, I was faced with a decision on what life path to follow. I have never regretted the decision to pursue music, for I have had a rich life as a performer and teacher. Still, the love of science was always present around the periphery. I kept reading, observing, and pondering about things scientific, albeit at the level of an avocation.

With my plunge into voice science a number of years ago, those two youthful passions have merged. Biology (and physics) have achieved an ever-increasing significance in my career, leading up to the writing of this book.

PROJECT BACKGROUND

This project officially began in spring 1996 during a conversation with the chair of the music department at Drew University, Dr. Norman E. Lowrey. We discussed my dream of having spectrographic capability in my voice studio at Drew to enable me to begin experimentation with the use of computer-generated analysis as feedback in voice training. At the time, spectrographic software was prohibitively expensive, and we talked about finding a donor for the funds to help make the idea a reality.

Several weeks later, Dr. Lowrey handed me a floppy disk and asked, "Is this the kind of thing you're looking for?" On that disk was a copy of freeware he had found on the Internet, a program written by Richard Horne called Gram.

Gram was a fully functional, professional quality spectrogram. I was astounded by its functionality and by the fact that it was free. Experimenting at home, I spent countless fascinating hours exploring the workings of my own voice, correlating what was on the monitor with the principles of voice science. Several months after this experimentation began, a donor agreed to provide the computer equipment needed to bring the technology into our voice studio at Drew University. We launched this project with the establishment of a small voice lab in the Music Department.

After setting up the equipment and performing some tentative first experiments, the project quickly verified my long-held idea that the spectrogram could be used as feedback in teaching voice. But, with all my faith in the efficacy of its use, I still hadn't realized the scope of its potential application. Soon, I was taking careful notes on how the screen images could be employed in the day-to-day workings of the voice studio.

About the same time, Gram's creator, Richard Horne and I began corresponding via e-mail about possible changes to the program that could improve its applicability in the voice studio. His willingness, enthusiasm, and dogged determination to provide improvements were, and continue to be, a major contribution to this field.

SOME PRE-PROJECT HISTORY

As a singer as well as a teacher of singing, I have always been deeply interested in the details of fine vocal technique. This interest in how things work (not just the voice, but *everything*) was a lifetime gift from my father, a mechanic of considerable talent and skill. On countless occasions, he admonished, "You can't fix a machine until you understand how it works." That admonition applied directly to the act of singing—while not a machine, the voice is still a biomechanical instrument that obeys the laws of physics. Understanding the instrument and the physics underlying its correct operation was absolutely necessary to my philosophy of vocal pedagogy.

Much of the understanding of fluid dynamics needed for the understanding of the voice came from an unusual source. My good friend, Antoine du Bourg, a gifted teacher of physics and music at the Pingry School, taught me to sail. Tony bases his philosophy of sailing pedagogy on the premise that one has to know the physics of *how* a sailboat works in its environment in order to sail well. He permeates days of sailing with discussions of fluid dynamics: vectors, the Bernoulli effect, trailing edge separation and vortex production, angles of attack, lift, laminar flow, pressure gradients, and the like. The summer I learned to sail with Tony coincided with the beginnings of my study of voice science, and the synergy of understanding these principles of physics—in both sailing and science of voice—helped my vocal study immeasurably.

In this initial study, I read the available literature on the voice, quickly discarding sources that weren't based on solid science. The centerpiece of my early study was Vennard's seminal work, *Singing, the Mechanism and the Technic* (1968). Vennard's work with Janwillem Van den Berg at the Voice Research Lab of the University of Groningen gave him access to spectrographic technology. His book is peppered with numerous spectrograms that illustrate principles of voice science and specifics about vocal technique, which made his writing about voice science so compelling and clear. At last, I had found a work on vocal technique that was reinforced with objective criteria, not just personal opinion. Years later, when real-time spectrography was possible, I began to wonder if it could be used as an objective feedback device in the voice studio. When I had my first hands-on experience with a working real-time spectrograph, albeit for 5 precious minutes, the ideas that led to this book came closer to the surface. But, alas, when I looked into acquiring the technology, the cost proved to be prohibitive.

Much later, while reading Titze's *Principles of Voice Production*, this intriguing paragraph appeared at the end of a short section on the spectrogram:

> Vocologists are encouraged to become familiar with a sound spectrograph. It is an important tool for analysis that can be used not only for research but also for instantaneous feedback (sic) in vocal training and therapy. (Titze, 1994, p. 165)

That encouragement from so distinguished an authority put the proverbial "icing on the cake" and rekindled my desire to find a way to obtain a spectrograph.

THE NATURE OF THIS BOOK

The primary audience for this book is singers and teachers of singing. They are the constituency that might be most able to use both the information and pedagogical approach found here. For those without a background in voice science, two chapters near the beginning of the book present the basic physics of sound and human vocal production. As the reader delves deeper into the book and encounters the spectrographic examples, many facets of vocal technique will be explored. *It is not the purpose of this book to give an overview of the many traditions of vocal pedagogy, but to teach the reader how the spectrogram can be used in service of his or her own pedagogical approach.* Therefore, when inspecting the detailed presentations in the text, please remember that the examples given are of techniques that are used in my studio. They are meant to teach the *use* of the technology, not necessarily the method. (I will admit, however, that I would not be displeased if readers decided to adopt some of those pedagogical principles.)

Another audience that may find the book useful is the community of vocal therapists and professionals in related disciplines who may not have an extensive background in the use of the spectrogram, the power spectrum, or EGG. As the reader explores the detailed vocal principles shown by the spectrograms, he or she might consider a reevaluation of the use of spectrographic technology in everyday practice.

Voice scientists may also be interested in what is presented here. In the chapters that deal with detailed spectrographic analysis of vowels and consonants, some theories are presented that have not as yet been researched in the lab. There are many explanations of technical solutions, buttressed by spectrography, that work in the practical day-to-day voice studio but may seem incomplete to the knowledgeable voice scientist. It is hoped that they might become intrigued with some of the issues raised and tackle the theories presented in their own laboratories. I have tried to be careful about labeling these areas of conjecture and apologize if I missed any.

THE CD-ROM

The CD-ROM that accompanies this book is a critically important addition. First, it contains a fully functional copy of the spectrogram program used throughout the book so the reader can experiment with his or her own voice. It also contains a demonstration copy of VoceVista, the new software that allows detailed power spectrum, waveform, and EGG work.

With these programs on the disk, the reader will be able to experience real-time analysis of every computer-generated example printed in the book. Thus, the static images in the text will come alive as "living" sound and sight. When working with the imagery on the CD, the reader will be able to explore the powerful features of the programs by manipulating analytical parameters and viewing the results.

MALE/FEMALE DIFFERENCES IN SPECTROGRAM OUTPUT

In a later chapter, we deal with the differences in the appearance of the spectrographic output that exists between male and female voices. While there are some spectrograms made with female voices, most images are of the male bass-baritone voice (specifically, the author's). Time constraints dictated by the publication schedule meant that the author had to provide most of the sung examples. Through constant experimentation over the years, I have learned to do many of the "wrong" things one hears in the voice studio and, during the intense 10-month period in which this book was written, it was easier to perform these examples myself rather than search out those who possessed the problems naturally, or who could be quickly maltrained to produce the examples.

FINAL THOUGHT

The writing of this book has been an exhilarating experience for it has forced me to codify years of thinking about the voice. It is hoped that this effort will help others learn about voice science, the potential for the objectification of the principles of the technique of great singing, and the wonderful opportunities we have if we utilize computer-generated analysis of sound in the voice studio. If we work to truly "understand how the machine works," our attempts to "fix it" can only improve and the craft of singing with it.

ACKNOWLEDGMENTS

This book has many godparents, people who listened to my quasi-evangelical preaching about the subject and who, each in his or her own way, had an impact on the outcome. Aside from those individuals mentioned in the Preface, there are many others who have been involved with the production of this book.

Contributors

Richard Horne occupies a special place in this list. If it were not for his programming talent and his knowledge of acoustics, this book and the field it espouses would never have happened. We thank him for writing Gram, for having the generosity to make it free for all to use, and for his talent and discipline in tailoring the software for use in the voice studio. His appendix on the software controls that make Gram so flexible is also most helpful.

Donald Miller and Harm K. Schutte

Robert T. Sataloff

Robert A. Volin

Katherine Verdolini

David E. Krebs

Ron Nair, my talented artist brother, for the illustrations in the first chapter, the design of the book's cover, and for his constant assistance and patience in helping me learn the intricacies of several graphics software packages that have been so helpful in preparing the figures for this book.

Official Readers

Raymond Kent, who in the beginning stages, helped purify the basic voice science chapters, including a gentle education on the difference between an artichoke and an avocado.

Robert T. Sataloff for perusing the initial outline and rough draft as well as for his faith in the project and his willingness to be vocal about it. This included an invitation to present these ideas in a workshop at the 27th Annual Symposium: Care of the Professional Voice in June of 1998. That presentation, and the reaction to it, constituted a major turning point in the decision to write and publish this book.

Thomas Murry, reader and Singular consultant who supported my original proposal for the publication of the book.

Linda Carroll, who pulled me back from the brink of phonetic and vocal heresy on several occasions and who did the most detailed reading during the early stages of the writing.

Donald Miller, friend and colleague, who takes great delight in putting ideas through a fiery crucible. Don has played a major role in moving my rhetoric from the absolute positives of a voice teacher to the levened rhetoric of voice science.

If there are errors of fact or concept in this work, it is no fault of these dedicated readers; any faults are totally mine.

"Unofficial" Readers

Those who helped read or clarify portions of the manuscript:

Johan Sundberg

Ingo Titze

Three Affiliate Artist Teachers in the voice group of the Drew University Music Department:

Laura Greenwald, for her advice on the project, as well as for her faith and encouragement on the efficacy of using spectrographic feedback in the voice studio. Thanks are also due Laura for providing the voice for some of the spectrograms used in the book.

Geoffrey Friedley

Kevin M. Kelly, Drew alumnus, once my protégé, now a fine voice teacher in his own right.

Lynne Olsen, friend and confidant, who understood and, in many ways, enabled my almost maniacal obsession with this book. Her many days of proofing, correcting the manuscript, and chasing down references enabled this project to stay on schedule.

Students Who Were Subjects in the Lab

Every voice student who ever watched the monitor and joined me in experimentation with the wonders of the spectrogram and its use in the voice lab.

Special thanks go to Amy Hutchins and Kristin Daily, who sang for some of the spectrograms found in the text.

Others Who Had Their Own Role in Seeing the Project get off the Ground

Dr. James W. Mills, professor at Drew University, who so generously funded the equipment to start our voice lab.

Pamela Harvey, whose freely given gift of her knowledge and enthusiasm has helped greatly. Pam also generously provided the stoboendoscopic videos found on the CD-ROM.

Jessica Sockel, Drew student and friend who wrote the CD-ROM included with this book.

The Staffs of Singular Publishing Group and So Cal Graphics in San Diego

Marie Linvill and the people at Singular who saw the need for the book and who backed the project to the hilt.

Editor, Candice Janco, my project maestra up to the production time, always there, gently pushing, making sure that the project stayed on schedule

Production Editor, Sandy Doyle, who performed the final edits and saved this neophyte writer on many occasions. Sandy was at the center of guiding this book toward whatever clarity and coherence the book has.

Kristin Banach, whose help in the illustration permissions was enormously appreciated.

Dana Wasserman, whose technical help, humor, and support helped more than she can know.

Freelance Production Editor, Randy Stevens, who did the production editing, interior book design, and proofreading.

Rosie Holub, Michelle Mason, Ruth Miller, and Cheri Blessing, at So Cal Graphics, for the valuable technical help with the art files and typesetting.

If I missed anybody in this long list, please forgive me.

CONTRIBUTORS

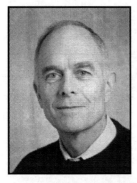

Donald Miller
Bass-baritone Donald Miller is an opera and concert singer, trained in the United States, Italy, and Germany. For two decades he taught at the Syracuse University School of Music, a position he left to pursue research on the acoustics and physiology of the singing voice at the Groningen (Netherlands) Voice Research Laboratory. Since 1984, he has regularly published scientific studies on the singing voice together with Harm Schutte. In 1996, he and tenor James Doing introduced the feedback program VoceVista at the national meeting of the National Asspciation of Teachers of Singing in St. Louis. His long-term project is a monograph on registers in the singing voice. He can be reached at d.g.miller@med. rug.nl

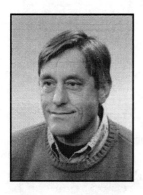

Harm K. Schutte
Professor Dr. Harm K. Schutte, M.D., Ph.D., is an ENT specialist/phoniatrician, with special interest in voice and speech physiology and pathology. He is a member of the Faculty of Medical Sciences, University of Groningen (Netherlands), as professor in voice physiology/medical voice and speech physiology (Phoniatrics and Voice Care). He directs the Groningen Voice Research Laboratory. His doctoral thesis was on the subject of *The Efficiency of Voice Production*, an aerodynamical study of normal and pathological voice production, under Professor Dr. Jw van den Berg. His research is focused on aerodynamic and acoustical phenomena in the professional singing voice, using physiological and acoustical investigation techniques.

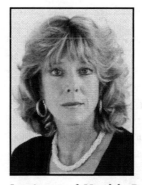

Katherine Verdolini
Katherine Verdolini, Ph.D., C.C.C., S.L.P., is Assistant Professor of Otology and Laryngology, Harvard Medical School; Associate Professor of Communication Sciences and Disorders, MGH Institute of Health Professions; and Research Associate and Singing Voice Specialist, Voice and Speech Lab, Massachusetts Eye and Ear Infirmary. She is a teacher of singing and member of numerous professional organizations including the American Speech-Language-Hearing Association, the American Psychological Association, the National Association of Teachers of Singing, and the Voice and Speech Trainers Association. She is the re-

cipient of a $500,000 award from the National Institute on Deafness and Other Communication Disorders to study cognitive and neurophysiological mechanisms of skill acquisition for voice. She further participates in several NIH-funded grants in basic voice science, basic cognitive and neuroscience, and clinical trials. She regularly presents her clinical and research work nationally and internationally.

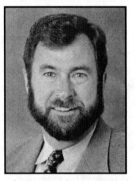

David E. Krebs
David E. Krebs is Professor of Physical Therapy and Clinical Investigation at the MGH Institute of Health Professions, Boston, Massachusetts, and Director of The Massachusetts General Hospital's Biomotion Laboratory. He also holds academic appointments in Orthopaedics at Harvard Medical School and Mechanical Engineering at the Massachusetts Institute of Technology. Dr. Krebs has more than 100 publications and has been awarded more than $4 million as principal investigator on federal and foundation research grants, primarily in the neural and biomechanical constraints of human locomotor control. Dr. Krebs received his B.S. in physical therapy and M.A. in applied physiology from Columbia University and his Ph.D. in pathokinesiology and physical therapy from New York University.

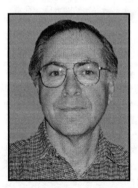

Robert A. Volin
Dr. Robert A. Volin is Associate Professor of Speech-Language Pathology at Lehman College of the City University of New York and is on the staff of the Speech and Hearing Department at Westchester County Medical Center. He has been an active clinical computer user since 1978. He is co-creator of the *Language Stimulation Software* series of clinical programs designed for aphasia rehabilitation. He has written about clinical computer applications and computer-assisted biofeedback, and has presented numerous workshops in the Northeast. He paddles his kayak whenever he can.

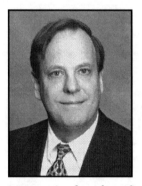

Richard S. Horne
Richard Horne is an electrical engineer and computer programmer with a long interest in audio spectrum analysis. His interest in audio spectrum analysis began as an amateur's interest in the identification of bird songs. Since the advent of powerful personal computers, Richard has created and continuously improved programs for analysis of the audio spectrum by anyone with a desktop computer. His freeware program, Gram, is widely used by amateurs and professionals around the world.

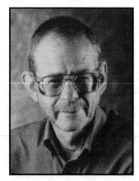

Ron Nair   Ron Nair designed the cover of this book and drew the illustrations in Chapter 1. He is a graphic artist and was educated at the Art Institute of Pittsburgh, where he earned an Associate in Specialized Technology Degree in December, 1982. He has held the post of Assistant Director of Education/Interim Director at and is currently an Instructor in the School of Design/Graphic Design at the Art Institute of Philadelphia. He teaches Computer Graphics, Electronic Design, Digital Imaging and Manipulation, Portfolio, and Typography. He also runs a graphics production company, Smudged Thumb Graphics, and can be reached at redd1@worldnet.att.net.

COMPANION CD

Two symbols are used during the course of this book to denote the presence of correlative material that can be found on the CD-ROM that accompanies the book.
🔘 Indicates the presence of a .wav or .vis file from which a figure shown in the text was produced. Use Gram to analyze the .wav files and VoceVista to analyze the .vis files. Information on running these files in the two programs included on the CD can be found in the CD's help section. Detailed information on changing Gram's analytical parameters during analysis can be found in Appendix C of the text.
🔘 Indicates the presence of an endoscopic video that can be found on and played from the CD-ROM. These videos give the reader a real time look at how the larynx functions during demonstrations of various points made in the text. To play these videos, you must have a Windows video player installed on your computer.

INSTRUCTIONS FOR RUNNING GRAM AND VOCEVISTA FROM THE COMPANION CD ROM

Minimum Hardware Requirements

To run Gram or VoceVista from the Companion CD requires a Windows 95/98 or Windows NT 4.0 computer with a 6x or higher CD-ROM drive, sound card, and at least 16 Mbytes of RAM memory

Running the Examples Found in the Book

The Companion CD is designed to run on most computers. Users should not need to install any files to their hard drives under normal operating configurations to view the files on the CD.

Starting the VTT Companion CD

To use the CD to view examples found in the book, use either Run (found on the Windows Start button) or My Computer (Windows Explorer) to locate the program icon (Vtt.exe) in the root directory of the CD. Once the VTT screen has appeared, use the on-screen menus to learn about the CD or view the files illustrated in the book.

Clearing the Example

After a file has been viewed, cancel Gram or VoceVista window by clicking on the cancel "x" found in the upper right corner of the Gram or VoceVista screen.

Resizing the Gram or VoceVista Example Screen

To resize either the VTT Companion CD screen or the Gram or VoceVista screen, use the normal Windows resizing functions found at the upper right corner of the respective windows.

Exiting the VTT Companion CD

To exit the VTT Companion CD, the usual Windows methods are available:

- cancel "x" in the upper right corner of the VTT screen
- alt/F4
- Exit under the VTT drop down file menu

Audio Playback

Gram

Once a Gram display has been generated by selecting a figure from the menu, the first scan of the file will be silent. To hear the file simultaneously with the display, audio playback can be started using the "Play" or "Play Wdw" buttons at the lower right corner of the Gram window. The "Play" button will play back the entire length of the recording. The "Play Wdw" button will play back only the portion of the recording that is visible in the Gram window. See Appendix C or the Gram help file (gram.hlp) for complete instructions.

VoceVista

Playback of the VoceVista display will begin automatically as the program is started. To replay the VoceVista display, press the spacebar. See the VoceVista help file (vvista.hlp) for complete instructions.

Installing Gram or VoceVista on User's Hard Drive

Both Gram and VoceVista are normally run directly from the Companion CD for analysis of the figures in the book. However, these programs can be copied to the user's hard drive and used independently in the studio for recording and analysis of voice.

To create an independent version of Gram, copy gram.exe, gram.hlp, and gram.cnt to any convenient directory on the hard drive. Create a desktop shortcut for gram.exe to allow Gram to be launched by a double mouse click on its desktop icon. Then, to analyze a recorded file, choose "File–Analyze File" from the Gram menu and select any of the wave (*.wav) files on the CD for analysis.

To create an independent version of VoceVista, copy vvista.exe, vvista.hlp, and vvista.cnt to any convenient directory on the hard drive. Create a desktop shortcut for vvista.exe to allow VoceVista to be launched by a double mouse click on its desktop icon. Then, to analyze a recorded file, choose "Project–File Analysis" from the VoceVista menu and select any of the VIS (*.vis) files on the CD for analysis.

Both Gram and VoceVista provide many different adjustments that affect the appearance of the spectrum displays. A thorough review of the book's Appendix C for Gram as well as each program's help file will be necessary to obtain the best performance.

Adjusting the Gram Display To Match the Figures Found in the Text

The spectrogram figures in the book have been adjusted to best reveal the spectral features under discussion. To recreate these figures on the computer screen may require some adjustment of signal processing parameters in order to stretch the image in the horizontal (time) or vertical (frequency) dimensions.

Gram uses the Fast Fourier Transform (FFT) mathematical technique in which frequency resolution is proportional to the width of the FFT data window (number of sampled data points). In general, choosing a larger FFT size increases frequency resolution and expands the vertical dimension of the display. Similarly, choosing a smaller time scale increases the time resolution and expands the horizontal dimension of the display. To make these adjustments to the Gram display, choose "File–Parameters–Change" from the Gram window menu. The "Analyze File" dialog box will then appear, allowing selection of FFT Size and Time Scale. See Appendix C and the Gram help file (gram.hlp) for complete instructions.

Since most of the examples found in the book were produced by the author, the Gram software is initially configured for display of the spectrum of the male voice. Because the pitch of the female voice is higher than that of the male voice, adjustments may be necessary to the Gram settings to ensure that the highest frequency components of the female voice are visible on the display. Similar adjustments may be necessary for any vocalization containing very high frequency components. Reducing frequency resolution will bring the higher frequency components into view in the Gram display window. When necessary, the frequency resolution can be reduced by changing the FFT width from the usual 1024 data points to 512 data points. Choose "File–Parameters–Change" from the Gram menu and choose FFT Size of 1024 for the male voice and 512 for the female voice.

Known Problems

This Companion CD is configured to run on most computers in the Windows environment. *Neither the author nor Singular Publishing Group, Inc. warranty the functionality of the CD for all possible computer configurations.* To help the user, some of the known problems encountered during beta testing appear below.

Conflicting CD-ROM Drives

If a machine has multiple CD drives, especially if one of them is a read-write

drive, the Companion CD may not run correctly. If the error screen

> **System Error**
>
> Windows cannot read from drive x: If this is a network drive, make sure it is working. If it is a local drive, check the disk.

appears after double clicking on the VTT.exe icon, take the following steps to use the CD.

- run the Tbl60run.exe file on the CD to run the Asymetrix ToolBook program
- choose "cancel" if a drive error message appears
- after a moment, the ToolBook "Open" dialogue box appears
- go to the "List Files of Type" box in the lower left corner, scroll down to and select "All files"
- go up to the "File Name box," scroll down to the VTT.exe file, double click and the CD will function normally

If users encountering this problem will be running the examples during multiple sessions, it may be advisable to utilize Windows Explorer to drag both the Tbl60run.exe and VTT.exe files onto the screen to create shortcuts to the CD.

Video Examples Will Not Play

Video compression must be turned on in the Windows environment. Consult Windows Help for instructions.

No Audio

Consult Windows instructions and the manual for any proprietary sound card for help in troubleshooting audio problems. In many cases, the only action required to receive audio is to turn up the volume on the machine or the speakers. Also, make sure that the speaker as well as the wave functions are not muted in any proprietary mixer program found on the computer.

Dedication

To my parents, William and Marcia Nair, who started all of this,

and

to my students, past and present;
you all taught me much more than I could ever teach you.

CHAPTER

1

SCIENCE AND THE VOICE PRACTITIONER: A STATUS REPORT

Voice teachers have been successfully train- ing great singers for hundreds of years. The means by which such training has been accomplished has led to the development of many traditions of vocal pedagogy. The tools used in these traditions have been based primarily on teachers' intuition about the voice and how it works.

Following World War II, especially in the years since 1980, rapid advances in the sophistication of analytical instru- mentation has permitted great advances in the scientific understanding of the work- ings of the human voice. Sadly, many of these advances in scientific understand- ing have not filtered down to the every- day teaching methods used in voice stu- dios. Possible reasons for this state of affairs will be discussed later in this chapter.

One purpose of this book is to encour- age voice practitioners to avail themselves of this great body of new scientific knowl- edge and to learn to apply it in their ped- agogical practice. (Throughout the book, the term **voice practitioner** will be used to connote anyone who has a high level involvement with the singing voice. The term is an all-purpose inclusive that applies to singers, voice teachers, voice coaches, vocal pathologists who work with singers, and so forth.) Anything that illuminates the mysterious process that we call singing has the potential of engendering greater numbers of highly trained singers, and in potentially less time than intuitive methods alone.

Another purpose of this book is to advo- cate the use of real-time computer-aided feedback in the voice studio, both as a means of speeding up the process of voice training and as a means of helping both teachers and students achieve a greater understanding of voice science. The personal computer is no longer a luxury item in our homes and businesses and many voice practitioners own powerful, fast machines that were the stuff of fantasy just a few years ago. At the same time, the cost of computer programs that can provide spectacular voice analysis in real-time has fallen dramatically. Thus, this new technological capability is within easy reach of the average voice practitioner.

A new world awaits anyone who is willing to consider the use of this technology in the voice studio. Its benefits fall in three principal areas:

- New multifaceted possibilities in the diagnosis and correction of vocal problems
- Improved communication between students and teachers on matters of technique because the computer can help provide a more objective analysis of the voice
- Increased knowledge about the nature of the human voice that can be gained from utilizing the graphical representation of the inner workings of the voice that appears on the computer screen as the singer performs

Any voice practitioner can learn to use computer-generated analysis with a minimal knowledge of voice science. As the practitioners' scientific knowledge deepens, the possibilities available to them in the utilization of the computer as an aid in the development of vocal technique increases dramatically.

Before moving on to the potential inherent in the use of both the new scientific knowledge and computer-analysis feedback, some exploration of philosophical and practical matters regarding both voice practitioners and voice scientists may be helpful.

CONSIDERING VOCAL TECHNIQUE AS A PRIMARY CONCERN

Many voice practitioners, even some graduates of established vocal pedagogy programs, appear unprepared, unwilling, or unable to take advantage of the impressive gains made in the voice-research realm during the last 20 years. Explanations of this state of affairs might be found in two areas:

- Confusion about the dual role of vocal pedagogy, which involves the training of both technical and artistic matters
- A widespread lack of communication between the fields of vocal pedagogy and voice science

The Technique Versus Artistry Confusion

When many voice practitioners talk about vocal pedagogy, there often is no clear distinction made between pedagogical functions concerning technique and those concerning artistry. These are two totally different but equally important facets in the process of training a fine singer. There is no doubt that matters such as style, ornamentation, phrasing, acting through diction, and all of the other *artistic* concerns that fall within the voice practitioner's responsibility are all crucial to the success of a singer. Without first gaining a sound technique, however, it is difficult to move on to those loftier artistic concerns. The great Lilli Lehmann (1903) wrote:

Technique is inseparable from our art. Only by mastering technique of his material is the artist in a condition to mold his mental work of art. (As cited in R. Miller in his chapter in Sataloff [1997, p. 309])

Without attention to the myriad details that constitute the sonic fabric of our art, our ability to emote and soar is compromised. Ultimately, great art is *enabled* by attention to countless details.

Nonetheless, many voice teachers, especially those who teach beginners, seem reluctant to admit the role of technical detail, as if such an admission would diminish their roles as trainers of *art*.

A Visual-Art Analogy

To clarify this issue, it may be easier to consider the technique-versus-artistry differential by examining it as it applies to the visual arts.

If a painter were given a limited number of colors and told that the colors could not be mixed to form new ones, that painter's ability to express ideas and emotions would be compromised. If a soft magenta—needed to express the innermost feeling of the moment—was missing from the palette, that moment and perhaps a great deal of the expressive potential of the art would be absent.

Another example may help to further illuminate the case. A Gothic cathedral, such as Notre-Dame in Paris, is an overwhelming visual and emotional experience. Our first reaction is to the totality of that visual experience. But, if we spend much time in the cathedral (especially if

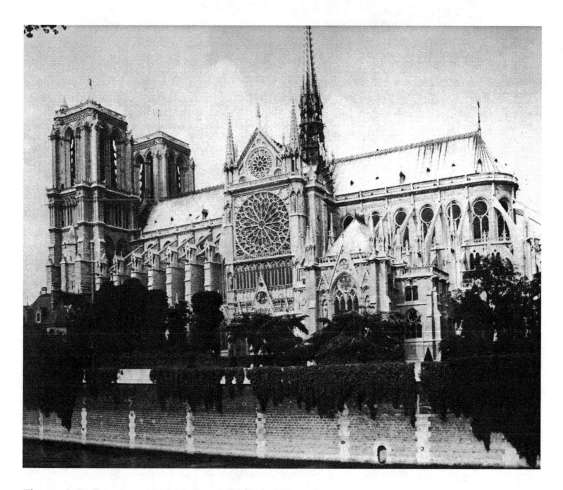

Figure 1–1. Exterior view Notre-Dame Cathedral, Paris, France.

that time is not spent looking through the viewfinder of a camera), details become evident in ever greater abundance. Those details may become more and more minute until the observer may be captivated by the third gargoyle from the left because it has a strange right eyebrow.

One still has the emotional reaction to the totality, the macro, but the experience is all the richer because of the micro world contained *within* the macro. The more detail that is perceived, the more the brain and the emotions will be engaged to experience the cathedral as an overwhelmingly rich experience.

It is the same in the vocal arts. A great singer must gather a palette of such exquisite depth of detail that any emo-

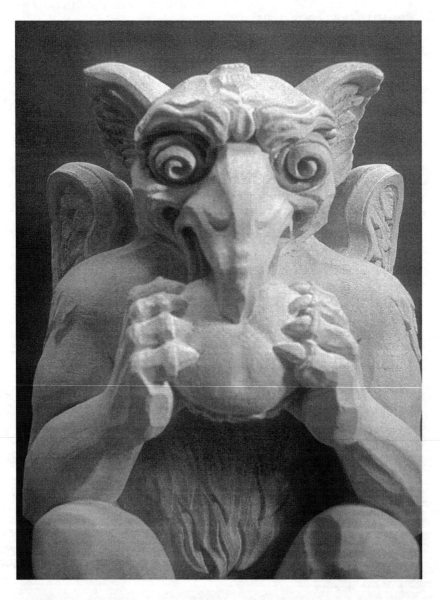

Figure 1–2. Gargoyle eating a cheeseburger. (Contemporary sculpture by Walter Arnold. Photograph reprinted by permission of the sculptor. Mr. Arnold can be found on the internet at http://www.stonecarver.com.)

tional or spiritual dimension required can be instantly summoned.

An internationally ranked singer held a masterclass a few years ago and was asked by one of the students, "How did you develop your wonderful 'ah' vowel?" The artist replied, "Which one?" and then proceeded to give a 15-minute demonstration of how to color that one vowel in dramatic situations where the different colors she had learned to use were employed with stunning, dramatic effect.

THE VOCAL PEDAGOGY PROFESSION

Our profession, long unregulated from without or within, seems to be on the brink of change. Some of that change has been brought about by greater numbers of graduates of vocal pedagogy programs. Other pressure for change may come from those pioneering voice teachers who are not graduates of contemporary vocal pedagogy programs but who, out of curiosity and dedication, continue to learn about their art as new information becomes available.

Historically, anyone who so wished has had the right to declare him- or herself a teacher of voice. Some of these individuals happen to be well-trained teachers taught by some of the greatest singers and vocal pedagogy experts of our time. There are also many great teachers of voice who understand their own voice intuitively and keep producing well-trained singers without the benefit of formal vocal pedagogy training. Still other voice studios are unfortunately staffed with teachers whose qualifications go no farther than the fact that they are able to sing well. Many have little or no understanding of how they sing so well and are mostly limited to the **model/imitation** method as their primary pedagogical tool.

This statement is not meant to denigrate model/imitation as a pedagogical tool. When all is considered, no matter how much voice science a teacher learns, model/imitation is likely to remain the primary pedagogical tool used in the voice studio. If more voice teachers were armed with a thorough knowledge of the anatomy, physiology, and physics of the singing process, they could explore a wider arsenal of pedagogical devices that might considerably enhance the traditional model/imitation technique.

Richard Miller (Sataloff, 1997) stated:

It is the responsibility of the singing teacher in a scientific age to interpret and expand vocal traditions through the means of current analysis so that the viable aspects of tradition can be communicated in a systematic way. The advantage of teaching singing in the era of the voice scientists is that today's teacher has the means of sorting through what is offered, both historically and currently, the vocal pedagogy smorgasbord, and of choosing rationally what is most nutritious, while discarding the garbage, of which there is plenty. Today's singing teacher has access to a greater body of solid information and rational tools than ever before. We owe it to our students to be able to take advantage not only of everything that was known 200 years ago, but also of everything that is known today. (p. 299).

Nothing that follows in this book is meant to deny the fact that traditional voice teaching, much of it intuitive, has produced countless great singers. The intent of this book is to explore the possibility of enhancing the teacher's intuition and, as a result, perhaps speeding up the process of the acquisition of first-rate vocal skills.

Moral and Legal Concerns

As of the writing of this text, there are still no professional licenses, minimal proficiency examinations, or government- or association-regulated standards for the profession of teaching voice.

Aside from the moral obligation to know everything we can and, in the physician's rubric, to do no harm, we must also consider political and legal trends in the recent past. The possibility of a voice teacher being involved in a liability action becomes more real with each passing day. A teacher who cannot answer a plaintiff's attorney when questions about vocal science and research begin to fly will be virtually defenseless. As a broad defense, voice practitioners will soon have to adopt the same kind of peer review and quality control that is currently standard in other professions such as medicine and speech-language pathology.

Robert Sataloff (1997) wrote:

At present, most teachers and music schools rely on very little beyond personal opinion to define good singing, healthy singing, successful training progress, or even a 'good voice' . . . . Clearly, objective voice assessment has been a boon to laryngologists and can be a valuable adjunct to the individual singing and acting teacher. Moreover, it may provide our first real means to define good, healthy singing, acting, and teaching and to help promulgate high standards of practice among those who choose to call themselves "voice teachers." (p. 757)

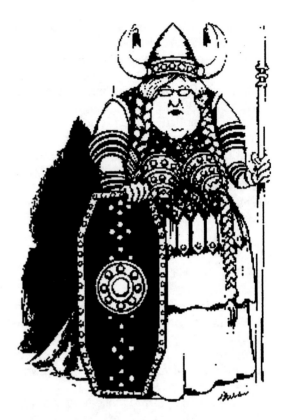

Figure 1–3. The singer. (Original line drawing by Ron Nair. Reprinted with the artist's permission.)

SCIENTISTS, SINGERS, AND COMMUNICATION

Both scientists and voice practitioners have long lamented a failure of communication between the two groups. Several prominent writers over the years have eloquently written about this problem. Although the situation has improved somewhat, it still has a long way to go.

Neither side is without blame in this dialogue, and to develop common solutions to the problem, we must spend some time discussing each side's problem with the other.

The Voice Practitioner's Viewpoint

When the subject of applying science in the voice studio is raised, many voice practitioners immediately respond with a litany of complaints. From their perspective, scientists assume that all voice professionals know the principles of physics and the mathematics that underlie current scientific understanding of the voice. In reality, not enough voice teachers know these principles in any depth, and to them, it seems as if the scientists are talking a foreign language.

Do Scientists Really Know How To Communicate With Us?

Part of the problem is seen as a real or imagined resistance on the part of many scientists to bring explanations of the complexities of vocal science down to a level understandable by the average voice practitioner. Such attempts at basic education often fall under the label of "popularization."

There also seems to be a subconscious feeling that scientists who popularize scientific concepts will be held in less regard by their colleagues. An excellent example of this is found in the difficulties experienced by the distinguished scientist, Carl Sagan. When he went on his crusade to bring difficult concepts of astrophysics to the general public in a form that could be understood by lay people, many of his colleagues criticized him.

Interestingly, Sagan is now held in higher regard because many young scientists today became scientists *because* of his popular crusade. As a result, we are beginning to enjoy a new generation of scientists who are not afraid to show excitement about their subject and who are not afraid to take the message of their work to the public. Popularization seems to attract less of a stigma than in the past. Perhaps it is within the ranks of these "Saganists" that we will find scientists who are more willing and able to explain the message of voice science to voice practitioners.

Jargon

Another problem voice practitioners often face when talking with scientists is terminology. Because most singers and teachers of singing do not have sufficient training in voice science, they often invent their own terminology. When trying to communicate with scientists, voice practitioners may encounter differences in terminology so pronounced that they are tempted to call for a translator! Because they have no background in biology or physics, even the most rudimentary scientific terminology seems cold and "anti-art."

Is This the Whole Picture?

Finally, even when a scientist delivers a very cogent explanation of a facet of the vocal model, a voice practitioner will quite often say something to the effect of,

"Well, that helps explain some things, but it doesn't go far enough. I feel other things happening in my voice." No matter how much the scientists discover and explain, voice research does not seem to come close to explaining the totality of what singers experience.

Part of the reason for the singers' sense that the model is incomplete may stem from the fact that most subjects used in voice experiments are not singers of international rank. Imagine a research study set up to explore the physiology of football players that used high-school level players as subjects. Although there would be many comparable traits, the strength, maturity, experience, and above all the physical endowments that enable a player to have a viable professional football career would be missing from the study.

Without research subjects from the ranks of world-class singers in the midst of robust professional careers, it is understandable that much critical information may be missing from the resulting vocal models, models that seem to leave too many unanswered questions when read by the professional singer.

Many scientists will, of course, take the time to consider what singers have to say (even if unscientific words such as "feel" appear in the discussion) and attempt further explanation. Some may even get new ideas for further research. Others too quickly dismiss the singing practitioner as outside the scientific "club" and therefore not qualified to comment on or propose research.

The same problem also occurs in communication between voice practitioners and medical doctors. While attempting to explain their vocal problems, singers describe sensations that they have spent a lifetime experiencing and studying. The doctor, who most often has no experience as a singer, often dismisses the singer's complaint as superfluous. How many doctors understand the chasm that exists between the operational parameters of the speaking and singing voice?

So, from the viewpoint of the voice practitioner, scientists seem to be unwilling or unable to come down from their lofty heights to talk about practical matters. To make matters worse, they insist on the use of a complex language that seems almost impossible to penetrate.

The voice practitioner may feel that the blame for the much-lamented lack of communication between scientists and singers must be laid at the feet of the scientists. Then when the scientists turn and point an accusing finger at the singer, the singer says, "Moi?"

The Scientist's Viewpoint

Lest the reader feel that this chapter is a diatribe against voice scientists, we will now turn our attention to the communication problem as seen from the voice scientists' perspective. From their position, the situation appears far different.

Voice Practitioners Don't Know Enough Science

When scientists attempt to communicate with singers, they are often met with a

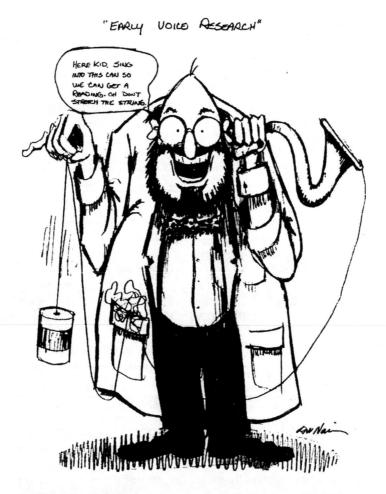

Figure 1-4. The voice scientist. (Original line drawing by Ron Nair. Reprinted with the artist's permission.)

frightful lack of scientific knowledge. To them, it appears that voice professionals do not wish to take advantage of the remarkable body of information scientists have discovered.

Scientists often have to stand and listen while voice practitioners proffer seemingly definitive answers—answers that the scientists know were proven false in the laboratory perhaps decades ago. To make matters worse, such ideas are often couched in subjective terminology. Voice teachers seem to want to hold on to their cherished assumptions and not take the time or effort to learn what the scientists have discovered.

Spurious and Inexact Terminology

Many singers freely employ terminology that, to the scientists, is excruciatingly inexact and subjective. There is no quicker way to lose credibility with a scientist than to start speaking the loose language of jargon. To the scientists, talk between a scientist and a voice practitioner, or listening to a discussion *between* voice practitioners, often sounds like the embodiment of "the emperor's new clothes."

Thus, from the scientists' viewpoint, the blame for the lack of communication must surely rest at the feet of the voice practitioners. When the scientists see singers pointing accusing fingers at the voice-science field, the scientists deny all charges, saying "Nous?"

Each camp remains on its own side of the divide, suspiciously eyeing the other like two prize fighters awaiting the bell to start a new round.

TIME TO CHANGE THE PARADIGM

This unfortunate situation will not be resolved until each side is willing to address the concerns of the other. D. Ralph Appelman (1967) stated the problem as follows:

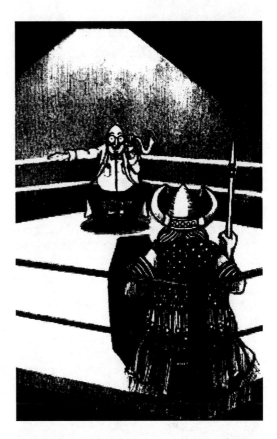

Figure 1–5. "Not talking, are we?" (Original line drawing by Ron Nair. Reprinted with the artist's permission.)

Vocal pedagogy cannot survive as an independent educational entity if the physiological and physical facts, which comprise its core, remain subjects of sciolism (superficial knowledge). Researchers must constantly interpret these scientific facts so that they might become realistic pedagogical tools that may be employed by future teachers of voice. (p. 5)

This situation will not improve until the voice profession makes a greater effort, both in everyday practice and in the training of future singers and voice teachers, to understand and incorporate scientific knowledge of the voice. The voice scientists cannot carry the burden alone.

Transforming the Nature of Our Dialogue

The Issue of Practicality

The longer one ponders the problem of communication, the more it appears an issue of practicality. The voice practitioner is engaged in the *practical* act of improving the singer's voice. At best, this is a difficult process involving considerable behavioral modification. Good voice teachers are continually searching for methods of accomplishing change in their students. Thus, the focus of the voice teacher is on *use* of knowledge, not acquisition for its own sake.

For scientists, the *acquisition* of knowledge is the primary goal. Pure research does not need to have application as a goal. When attending conferences, voice practitioners often react to a scientific presentation with the thought, "That's all very interesting, but how can we apply it?"

This is a classic conundrum. Many scientists don't know enough about the highly trained singing voice to offer suggestions on how to employ the results of their research to good effect in the voice studio. At the same time, voice professionals—sensing no immediate practical application of research results—do not see the need to spend time and effort learning enough to understand the available scientific knowledge. Until both sides work on the practicality issue, little mitigation of this communication problem will occur and little of the great body of scientific knowledge will find its way into the voice studio.

Formula for Change

A possible formula for a change includes the following:

- More scientists must extend an effort to translate their complex research in a way that can be grasped by people who do not have the benefit of a deep scientific background. We need more "Carl Sagans" in the field of voice science.
- More voice professionals must take the time to learn what has been discovered and to energetically take those discoveries into the voice studio. We must find ways to practically apply the lessons learned from science.

More scientific study using artists of professional rank as subjects is necessary. Admittedly, it is difficult to procure research subjects due to the performance schedules of ranking singers, but scientists need to make greater effort in this direction.

Some research has utilized recordings in lieu of live subjects. While not an ideal solution, it is better than working primarily with singers of more modest attainment. One laboratory that has taken this approach is the Voice Lab at the University of Groningen. They have been conducting a computer-aided study of the recordings of world-ranking singers in an effort to understand strategies by which tenors of professional rank move between their middle and upper registers. In a paper that reports the results (Miller & Doing, 1998), distinct vocal strategies utilized by professional singers have been revealed. Perhaps no study of less gifted or less trained tenors could have given voice practitioners as much insight.

Later in this book, the principal author of that paper, Donald Miller, will thoroughly explore two of the three principal computer-based feedback technologies now available for use in the voice studio (power spectrum and EGG).

Until similar studies of internationally ranking voices are undertaken—studies that utilize both recorded *and* live performances of artists of rank as subjects—well-trained, talented singers will not have many of the answers they seek from voice science.

- Singers of international rank must make themselves available as subjects for research. As long as voice scientists are forced to use amateur subjects, there will be too many missing or erroneous answers in the models.
- There must be more dialogue between scientists and voice professionals centered on finding practical applications for the body of research at hand. Until these points of commonality are found and applied, neither side will have much reason to communicate with the other.
- Both voice professionals and voice scientists must work toward the goal of employing analytical instrumentation, long available in the scientific field, as a practical solution for both the diagnosis of vocal problems and as a source of feedback that can be employed in the behavioral modification process of voice teaching.
- Voice practitioners and voice scientists must work together to develop a terminology that will be effective and accurate, both in discussions between singers and scientists and within voice studios as well.

One only needs a quick perusal of Cornelius L. Reid's *A Dictionary of Vocal Terminology* to realize the astounding number of terms currently used in voice studios. His dictionary contains only the most common terms and attempts to group synonyms together under the heading of the most common or logical word used for that definition. One is struck by how many words can be used for the same concept. The words found in Reid's dictionary are just a small sampling of what one could find by going from studio to studio. With no standard terminology, the vocal pedagogy field is hamstrung when intraprofessional communication is attempted. The result is a sort of Tower of Babel in which miscommunication is quite often the result.

Toward a Standardized Terminology

As Richard Miller (Sataloff, 1997) wrote:

There is a body of information that ought to be drawn on by anyone who claims to teach anything to anybody. No one can know it all, but we must be willing to modify what we do know as information expands. Demythologizing the language of vocal pedagogy is part of that process. (p. 300)

This new standardized terminology must be based on objectivity and not the subjectivity that underlies much of the vocal terminology of the past. Much of this needed terminology already exists in the field of speech and voice pathology.

Such a standardized terminology for the voice profession might encompass the following three classes of vocabulary.

Type 1: Terminology Already Existing in Speech and Voice Science

Type 1 is the great body of scientific terminology already in use in speech and voice science fields, which can be used equally well in the voice studio or at a scientific conference.

Type 2: Usable but Not Advisable in the Studio

Type 2 is terminology needed for scientific discussion but not required or desirable in the working voice studio. Such terminology might overburden the typical student/teacher relationship in the voice studio, but terminology is critical to attain the specificity needed in any discussion between voice scientists and voice practitioners.

Type 3: New Terminology Needed Where Speech and Song Techniques Diverge

Type 3 is a small body of terminology, agreed on by both groups, that must be created to take the differential between the technical needs of the speaking and singing voice into consideration.

SUMMARY

This book attempts to encourage voice practitioners to embrace the findings of voice science and to modernize our profession with the use of readily available technology. The book will:

- Introduce the basic concepts and terminology of voice science needed to explore the use of voice-analysis technology in the voice studio
- Employ a scientific terminology that is usable in the voice studio
- Call attention to the sometimes great divergence between speech and singing techniques
- Teach the elementary use of computer-based, voice-analytical technology
- Promote the use of computer-based, analytical equipment as feedback to accelerate the development of singers
- Suggest to both scientists and singers the types of practical solutions that can benefit from the application of such technology

All of these goals, taken together, are an attempt to move both voice practitioners and voice scientists toward a state-of-the-art vocal pedagogy in which our next generation of singers can flourish.

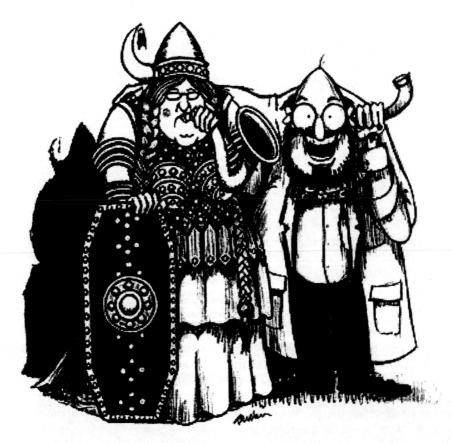

Figure 1–6. "Perfect harmony." (Original line drawing by Ron Nair. Reprinted with the artist's permission.)

2

ONGOING EVOLUTION: ADDING TO THE VOCAL PEDAGOGY ARSENAL

To understand the rationale behind the inclusion of the computer in the voice studio, a review of traditional vocal pedagogy methods is in order. The use of computer analysis is not a radical departure from tradition, but can be viewed as a logical step in its evolution.

TRADITIONAL METHODS: MODEL/IMITATION

Traditionally, much of voice teaching has relied heavily on the model/imitation method where, in an attempt to correct vocal problems, the teacher would sing a model of the desired sound and the student would attempt to replicate it.

Through repetition and small incremental adjustments, the student experiences the sound and feel of the correct model and eventually makes the technique habitual. It is a slow but effective behavior-modification technique that has been used successfully to train legions of singers throughout the history of vocal pedagogy.

Vocal Pedagogy Is Behavioral Modification

Vocal pedagogy, is in fact, a form of a behavior modification. The combination of verbal and aural **feedback**, together with constant repetition, permits students to gradually modify their neural-muscular skills to produce a final product that is often far removed from speech norms (more about this in Chapter 4).

The acquisition of motor skills often requires our brain to compare the "before and after" during the learning process. As one learns the position of a control on the dashboard of an unfamiliar car, for example, he or she may reach for the switch, miss it, and then look to see where the control is located. After calculating how to correct the motion, the individual attempts the task again. During this repetitive process, the brain utilizes the comparison to build a **muscle memory** of what the arm and hand must do to locate the control. With sufficient repetition, one can eventually locate the switch with little or no visual input.

The model/imitation pedagogy should work in the same way, but singers encounter two major impediments to its success:

- For the most part, there is no visual input to help the learning process. Most of the target behaviors for the singing musculature are internal, not external where singers can see them.
- Singers' internal perception of their own sound is *markedly different* from the external reality experienced by listeners.

The Singer's Internal Aural Perception

The first time people hear their own voices on a tape recorder, they universally react with a statement such as, "Please tell me that that is not the sound of my voice!" (Are you laughing or smiling right now in the memory of that moment?)

There are two reasons why our voices sound so different in our heads from the way others hear them. First, sounds leaving the mouth reach the ears, which are *behind* the end of the vocal tract (the mouth), with varying degrees of success.

The determinant of what reaches the singer's ears is frequency dependent. Additionally, Johan Sundberg (1987) wrote,

There is one more reason that a voice sounds different to speakers and listeners. The sound from our voice organs propagates not only in air but also within the tissues of the speaker's body . . . part of the sound one perceives of one's own voice has traveled directly from the vocal tract to the hearing organs by so-called bone (as opposed to air) conduction. The bone-conducted sound differs from the air-conducted sound in one important respect; at high frequencies, bone-conduction is less efficient than air-conduction, so that the received spectrum of a bone-conducted sound falls off toward higher frequencies at a 6 dB/octave faster rate than airborne sounds. (p159)

When the instructor, through much hard work, finally succeeds in enticing an acceptable vocal sound from the student, that singer may well perceive that sound as "wrong." It doesn't match the internal norm of the student's speech experience. If the difference in the production is found in the higher frequencies, the student may not hear the difference at all. This means that no matter how much the subject wants to believe the teacher, the student's own perception of the product emanating from the mouth will not be confirmed by the subject's aural processes.

Elementary Feedback and the Internal Perception Problem

The idea of utilizing feedback in a voice studio is by no means new. Even the simple spoken encouragement, "That's right. Do it again that way," is a form of feedback. Teachers have long used mirrors, tape recorders, and more recently, video recorders to offer their students additional tools to aid in their vocal and artistic development.

External "Ears": The Tape Recorder

When portable tape recorders first came into common use, voice teachers and coaches slowly accepted them into the pedagogical process. Today they are almost universally accepted, and we have gained a powerful aid in the battle with the singer's internal perception. When students hear a tape recording of their performance, they begin to perceive the differential between their distorted internal image and the sonic reality outside their bodies.

The tape recorder does have one great limitation; it can only present its view to the student *after the fact*. To be truly effective, such aural feedback should be in **real-time**, that is, the singer would benefit greatly if he or she could instantly hear the results. (The tape recorder can, in fact, be used in this way. See Chapter 6 for details.)

Adding the Eyes to the Equation

Many voice teachers use a mirror in their everyday teaching because it enables students to use their sight as a source of additional information during the learning process.

An instructor may point out repeatedly that a student's mouth aperture is not sufficiently open for the production of a certain vowel. If the student has a poor physical sense of his or her mouth opening, such verbal admonitions may not be sufficient to correct the problem. By looking in the mirror, the student can see and correct the problem. As the problem is corrected by visual means, the student will also learn the change in the sound and the feel of the production that accompanies a wider opening.

At first glance, the mirror may be regarded as a minor source of feedback because most of what we need to change is internal, and therefore invisible. After much experience, many teachers realize that subtle evidence of internal processes does present external clues that can be used in the behavioral-modification process. One may recognize that tension visible in the eyebrow region may be a telltale sign of concurrent velar tension. The tension in the velum cannot be seen, but the telltale eyebrow can. Having the student watch for the sign of the unwanted behavior can speed up the learning process. Even at its most sophisticated level, however, the use of a mirror (or in some state-of-the-art studios, a video camera) is still limited in its scope as a device to aid the acquisition of a fine singing technique.

TECHNOLOGY: THE EYE/EAR COMBINATION

Sound analysis technology has been in existence for approximately 50 years. This technology, beginning with the use of the oscilloscope and now utilizing sophisticated computer software, can present our eyes with graphic evidence regarding the nature of the sound being analyzed.

Ingo Titze (1994) encouraged the use of such analytical technology:

Vocologists are encouraged to become familiar with a sound spectrograph. It is an important tool for analysis that can be used not only for research but also for instantaneous feedback (sic) in vocal training and therapy. (p. 291)

At the time he wrote this intriguing encouragement, such technology was out of financial reach for the average voice practitioner and was found only in research laboratories. Beginning in 1994, however, the cost factor that kept the technology out of the voice studio was solved with the introduction of a freeware program posted on the Internet. This program, which can be found on the CD accompanying this text, will be explored in detail later in the book. With the technology now well within the studio budgets of most voice teachers, it is time for vocal practitioners to consider the possibilities of employing the technology in their vocal practice.

Why Should We Use Technology?

Let's go back to our switch-on-the-dashboard analogy. What if the driver could not see the target switch? The process, through trial and error, would be a long one until the driver found the switch by accident enough times to learn its position in space. But what if the driver had a computer-generated graphic representation, not a realistic photo image, but a schematic graphic that would indicate how far the user's hand was from the switch and in which direction. Success would be possible in a time frame approaching that accomplished through direct visual/tactile input.

If a singer's ear is predestined to "miss the target" because of a distorted aural image, why not present a graphic analysis of the sound, as it is occurring in the room, which allows the use of sight to the guide the ear?

How Can the Eye Guide One's Hearing?

Musicians describe hearing a familiar piece of music with totally "new ears" once they listen to that work with its score in front of them. Details never before heard, once spotted by the eyes, become apparent to the ears. Musicians continue to hear those newly acquired details even after the visual stimulus of the score is removed. In a real sense, the musician's eye guides the ear toward a more intimate knowledge of the sonic landscape of the work.

This same phenomenon can occur in the voice studio. Minute gradations of

sound, not immediately apparent to the student's ear, suddenly become audible when the eyes perceive the visual evidence revealed by a computer sound analysis program. With proper guidance, the singer will soon be able to recognize the aural evidence without the aid of the visual clues provided by the computer.

Most singing technique involves internal structures that neither the teacher nor student can see. Any window into that internal process can potentially be of enormous help during the learning process.

Why and What

The use of feedback provided by contemporary digital technology has the potential to provide just such a window. It can greatly accelerate the learning process by providing quantifiable information to both student and teacher. As the student learns to hear and sense the "feel" (muscle memory) of good vocal production in ever-greater detail, the teacher can begin to introduce anatomy, physiology, and basic concepts of physics. In this way, the student not only can begin to hear subtle differences, but can understand *why* the differences occur and how to correct them.

DIGITAL FEEDBACK IN REAL-TIME

Earlier, this text cited the use of the mirror in the voice studio as an excellent auxiliary aid because it provides the singer with visual feedback in *real-time*. As a vocal task is executed, the singer receives a seemingly simultaneous external view of his or her performance.

Today's computers can also deliver a visual representation of software-produced, acoustic analysis in real-time. The information contained in the resulting graphic can then be correlated with the causal effects of the singer's use of the anatomy and physiology.

Voice practitioners now enjoy the availability of computer-based software programs that are both affordable and readily available. These programs can analyze the human voice in numerous ways and display the results on a computer monitor. Even though this technology is available, it is seldom employed in the voice studio, either because the teacher is not aware of its existence, or because the teacher has heard about it in the past, but felt that the technology was too expensive. It is now time to consider the inclusion of the computer into the vocal pedagogy process.

BRINGING THE COMPUTER INTO THE VOICE STUDIO

It is fascinating to watch the reaction of voice practitioners as they experience state-of-the-art computer technology used in the vocal pedagogy process for the first time. Their reactions fall into one of two general groupings, pros and cons.

Pros

Connecting Sight with Hearing

Many voice practitioners respond enthusiastically to the idea of computer programs that analyze the human voice. They become instantly immersed in what they see and begin to identify components shown on the screen with what they are hearing and feeling. For those teachers, there is a fascination with the ability to compare what they are hearing with the information coming from the computer. The possibility of being able to *quantify* what is being heard is instantly apparent.

Improved Communication With Other Professionals

A second reaction usually follows as teachers realize that by indicating a tell-tale visual sign on the computer graphic, a student or a colleague can be guided to see and hear exactly what they are hearing. This allows them to discuss and analyze the root physiological cause for that particular sonic event. Both parties can see the same evidence objectively, removing the potential barrier that might have been present had they employed only the subjective sense of hearing.

Accelerated Learning With Digital Analysis

A third reaction often found in this group is the realization that the technology also may enhance their own learning about the voice. One colleague, who had just completed a doctorate in vocal pedagogy, exclaimed, "I am understanding, for the first time, things about acoustics and physiology that I have been 'learning' for years. It all just came together!"

Cons

Other practitioners have a decidedly negative reaction to using the computer in the voice studio. In this group, two immediate objections are commonly heard: "I don't need a machine to replace me!" and "The computer has no place in art."

Fear of Replacement

The profound fear of being replaced by a machine is a valid concern in our contemporary society, given the fact that most professions have changed radically since the advent of the computer. The arrival of advanced technology has fostered much beneficial change, but the cost has been high as countless jobs and careers have been lost.

When it comes to the craft of teaching voice, the fear of replacement by a machine is groundless. The trained human ear is far better equipped to help a voice student than any computer could ever be. As human beings continue to learn about the voice, we often feel humbled by the ability of the ear (in tandem with the brain) to hear and interpret the sounds around us. As we learn more about the complexity and subtlety of our hearing, the sheer elegance of the system may become overwhelming. We also may sense the enormity of what we still do not know. As a skilled voice teacher works with student after student, year after year, that teacher's ability to analyze what is heard becomes staggering in its breadth and specificity. Robert T. Sataloff (1997) has noted:

The best acoustic analyzers are still the human ear and brain. Unfortunately, they are still not very good at quantifying the information they perceive, and we cannot communicate it accurately. (p. 756)

The last part of Sataloff's statement points to the reason why rather than fearing the technology, we might benefit by embracing it. We tend to hear sound as a totality and must work hard to hear the complex constituents of each sound. This is the very area in which the computer excels.

No matter what level of sophistication computer technology achieves, human beings will still have to interpret the display, correlate it with what is being heard, and then decide on the best course of action for the student.

A Computer Has No Place in Art

Many voice practitioners also believe there is no room for the computer in art. The problem with that statement is that it mixes two totally different but necessary facets of the artistic process, a subject discussed in Chapter 1. On one hand, the premise is correct: In the areas of emotional expression and human spirit that are the hallmark of great art, there is little, if anything, that the computer can

contribute. There is more to the artistic process, however, as we must spend countless hours engaged in the task of amassing the "raw materials" of sound that enable a great artist to convey the emotions and spirit that we recognize as art. It is in this area, technique building, where the computer can be of enormous value.

Unspoken Negatives

Finally, there are two other reasons why a voice practitioner may be unwilling to consider the use of a computer in the studio. While one might hear the two objections discussed above, one rarely hears a voice practitioner admit to the next two excuses.

Incomplete Knowledge About the Workings of the Voice

Voice practitioners may not consider the use of computer-aided voice analysis because its use requires a fair amount of scientific knowledge about vocal production. If practitioners lack this knowledge, they may be reluctant to consider the use of a computer, fearing it will reveal that lack of knowledge. The potential embarrassment of admitting this lack of knowledge may outweigh the natural curiosity and joy of learning that should be the standard reaction to a new learning and teaching tool. The only answer to this dilemma is for the person demonstrating the technology to introduce it slowly, starting with basic precepts. Once a solid base has been established, the practitioner may be comfortable moving deeper into the scientific depths. As a voice practitioner becomes more comfortable with the technology and realizes its potential benefits, the embarrassment objection can be quickly overcome.

The "I've Already Got the Answers" Reason

One is even less likely to hear this final objection spoken: "It was good enough for my teacher, Madame Olga, so it is good enough for me." Surprising as it may seem, this problem does exist, with more frequency than voice practitioners would like to admit. Some of these practitioners produce excellent singers from their studios. But most do not. Both types of teacher can benefit from an infusion of more knowledge and contemporary feedback aids. Their students may be better trained in the end and in a shorter time frame than they would have experienced prior to their teacher's acquisition of new knowledge. So much has been learned about the workings of the voice, especially during the last 20 years, that "Madame Olga's" technique may become even more lustrous with the addition of some of that knowledge.

THE COMPUTER AS AN ADJUNCT TO THE BRAIN/EAR COLLABORATION

Present-day computerized analytical technology is breathtaking in its ability to represent sound. As it weaves a graphic representation of the sound on the monitor, it can uncover hidden details in the totality of what our ears perceive. In so doing, it allows us to perceive critical aspects of sound that we might not otherwise hear.

As wonderful as the technology is, it cannot diagnose vocal problems by itself. It can only confirm what a good teacher should already be hearing or sensing while possibly adding further information that may aid in the diagnosis and solution of a student's vocal problems.

Digital Analysis as a Studio Tool

The reasons voice practitioners should consider including the computer as an adjunct in the studio are threefold:

- The student's ability to correlate what is heard with what is sensed in his or her voice can be greatly accelerated through the use of visual feedback. Many times, students are incapable of hearing what voice practitioners are trying to tell them about their vocal production. As students—with the teacher's guidance—become more adept at reading the computer graphics, their ability to hear detail in their vocal production may be substantially enhanced. We will discuss this in greater depth near the end of this chapter.

- It provides objective confirmation of what the teacher perceives and presents. As a voice teacher watches the computer graphics in real-time and correlates them with what is heard, he or she quickly learns to recognize visual images that represent the student's technical problems. By pointing out the graphic signatures of elements that have raised the teacher's concern, the student gains objective verification of what the teacher conveys during the session. The opposite is also true: desirable aspects of the student's vocal production can be seen as well. By pointing out evidence on the monitor that represent improvements in technique, the teacher gains a powerful adjunct in the process of positively reinforcing continued growth.

- The teacher's knowledge of the voice becomes more objective through the use of digital analysis. As increasingly subtle constituent details of a singer's technique are perceived, questions naturally occur: "What is causing that minute shift in the graphic? Can I replicate that image and sound with my own voice? What can I tell the student to change in the voice to make the image, and therefore the sound, better?" In this way, the teacher will build a mental "database" of technical solutions that correlate with the evidence on the monitor. The utilization of this database can considerably speed up the elimination of technical problems in the student's voice. Not only will the student improve, but a better, more versatile, voice teacher will result as well.

GOALS

We can summarize the need to bring voice science into the studio via computer technology with the following goals:

- Objectification of the concepts of vocal production, both in terms of physics and physiology
- Objectification of teaching methods for the correction of vocal faults (both the student and the teacher can observe, as well as judge, the efficacy of a teaching technique)
- A standardized, more objective terminology for use in the voice studio (it is hard to continue the use of jargon when faced with the objectivity of what is observed on the monitor)

SUMMARY

Although it may be comfortable for voice practitioners to cling to their cherished models from the past, we now live in a time where knowledge is abundant, knowledge that can shed much light on our craft. We have an obligation to accept its presence and to use it to the fullest of our ability.

The great Herbert Witherspoon, director of the Metropolitan Opera Company in the 1930s, who had a huge influence on vocal pedagogy expressed:

The singing voice is an acoustic instrument that must be produced naturally in accordance with the laws of physics, and . . . the singing voice is primarily a physical instrument that obeys the laws of physical function (Miller, R., 1986, p. 310)

Those precepts are as true today as they were when Witherspoon first presented them in 1925. The difference is that the post-World War II explosion of knowledge, combined with the availability of computer-driven means to explore the voice, should compel voice practitioners to take Witherspoon's words to heart by learning to employ all the new tools available to them.

CHAPTER

3

THE NATURE OF SOUND

PEELING THE ARTICHOKE

Studying the physics of the vocal instrument is a little like studying an artichoke. It is easier to understand the concept of the vegetable if one sees it whole before laboriously peeling it, leaf by leaf. When explaining sound, many authors rapidly discard the outer layers to get to the good parts. As a result, the reader is often confused because the author has plummeted to the depths of the subject before the reader has a firm grasp of what constitutes the totality of an artichoke.

As with the artichoke, we want to understand sound as a whole before beginning its dissection. In this chapter and the next, we are going to attempt to show the concept of the whole "plant," and then slowly peel the outer "leaves," but only so far, far enough for the reader to understand the ensuing discussions of the analytical technology. What follows is intended as a re-

view for the voice practitioner, not an in-depth discussion of the physics of sound.

Should the reader wish to go on peeling this "artichoke" until its heart is reached, a suggested reading list can be found after the References, toward the end of the book.

WHAT IS SOUND?

Definition

Sound is the movement of a specific type of energy through a medium, such as air. For a sound to exist, three physical factors must be present:

- an elastic material
- an energy source to distort that material, and
- an elastic medium to convey the resulting energy outward from its source.

An Elastic Material

There must be a generator of sound—a source that is made of a material that has elasticity. A material is said to have elasticity when its shape can be deflected away from its resting state, and then, when force is no longer applied, the material will return to its original state. An excellent example of elasticity is a rubber band. If one applies force to the material, it will distort (stretch) away from its resting state (its original shape). Once the application of distorting force ceases, the rubber band will return to its resting state. If one exceeds its limit of elasticity (its ability to distort without structural failure), its structural integrity will fail. That is why a glass, which has minimal elasticity, is easily broken.

Application of Deflective Force

If the material is sufficiently elastic and a suitable deflective force is applied, it will display another attribute, the ability to vibrate. Once it is distorted from its resting state, it will reverse direction, trying to return to its resting state. But inertia (the tendency of an object in motion to stay in motion or an object at rest to stay at rest) causes the material to continue traveling past its point of rest in the opposite direction. At some point in that travel, its elasticity will cause it to rebound back toward its resting state. This movement of the elastic material is called **vibration**. One complete execution of this motion, starting from the resting state, moving to the side in one direction, rebounding to the other extreme, and then returning to the resting state is called a **cycle**.

The description in the preceding paragraph illustrates **simple harmonic motion**. In the real world, there is an opposing physical factor that removes some of the energy of vibration during each cycle, a state called **damped oscillation**. During each cycle, friction and other factors gradually dissipate some of the energy,

and thus, the maximum point of deflection will become correspondingly shorter during each succeeding cycle. Ultimately, the material will return to stasis—its resting state.

Picture a child on a swing. The application of force causes the swing to move in its arc. If the force is removed, the swing will eventually lose all of its energy and come to a standstill. A cymbal is another example. It is made from a material of such elasticity that it loses little energy during each cycle, thus it possesses the ability to vibrate for a long time without requiring the application of additional force. If one continues the application of force, the vibration will continue as long as the force is present. This is a state called **sustained vibration**.

A Sound Source: A Deflective Force Acting on Elastic Material

These two factors together, deflective energy applied to an elastic material, constitute a **sound source**. Most musical instruments, the voice included, possess sound sources and accompanying energy-delivery systems that have the ability to sustain vibration. In the voice, as long as a pressurized air stream continues to impart deflective force to the vocal folds (the human sound source), the vibration (called **phonation** in the case of the voice) will continue.

A Medium To Convey the Generator's Energy to Its Environment

Elasticity in the Conductive Medium

When the generator is in motion, it imparts its energy to the medium around it. This medium, too, must possess the property of elasticity. In the case of speech and song, the conveying medium is air. Other conveying media can be water, wood, and even stone. Anything that has elasticity and can be displaced from its resting state by energy pulses created by a sound source can be a medium. Of course, some materials do a better job of conveying energy than others.

The molecules that make up the conveying medium act in sympathy with the generator. Whatever the motion of the generator, the molecules in the conveying medium do likewise. As the generator moves outward, it creates a wave of pressure in the conveying medium. This pressure wave is a momentary increase in density of molecules called **compression**. As the tuning fork reverses its travel and goes the opposite way, a **rarefaction** occurs. This phenomenon can be easily seen in Figure 3–1.

Air as a Medium

When we phonate, we use air as our conveying medium. Air is elastic, another way of saying that its molecules tend to want to remain in the same place. If a molecule is displaced from its resting state, it will im-

part its energy to the next neighboring molecule and then return to its previous position in space. As the sound source oscillates back and forth, it will first create a compression wave (higher density of air molecules). Then, as it moves in the opposite direction, it leaves an area of rarefaction (lower density of molecules). The molecules of air move micro distances during this transfer of energy, always returning to their original position (again, see Figure 3–1 for a representation of this phenomenon).

While the first molecule adjacent to the vibrating sound source is returning to rest, its neighboring molecule displaces and passes its energy on to its neighbor until all of the molecules in the medium have received and passed on the energy.

It is important to understand that there is no permanent movement of molecules to another point in space during this process. If such movement did occur, one could feel a refreshing breeze in front of a stereo speaker, and a symphony orchestra might generate a strong wind. Of course, this doesn't happen; the molecules briefly displace and then return to their starting point.

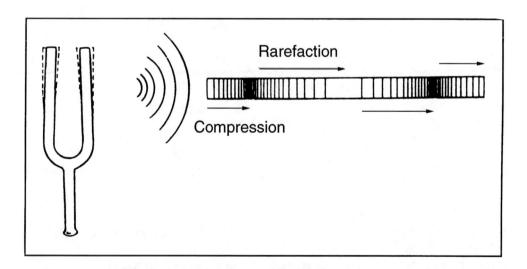

Figure 3–1. Drawing of a sound wave produced by a tuning fork, showing compression resulting from the right swing of the tine and rarefaction as it swings to the left. (From *Vocal Health and Pedagogy* by Robert T. Sataloff, 1998, p. 67. San Diego, CA: Singular Publishing Group. Copyright 1998 by Singular Publishing Group. Reprinted with permission.)

To visualize the phenomenon of energy transfer, picture the familiar "human wave" as performed at sporting events. It is initiated when one person stands up and quickly sits back down. As the adjacent person senses the first person's motion, he or she performs the identical motion. This energy transference, a wave, will run its course through the crowd until the person farthest from the initiator has stood up and sat down. During this wave, people do not move from their lateral position in the crowd, but from a distance, it is an impressive display of transmitted energy. It is almost the equivalent of the transmission of sound energy. (The human wave is not exactly like a sound wave because the energy of one person is not being transferred directly to the next. If, instead of standing, each person rocked to the side and then returned to his or her original upright position, this analogy would be more precise.)

The Tree in the Forest Conundrum

When one discusses the definition of sound, someone will invariably ask the famous philosophical question, "If a tree falls in the forest and no one is around to hear it, is there sound?" The scientific definition is not dependent on a hearing organism being present. A simple example should suffice to clarify the point. If a person blows a dog whistle, he or she cannot hear its sound because it lies above the range of human hearing (c. 20,000 pulses per second). Nearby dogs can hear it and respond accordingly. Just because one individual can't hear it doesn't mean that sound is not present. While this answer may not satisfy the philosophers, it will suffice for our purposes.

A more entertaining question arises during science-fiction films that are loaded with the wonderful sound of roaring engines and firing weapons. Such sound is not possible in the vacuum of space because there is no medium to convey the vibrations.

Once the two conditions exist—a sound source excited by the application of energy and the concomitant transmission of that energy through a conveying medium—sound will occur.

ATTRIBUTES OF SOUND

Moving past the purely theoretical definition of sound, we must briefly discuss the sounds that humans can hear. In a healthy human with excellent hearing, those sounds consist of pulses of energy that are generated in a range of 20 to 20,000 hertz (named after Heinrich Hertz, the discoverer of the principle of electro-magnetic waves). A hertz (or, to use the commonly used abbreviation, **Hz**) consists of one complete displacement cycle of the sound source (see Figure 3–2). Remember, a cycle is the movement of an elastic mass from the point of its state of rest to one extreme of deflection, returning past the resting point to the other deflective extreme and back to its point of rest.

Just as the conveying medium (air) must possess the property of elasticity, our eardrums, our receiving device, must also be elastic to be capable of reacting to the arriving pulses of energy. After each pulse of energy deflects the eardrum, it must return to rest, ready to receive the next pulse. As our eardrums are displaced, that displacement is converted, through a delicate linkage in the middle and inner parts of the ear, into minuscule impulses that travel up our auditory nerves to the brain. In the brain, those neuro-impulses are interpreted as sound.

Frequency and Pitch

The number of times per second that the vibrating medium executes a complete vibratory cycle is called its **frequency**. When our ears react to a specific number of pulses per second, we *perceive* that sound as having a pitch. The higher the

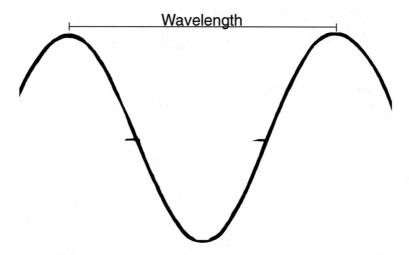

Figure 3–2. Drawing of one cycle of a pure tone. (Adapted from *Vocal Health and Pedagogy* by Robert T. Sataloff, 1998, p. 67. San Diego, CA: Singular Publishing Group. Copyright 1998 by Singular Publishing Group. Reprinted with permission.)

frequency of the cycling, the higher we perceive its pitch. An object vibrating at 440 Hz will be perceived as "middle A" on the piano. If another object vibrates twice as fast, 880 Hz, it would sound the "A" above "middle A." A frequency of 220 Hz would produce the "A" below "middle A."

Figure 3–3 depicts time as distance. Within the same distance (time) on the drawing, the sound on the right has more cycles than the one on the left per given unit of time. Therefore, the sound depicted on the right would have a higher number of cycles in the same amount of time and would be perceived as higher in pitch.

Amplitude

The amount of force applied to the sound generator introduces another variable, **amplitude**. Humans perceive changes in amplitude as changes in loudness. If one increases the amount of deflective energy to the vibrational process, a correspondingly greater distortion of the sound-generating material will occur. As the vibrating material swings in a larger arc, it will displace the neighboring air molecules

with more force. When that increased force finally reaches the ear it will cause a correspondingly greater displacement of the eardrum, which will cause the resulting nerve impulses to the brain to be more intense. As a result, the brain will process this increase as a louder sound. This relationship can be clearly seen in Figure 3–4; both sounds have the same number of cycles for the given amount of time (i.e., they are the same frequency), but the one on the right has far greater amplitude because its displacement from its resting place is greater.

Let us apply the concept of amplitude to a musical instrument, the piano. If you strike a key and keep it depressed the string will continue to vibrate. The pitch will not change, as the speed of the string's travel will remain constant. Just like the child on the swing, however, the string will gradually lose energy with each successive cycle. Its ever-decreasing arc will result in continually lessening amplitude, and our brain will experience the sound as getting softer. Ultimately, the string will resume a resting state, and no sound will exist. The principles of vibration of the vocal folds are the same; the

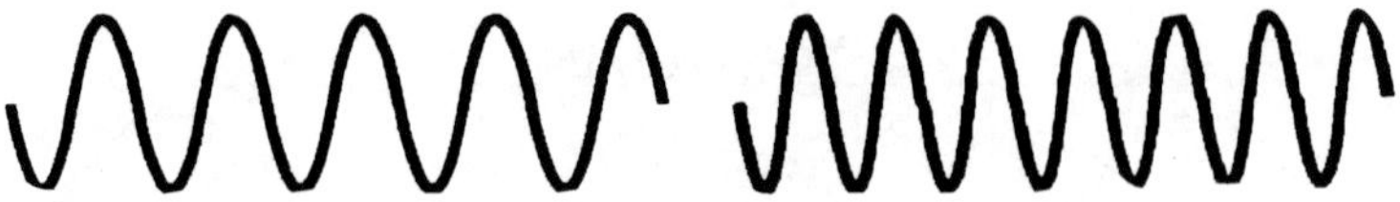

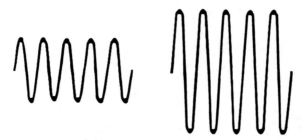

Figure 3–3. Waveform of sounds of differing frequency but the same amplitude: lower frequency (left), higher frequency (right).

Figure 3–4. Two sounds of the same frequency. The sound at the right has greater amplitude.

amount of energy supplied by the pressurized air stream will translate into relative amplitude and not affect the pitch.

Readers should note the distinction between frequency and pitch as well as amplitude and loudness. The concept of frequency and amplitude can be measured precisely with laboratory instruments; pitch and loudness are perceptions sensed in the brain.

MUSICAL TONES VERSUS NOISE: HARMONIC STRUCTURE

The sounds produced by a sound source may be perceived as musical tones or as noise. In this context, we are not defining musical tones as pleasing and noise as displeasing. Since two listeners may differ drastically in their opinion of the difference between music and noise, we must employ an objective definition, one that can be quantified according to principles of physics. A cymbal is a noise by definition, but its sound may be perceived as pleasing by many listeners. The acousti-

cian's objective definition hinges on whether the vibrations are **periodic** or **aperiodic**. Since the cymbal's vibrations are aperiodic, the instrument, which can be so pleasing when played softly and so thrilling when played loudly, is a noise.

Periodic Vibration

A periodic vibration is one in which a definable acoustical structure recurs at equal intervals of time. The graphics shown in Figure 3–5 are **waveforms** (a representation of amplitude vs. time with time represented on the x-axis and amplitude on the y-axis). Compare these two waveforms. The one on the left was produced by a tuning fork and represents a simple periodic vibration; the same simple pattern repeats every cycle. As a tone quality, it is rather boring. On the other hand, a musical instrument's waveform appears far more complex because much more happens during its vibration. The waveform on the right was produced by a voice, and the complexity of its graphic suggests that it might be more interesting to the ear than the simple periodic vibration.

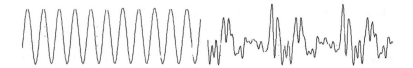

Figure 3–5. A simple wave (left) and a complex periodic wave (right).

Fortunately, virtually all objects vibrate in this more complex way, which causes the sounds we hear to be richer and far more interesting than that produced by a simple periodic vibration. Just as the myriad of detail that we perceive in visual art, such as a Gothic cathedral, can keep our brain occupied for long periods of time, this type of vibratory pattern functions in the same way. This mode of vibration is called **complex periodic vibration** to denote that the vibration is a far more complex vibratory phenomenon than a simple sine wave.

A complex periodic vibration is principally comprised of two simultaneously occurring components:

• The vibration that involves the entire mass of the object, which is the largest and slowest, is called the **fundamental**. Since this wave is the largest, it will be the lowest and loudest sound heard from the object and is the pitch that humans perceive.

• While the full mass of the sound generator is producing the fundamental, its mass is also dividing and oscillating in ever-smaller subdivisions of the whole, producing a complex series of vibrations. These subdivisions are smaller so their amplitude is less (softer), and their periods are faster (higher pitched). Such subsets of the complex vibrational pattern are called **harmonics**.

Harmonics, Overtones, and Partials

Harmonics

Harmonics is the preferred term for this complete series, but it is easy to confuse it with two other words, overtone and par-

tial, that may be applied to these tones. All of the tones in a complex periodic vibration are numbered sequentially upward through the higher frequencies. The difference in term usage lies in whether or not the fundamental is included in the series or is just the foundation for the series.

Overtone

The word **overtone** is synonymous with harmonic. The numbering system is the same for harmonics; the fundamental stands by itself and the complex tones above it are called **overtones** (remember this distinction by focusing on the "over" part of the term). As was the case with harmonics, the numbering of overtones begins with the first overtone above the fundamental.

Partial

The word **partial** denotes the fundamental and harmonics as a unified system. When referring to partials, the fundamental is the first partial and the numbering goes up through the harmonics from there. Many musicians tend to use the word partial synonymously with harmonics, a usage that is incorrect according to the strict scientific definition. The term partial, when used correctly, includes not only the harmonic partials (those coinciding with the overtones of a music sound), but nonharmonic overtones as well (such as those occurring in bells and the unstructured partials of noises).

Table 3–1 shows the mathematical relationship implicit in the harmonic series as well as the relationship between the use of the terms harmonic, overtone, and partial. In musical tones, the harmonic series

Table 3-1. Table of the harmonic series based on a fundamental of low C (C_2).

Harmonic or Overtone Number	Fundamental or F_o	Frequency of the Previous Harmonic		F_o value		Frequency of the Resulting Harmonic	Nearest Tempered Scale Frequency	Number of the Partial
11		719.4	+	65.4	=	784.8	G_5	12
10		654	+	65.4	=	719.4	F_5	11
9		588.6	+	65.4	=	654	E_5	10
8		523.2	+	65.4	=	588.6	D_5	9
7		457.8	+	65.4	=	523.2	C_5	8
6		392.4	+	65.4	=	457.8	$B\flat_4$	7
5		327	+	65.4	=	392.4	G_4	6
4		261.6	+	65.4	=	327	E_4	5
3		196.2	+	65.4	=	261.6	C_4	4
2		130.8	+	65.4	=	196.2	G_3	3
1		65.4	+	65.4	=	130.8	C_3	2
	65.4						C_2	1

constitutes a fixed mathematical relationship to the frequency of the fundamental. In this example of the harmonic series produced by C_2 (the C two ledger lines beneath the bass staff),[1] the frequency of each succeeding harmonic is obtained by adding the frequency of the fundamental to the harmonic preceding it. Virtually all musical instruments possess this relationship of harmonics to fundamental. These frequencies of the harmonics correlate with the pitches given in the "Nearest Tempered Scale Frequency" column.

Aperiodic Vibration: Noise

Noise is a difficult phenomenon to define in scientific terms. One could make an attempt by stating that a noise is an aperiodic sound and has no definable fundamental or harmonic structure above it (the mathematical structure defined in the previous section). A noise may suggest an area of pitch or resonance, but such characteristics are not measurable with much specificity.

This definition is fine up to a point. As we will see later, it is too simplistic, as it does not account for the role that individual perception plays in the definition of noise. The next illustration (Figure 3–6) shows the power spectra of two sounds, a voice on the left and a cymbal on the right.

This type of computer-generated graphic display, called a **power spectrum**, divides the sound into its constituent frequencies (*all* frequencies, whether they are periodic or aperiodic). Thus, it can be used to study all sounds, not just musical ones (much more will be said about power spectrum analysis later in this book). For

---

[1]Pitches are labeled from the lowest note on the standard piano keyboard (C_1 at 32.7 Hz, the next C is C_2 at 65.4 Hz, and so forth).

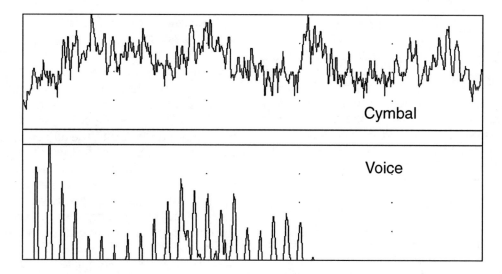

Figure 3–6. Power spectra of a complex periodic vibration (musical tone) and an aperiodic sound (noise). 💿

now, it is sufficient to know that a power spectrum graphically represents a sound at a given point in time, a sort of aural snapshot.

The x-axis shows a sequence of analyzed frequencies. As one scans from left to right, the frequencies portrayed get higher. On the y-axis one can read the amplitude of each frequency. The higher a peak that represents a harmonic appears on the graph, the louder it sounds. In this way, the relative strengths of frequencies in the sonic spectrum can be seen and measured.

Using this tool, one can see with the eyes what the ear hears, ascertain the location of the constituent harmonics, note differences in amplitude of harmonics, and identify harmonic patterns if they are present. Although the human brain comprehends the totality of the sound, the computer excels at determining the microelements that make up the sound.

As one can see, the sound of the cymbal is a ragged mass of frequencies with certain ones peeking out of the chaotic mess. The vocal spectrum, on the other hand, has a clearly defined harmonic structure that is readily perceived and quantified.

In the first paragraph of this discussion, the cymbal was cited as a noise because of its aperiodicity. Although we may *perceive* its sound as beautiful or intensely interesting, it is still aperiodic. If we ignore the personal perception factor, our simple definition still works; the sound of a cymbal is a noise because it has no periodicity.

Pause To Review

The phenomenon of sound is a chain of energy transference:

- Energy is applied to the sound source.
- In response, the generator vibrates.
- Those vibrations excite the air around the generator, causing waves of energy to ripple outward.
- The ripples impact on our eardrums and are converted into signals our brain can interpret as sound.

If this energy-transference chain is intact, we have sound present. Now, let's add another critical facet to our understanding of musical sounds, resonance.

RESONANCE

Thus far, we have only dealt with the sound source. There is another important component found in almost all musical instruments, the resonator. In most instruments, a **resonator** (something that can **resonate**) is placed between the sound source and the conveying medium, the air. This resonator strengthens the sound generated by the source, and in the process alters its tone. Without the action of the resonator, most sound sources would be unusable as musical instruments.

The word resonance and the related word, resonator are used freely by musicians to describe the working parts of their instruments that define and enrich the sound source. In everyday conversation, nonmusicians use the variant word resonate: "That canyon resonated with the sound of the birds," or "That idea just doesn't resonate with me." For such a common concept, finding someone who understands it or can explain it in acoustic terms turns out to be surprisingly difficult. However, the everyday examples given previously contain strong clues. In the first phrase, the acoustical environment in the canyon *enhanced* the sound of the birds; the second actually says, "I'm not in *sympathy* with that idea."

Two Different Kinds of Resonator

General Resonator

One reason it is difficult to properly define the term resonance is that we use the word resonator for two different types of acoustical processes. One is the *general resonator*, like the soundboard of a piano that reacts with vibrations of any pitch and reinforces the sound by presenting a larger vibrating surface to the atmosphere. This type of resonator transfers the source's energy to the conveying medium more efficiently than the sound source alone.

A Specific Type of Resonator: A Cylinder Closed at One End

The type of resonator that most closely approximates the model of the human voice is a tube, open at one end and closed on the other, that encloses an air mass. Since air is elastic, the air contained within such a resonator will vibrate when it is exposed to another vibration of a certain pitch. That certain pitch must have a mathematical relationship between the air mass in the resonator and the **wavelength** of the sound vibrating nearby. The wavelength is the distance a sound wave must travel to complete one full cycle as it moves outward from the sound source and into a medium (see Figure 3–2). For a sound with a frequency of 500 Hz (slightly sharp of B_4 on the piano), one complete cycle will have a wavelength of 68.8 cm of linear air space. It must travel that distance before the next wave can move outward. (Wavelength is calculated by dividing the nominal speed of sound by the frequency.)

Sympathetic Vibration and Resonance

Physicists discovered that an enclosed air mass will resonate (sympathetically vibrate) when the length of the resonator (and its enclosed air mass) equals one-fourth the wavelength of the nearby sound. One-fourth of the wavelength of the example 68.8 cm equals 17.2 cm. Using the value of 17.2 cm as an example of a resonator is pertinent because it falls within the range of the average length of the male vocal tract (17 to 20 cm). Thus, any sound that has the frequency of 500 Hz or any of its harmonic multiples will cause that resonant air mass to vibrate in sympathy and to add its own acoustical properties to the original source sound. An adjacent frequency above or below 500 Hz may cause the air in the tube to vibrate in sympathy, but not with as high an amplitude as the pitch that matches the natural resonance of the tube.

This same resonator will also resonate when excited by pitches that are odd multiples of the resonance of 500 Hz (1500, 2500, 3500 Hz and beyond). When sound from the source passes through the resonator, those frequencies that are in tune with the resonance will receive a boost in amplitude, and the others will be attenuated (softened) or even canceled. In this way, a resonator acts as an acoustic *filter* or lens, helping some frequencies and hindering others.

Wind instruments (woodwinds, brass, and the human voice) all employ such a resonator. It is important to note that the resonator does not *impart* energy to the air as the sound generator does but merely reacts to, and vibrates with, the acoustical energy already present.

The interaction between the sound source and its helper, the resonator, can be easily observed in wind instruments. If one blows on an oboe reed without the body of the instrument attached, a high, unpleasant screech will result. When the oboe body (the resonator) is attached, the

sound of the instrument changes radically (Figure 3–7).

TIMBRE

We have seen that musical instruments (including the voice) emit sounds comprised of complex periodic vibrations. These instruments produce sounds that are comprised of both a fundamental (the pitch we hear) and an extensive series of harmonics above the fundamental. Each type of instrument, be it a voice or a violin, has its own basic acoustical signature based on the *relative amplitude* of the constituent harmonics within the general pattern that is recognized as musical tone. The unique tonal quality peculiar to each instrument—or even more subtly, between two instruments of the same type—is called **timbre**. These differences are produced mostly by the resonator, which can alter the amplitude of the harmonics found in the originating pattern of the sound source; some of the harmonics are amplified, some are attenuated, and some are canceled out.

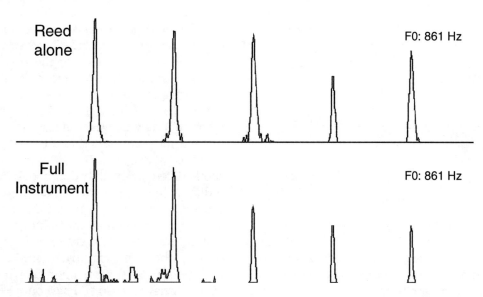

Figure 3–7. Spectra of an oboe reed alone and with the resonator attached. 💿

Differences Between One Instrument Type and Another

To recognize the aural difference between various types of instruments, the human brain converts highly complex sounds into neural impulses. The brain uses these impulses to compare different sounds by analyzing the differences in the amplitude of the individual harmonics present in the sound. Instrument "X" may have a strong 1st and 5th harmonic, while instrument "Y" may produce a pattern that emphasizes harmonics 2 and 6. Such a difference in harmonic amplitude can be seen in Figure 3–8, which shows the spectra of a cello and a baritone performing the same pitch.

When the brain analyzes these amplitude patterns, it consults its memory bank of sound patterns and compares incoming signals with its stored patterns. When the brain matches an incoming signal produced by a voice to its stored voice pattern, it recognizes the sound as that of a voice.

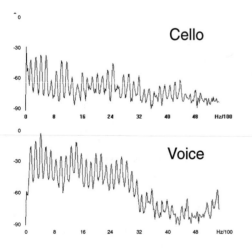

Figure 3–8. Spectra of a cello and a singer (baritone) performing the same frequency showing the differences in amplitude of the harmonics. **CD**

Differences Within the Same Instrument Type

What about singers or instruments of the same type? How do we distinguish between two individual voices even though they have the same general timbre? For example, two baritones singing the same pitch should have the same harmonic pattern visible in their spectra. How can the brain distinguish between two different voices? The answer is found in subtle differences of the amplitude of the harmonics that make up the recognizable pattern for the baritone voice.

Figure 3–9 shows the results of two baritones singing the same pitch. Both have the same recognizable pattern of strengths and weaknesses in their harmonic structure that tells the brain that we are hearing two examples of the human baritone voice. Within the patterns of the two voices, however, there are minute variations resulting from differences in the size, shape, and density of the anatomical structures comprising their vocal instruments. The human brain not only recognizes the pattern comprising the human voice but also differentiates between the patterns of two voices of the same type.

This ability to recognize small differences in a larger common pattern has a corollary in the sense of sight. When most people look at different car models from the same maker, there is a set of visual signals that first tells the brain the objects are cars (not trucks). Then the brain recognizes a commonality between all the models of one manufacturer allowing it to recognize that it is by maker X. There are also more subtle differences within the model line of maker X (a piece of trim or a differently shaped headlight) that gives the brain the information to identify individual models within that manufacturer's line of cars. To do this, the brain employs a similar sequence of pattern recognition as when it distinguishes between two baritones.

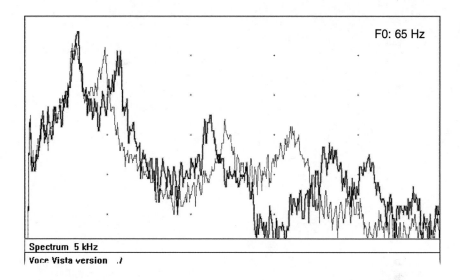

Figure 3–9. Spectra of the formants of two men singing the same frequency. The dark line represents the spectrum of a bass-baritone; the light line is that of a lyric baritone. Notice the subtle shifts in formants. ⓒⒹ

SUMMARY

More information is required before computer analysis as an aid in the voice studio can be discussed. This chapter has just touched on the basics of the physics of sound. The next chapter will build on these basics as it deals with the specific type of sound produced by the unique human vocal instrument.

CHAPTER

4

THE PRODUCTION OF VOCAL SOUND

THE MIRACLE OF OUR VOICE

Few people ever pause to consider the miracle of speech and song. If one takes the time to do so, the miracle—actually a constellation of miracles—is revealed in all its elegant complexity. The experience can be both humbling and exhilarating.

Among these miracles is the ability to produce the unique timbre that distinguishes one voice from all others and simultaneously produces the multitude of speech sounds required for language within that distinct timbre. To accomplish this, two simultaneous actions are required:

• The creation of sound by our vocal sound generator, the **larynx**. This organ creates the pulses of energy that become the raw materials of the final vocal product. Once the sound has been created, it radiates upward through the vocal instrument.

• Resonation of that sound within all our enclosed air spaces, from the top of the vocal folds up through the openings of the mouth and nose. As the sound travels upward, it is filtered and considerably modified. If humans did not possess this resonator, the sound produced by larynges (plural of larynx), would be almost useless for the production of language as humans know it. To understand the sound-making process, we will build on the basic principles discussed in the previous chapter. A solid understanding of the physics of the human voice will be essential to the understanding of the material in the chapters that follow.

THE LARYNX

The human larynx, shown in Figure 4–1, is a collection of cartilage, ligaments, and muscle. The **vocal folds**, the structures that actually make sound are located in the center of the larynx. They are comprised of two bands of muscle covered with **mucosal** tissue. While the vocal folds provide the source vibration for speech and song, they actually perform two more basic but critical functions, which are explained in the following sections.

NONVOCAL LARYNGEAL FUNCTIONS

First, the vocal folds constitute a gateway structure that functions as a valve, which can:

- help prevent the inhalation of foreign material and prevent it from reaching the trachea and lungs. The vocal folds can also aid in the expulsion of the for-

eign matter by the execution of a reflexive **cough**, and
- close completely to hold air in the lungs when support for the main torso is needed to facilitate the lifting of heavy objects or aid in waste elimination by helping musculature deliver downward force.

Creation of Vocal Sound

Second, on a much higher level, the vocal folds act as a sound generator for the speech and song processes. While most animals high on the evolutionary chain possess the ability to phonate, humans may be unique in their ability to produce complex language. At some point in our evolution, the human brain developed the ability to both conceptualize language and employ the vocal tract to produce sounds to communicate that language. Humans have evolved a form of communication that involves the highly complex manipulation of the anatomical structures from the pelvic floor all the way to

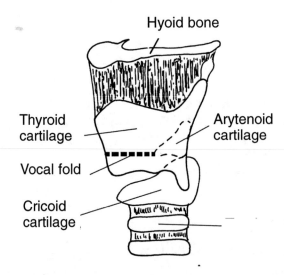

Figure 4–1. The principal structures of the larynx. (From *The Speech Sciences*, by R. D. Kent, 1997, p. 103. San Diego, CA: Singular Publishing Group. Copyright 1997 by Singular Publishing Group. Adapted and reprinted with permission.)

the oral and nasal openings. Our ability to communicate with each other in complex language (in the form of both speech and song) is one of the chief attributes that sets the human species apart from the rest of the animal kingdom.

All of these laryngeal functions, valve and sound generator, are accomplished by muscles that move the vocal folds toward the centerline of the larynx. When the lar-

ynx is not in active use as a valve or sound producer, the vocal folds are parked in an at rest position that can be opened to permit the free passage of breath to and from the lungs. When we employ our vocal folds as a valve, they move together to completely seal the airway. When we wish to phonate, they are held slightly apart. Figure 4–2 shows the vocal folds in these basic configurations.

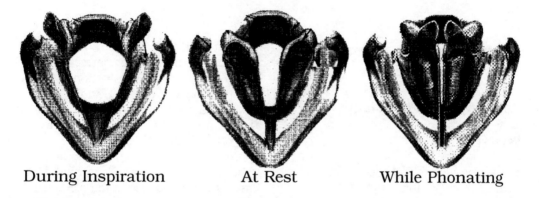

During Inspiration   At Rest   While Phonating

Figure 4–2. Vocal folds viewed from above in inhalation, rest, and phonating configurations. (Adapted from *Vocal Health and Pedagogy* by Robert T. Sataloff, 1998, p. 15. San Diego, CA: Singular Publishing Group. Copyright 1998 by Singular Publishing Group. Reprinted with permission.)

A Short Treatise on Throat Clearing

The prevention of the inhalation of foreign matter is among the most important functions of the larynx. The first line of defense in accomplishing this protective task is the flap that sits at the top of the larynx, the **epiglottis**. When one swallows, the epiglottis seals the top of the larynx to keep the food or liquid from going into the larynx and onward, down into the trachea and lungs. Inhalation of foreign matter into these organs could be life threatening, as blocked airways impair or destroy the ability to take in oxygen.

As swallowing is initiated, the epiglottis seals the top of the larynx just before the swallowing motion reaches the laryngeal area. But this task is not always timed precisely. When coordination fails and material passes into the larynx, highly sensitive nerves in the area sense danger and signal the abdominal muscles to expel air with considerable force. This act of potentially lifesaving desperation is a reflex action known as **coughing**.

When singers "clear their throats" to expel **phlegm**, the body functions much as it does in a cough. No matter how many times laryngologists and voice teachers

(continued)

implore singers not to clear their throats, the practice continues because it is basically an unconscious reflex action and difficult to control.

However, this clearing action can potentially damage the vocal folds. It often causes **edema** (swelling), and, at worst, can contribute to the development of vocal nodules (growths). The damage can result in impaired vocal production ranging in intensity from mild to severe called **dysphonia**.

Voice practitioners must constantly reinforce the importance of substituting a "hard swallow" for an irritating short cough. The CD that accompanies this text includes a short video clip showing the larynx as the throat is cleared ((cd) Video 4–1).

Fundamentals of Vocal Fold Vibration

Anatomy and Physiology

Vocal Folds

The sound-generating vocal folds are suspended in a "V" formation in the middle of the larynx. To form this "V," each vocal fold is attached to an **arytenoid** cartilage at the back of the larynx. Both folds are attached to the thyroid cartilage in the front (see Figure 4–1). The variable space between the vocal folds is called the **glottis** (note that the glottis is a *space* and not structure).

Arytenoidal Movement

The arytenoid cartilages and their accompanying musculature are capable of an amazing variety of motions that place the vocal folds in dynamically different configurations. These motions alter both the aperture of the glottis and the length of the vocal folds. (Refer to Figure 4–2 to view some of the possible arytenoid configurations.)

Glottal Position for Phonation

For the generation of sound to occur, the vocal folds must be placed in a stance where pressurized airflow from the lungs can cause the folds to vibrate. As long as the folds remain in the correct proximity for phonation, the application of pressurized airflow will create sound.

Should inhalation for additional breath be required, the arytenoids move away from the centerline, opening the glottis to permit the free flow of air. Should further phonation be required, the glottal aperture is again reduced to the configuration that permits phonation. In this text, the term **glottal focus** will be used to denote the degree of aperture separating the vocal folds.

Initiating Phonation

As we have seen, a deflective force must be applied to an elastic body for vibration and the consequent creation of sound to occur. In the case of the voice, the sound-generating bodies are the vocal folds, and the deflective force is pressurized air from our lungs.

Subglottal Pressure

The body must pressurize the air in the lungs and push it through the restricted area of the glottis. The pressure beneath the vocal folds, **subglottal pressure** (sub = below), must be higher than it is in the area above the glottis, **supraglottal** (supra = above), in order for phonation to occur.

When the vocal folds are in the narrow glottal focus in which phonation can occur and pressurized air from the lungs is applied from below, a phenomenon called the **Bernoulli** effect occurs.

The Bernoulli Effect

The *Bernoulli* effect is named after Daniel Bernoulli (pronounced "ber-nool-ee" or, in IPA,[1] /bɜ·nuli/), an 18th-century Swiss mathematician and physician who developed the kinetic theory of fluids (in physics, gas is considered a fluid).

Bernoulli discovered that when a gas traveling through a tube encounters a restriction, it both speeds up and experiences a drop in pressure at the point of restriction. Watching sand run through an hourglass may help clarify the concept of the Bernoulli effect. As the sand flows down through the glass, the sand in the wide tube at the top moves slowly and is densely packed. When the sand reaches the narrow waist of the hourglass (the point of restriction), it both speeds up and experiences a lowering of density (pressure).

In the human voice, this point of restriction is the narrowed glottis. When air, under pressure from the lungs and abdominal area, is forced through this smaller aperture, a low pressure (suction) develops between the vocal folds. The folds are pulled inward in response to this suction until they meet at the centerline (Figure 4–3).

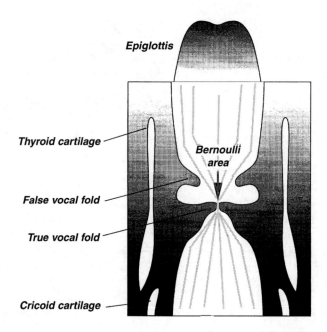

Figure 4–3. Schematic of airflow in the voice including the Bernoulli effect. (From *The Speech Sciences*, by R. D. Kent, 1997, p. 106. San Diego, CA: Singular Publishing Group. Copyright 1997 by Singular Publishing Group. Adapted and reprinted with permission.)

[1]Speech and singing sounds in this book will be represented by the symbols of the *International Phonetic Alphabet* (IPA). You will find a complete listing of all the IPA symbols for American English (as well as common sounds utilized in the principal singing languages other than English) in Appendix A at the end of this book. The reader is urged to become fluent in IPA, as its use facilitates understanding and communication between voice practitioners.

Myoelasticity Joins In

The Bernoulli effect sets up a chain of actions that help create and sustain vocal fold vibration. When the vocal folds close, the pressure of the subglottal airflow from below forces them apart again. Once they are apart, a combination of the Bernoulli effect and vocal fold **myoelasticity** pull the folds back toward closure at the centerline. Myoelasticity means muscle elasticity (myo meaning muscle, and elastic, indicating that the muscle will return to its resting state after it has been stretched).

When the vocal folds meet at the centerline, the cycle begins again as subglottal air pressure builds up and the vocal folds are moved apart. The full cycle of the parting and returning forces (Bernoulli/myoelasticity and air pressure) is illustrated in Figure 4–4.

How Much of a Role Does the Bernoulli Effect Play?

Most scientists agree that the Bernoulli effect plays some part in the process of bringing the vocal folds toward the centerline during each vibratory cycle. Scientists have recently theorized however, that the Bernoulli's importance in maintaining vocal fold vibration may have been overestimated. Significant contributions stem from myoelastic forces in the folds, from the acceleration of the airflow through the glottis, and from the sluggish response of the vocal tract to this airflow.

If the Bernoulli effect were not a factor in this phenomenon, all vocal initiation might have to begin with a full closure of the vocal folds, an action called a glottal stop (a type of initiation that can lead to vocal fold injury). In addition, if only the myoelastic effect were available to help return the vocal folds to the centerline, that return might be less efficient, possibly affecting one's ability to sustain vibration. For explanations in greater depth, the reader is urged to consult Titze (1994).

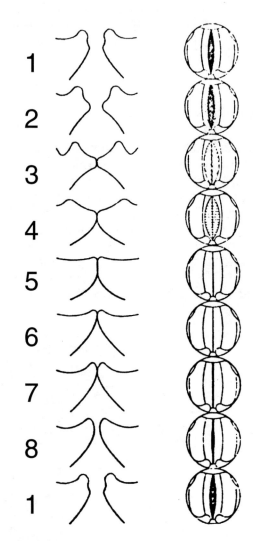

Figure 4-4. A full cycle of the vocal folds. (From *The Science of the Singing Voice* by Johan Sundberg, 1987, p. 64. DeKalb, IL: Northern Illinois University Press. Copyright 1987 by Northern Illinois University Press. Reprinted with permission.)

Creation of Vocal Sound

Each time the vocal folds meet, air pressure is built up and then released as the folds are forced apart again. As the folds part, a puff of pressurized air is released into the airway of the singer where it radiates upward and then emerges from the mouth. Each puff represents a complete vibration of the vocal folds, and the number of times per second these puffs occur determines the frequency of the sound. If the vibratory cycle emits 440 puffs of air per second, we perceive the pitch of those pulses of energy as middle "A."

The CD that accompanies this text contains a short video of the vocal folds vibrating in apparent slow motion (CD Video 4–2). The instrument that captures these remarkable images is called a stroboendoscope (strobo, because it uses a strobe light that is timed with the cycling of the vibrating vocal folds, endoscope because it is an image-conveying tube that can be inserted into the body to permit doctors and scientists to view a physiological or anatomical point of interest). (CD Video 4–3. Endoscopic views of the production of high, middle, and low pitches. Note the stretching and thinning of the vocal folds for the high pitch and the shortening and thickening of the folds on the low pitch.)

The previous chapter explained how the relative amplitude of the harmonics found in complex periodic vibrations allows the brain to differentiate between a voice and a cello, or even between two voices or instruments of the same type. With regard to the voice, these minute variants are mostly the product of the resonating system.

VOCAL RESONANCE

The sound created at the vocal folds must travel through the air-enclosing structures found between the top of the vocal folds and the openings of the mouth and nose. This area includes the top portion of the larynx (above the vocal folds), the pharyngeal cavity, and the oral and/or nasal cavities (Figure 4–5).

These areas form a resonator, open at one end (the mouth and nostrils), and

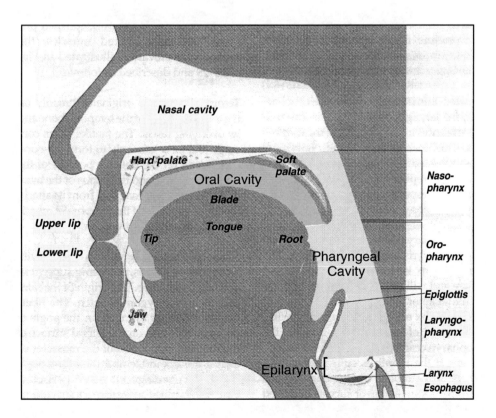

Figure 4–5. Sagittal view of the vocal system with the resonance spaces shaded. (From *The Speech Sciences,* by R. D. Kent, 1997, p. 167. San Diego, CA: Singular Publishing Group. Copyright 1997 by Singular Publishing Group. Adapted and reprinted with permission.)

closed at the other (at the vocal folds). Since the folds spend a considerable amount of each cycle in the closed position, this end of the resonator can be considered closed in terms of acoustics. All of the resonant structures are interconnected, and they function collectively as the human vocal resonator. Without this resonator, the sound emitted by the larynx would be feeble, possessing none of the qualities recognized as the human voice. Without the resonating system, humans would lack the ability to produce language as well.

Our Malleable Resonator

The human resonator is unique among musical instruments as it can be reconfigured in an astounding variety of shapes. Figure 4–6 shows a few of the shapes that

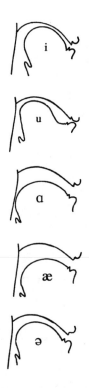

Figure 4–6. Views of various human resonator configurations. (From *The Speech Sciences,* by R. D. Kent, 1997, p. 335. San Diego, CA: Singular Publishing Group. Copyright 1997 by Singular Publishing Group. Reprinted with permission.)

the vocal resonating column can assume. Joan Wall and Robert Caldwell (1996) describe these as "trumpets designed by Dr. Seuss" in their video about the vocal tract. Humans reshape their resonators by the use of **articulators**, which are the movable parts of our anatomical structures, such as the musculature in the walls of the pharynx or the tongue.

Reshaping the Vocal Resonating Spaces

You can perform a simple demonstration to experience the reshaping capacity of your vocal resonating spaces. Open your mouth and gently flick a finger on your cheek, toward the back and just in front of the vertical part of your mandible (the jaw bone; the vertical structure is called the ramus). Don't make any sound with your vocal folds. The intent of this exercise is to explore only vocal resonance, not sound generated at the vocal folds. As you flick a finger against your cheek, you will hear the air in your oral (mouth) and pharyngeal (throat) cavities resonate a pitch. (If you have the ability to "cluck" your tongue, you can use that noise instead of the flicking finger.)

Repeat this exercise, but this time, reshape your oral cavity by forming a different vowel each time you make the sound on your cheek. As you do this, your articulators will create different "pitches" caused by changes in the size and shape of the cavities.

Source-Filter Theory

An elegant explanation of how the vocal resonator works can be found in the *source-filter theory* (Fant, 1960). Fant proposed that human vocal resonators act as an acoustical lens. As the sound source leaves the vocal folds, it is filtered by the vocal tract resonance. This resonance imprints its own acoustical "personality" on the sound source's harmonic spectrum. Based on the size, shape, and density of the walls of the enclosure, resonators can have one of four effects on the harmonic spectrum of the source sound. The filter can:

- amplify (make louder),
- attenuate (soften),
- nullify (cancel), or
- pass the sound through without any alteration.

Chiba and Kajiyama (1946) conducted the initial work on this concept, but it was not widely disseminated due to the political conditions that existed just after World War II. Gunnar Fant's book, from which the name of the theory is derived, has had wide influence; other researchers have further refined this theory (especially Johan Sundberg). Its explanation of vocal tract resonance and the role it plays in shaping our vocal production explains a significant portion of the acoustical phenomena that we encounter. (Other work on nonlinear models, such as that by Teager and Teager [1992] and others may help to fill existing gaps in our knowledge in the future.)

The Acoustical Lens

Since one of the goals of this book is to further the use of visual input to help vocal practitioners understand sound, the relationship between the resonator and the sound source might best be explained in terms of sight. One can compare the vocal resonator to an optical lens. When light reflects off an object, our eyes convert it into neural impulses that our brain can image as a "picture" of the object. If an optical lens is placed between the object and the eye, the image that we perceive will change because the lens alters the

incoming light. As long as the various lenses are not too distorting, the object will remain recognizable, yet altered according to the properties of the lens. Each change in lens shape will imprint its own distinctive visual "personality" on the image.

It is much the same with the acoustical lens formed by the human resonator. Every time the brain shifts the configuration of the resonator articulators (a change in lens shape), the size and shape of the resonator changes and produces its own acoustical effect (Figure 4–7). The

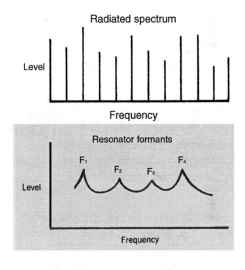

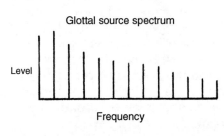

Figure 4–7. Schematic of the source filter theory showing a schematic power spectra of the glottal source (bottom), the resonator formants (middle), and the resulting radiated spectrum (top). The formants in the middle schematic filter the spectrum values coming from the source and produce the radiated spectrum. (Adapted from *Vocal Health and Pedagogy* by Robert T. Sataloff, 1998, p. 48. San Diego, CA: Singular Publishing Group. Copyright 1998 by Singular Publishing Group. Adapted and reprinted with permission.)

result of this collaboration between sound source and resonator is that the listener's brain acquires enough information to enable it to identify the individual producing the sound as well as perceive the various effects of the changes in filtration. These changes are recognizable as the various acoustical components needed for language production. Each unique articulator-induced shape possesses its own acoustical signature. The effects of the articulative reshaping of the vocal resonator will occupy considerable attention in later chapters as we explore the vocal production of singers with the help of computer analysis.

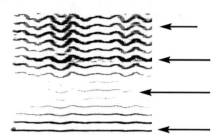

Figure 4–8. Spectrogram of vowel /i/ showing the horizontal strata which represent individual harmonics. Note the differences in intensity of the lines denoting the varying amplitude of the harmonics. **CD**

Vowels and Formants

When a resonator reinforces an area of the spectrum of the sound source, the area of reinforcement is called a **formant**. There can be multiple formants at various frequency regions in the sonic signature of any complex periodic sound.

Spectrogram: Another Way To Digitally Image Sound

A type of computer analysis—called the **spectrogram**—will allow for better understanding of formants. This type of analysis will form a major portion of the subject of this book. A spectrogram is similar to the power-spectrum analysis seen in Chapter 3. This type of graphic representation presents the acoustic analysis as follows:

- the X-axis represents time,
- the Y-axis represents frequency, and
- the color intensity of the lines represents amplitude. Each horizontal line in the displayed signal represents a different harmonic in the sound spectrum.

Thus the spectrogram shown in Figure 4–8 is actually a three-dimensional graph, revealing three analytical parameters in-

stead of the two shown in a power spectrum. A line or collection of lines of high intensity at one place on the graph *probably* indicates the presence of a proximate formant.

One can see evidence of formants in the spectrograms of two vowels, /i/ (Figure 4–8), and /a/ (see Figure 4–11). Tongue shape is the principal agent for the change of resonance that creates these two vowels. The physical shift in the resonating column is actually far more complex than just a tongue shape; other anatomical structures—such as the velum, the pharynx, and the jaw—play important roles as well. For now, the discussion will concentrate on the tongue.

The vowel /i/: A Front Vowel

To produce the vowel /i/, the tongue assumes a position that is forward and up in the oral cavity. This results in the creation of a small resonance area high in the front of the oral cavity. Simultaneously, a large resonance area is created in the pharynx. Since the apex of the tongue is forward in the mouth, it is called a **front vowel**.

In the spectrogram shown in Figure 4–8, one can see that the first formant (F_1) is low (indicated by the lowest arrow). In fact, it is the lowest formant of the vowel series that we call the front vowels. The middle arrow shows the relatively high F_2. The **singer's formant** (SF) is indicated by the upper arrow and is a combination of F_3 and F_4 (more information about this critical subject will be found later in this chapter).

Note that the symbol for formants is a capital F, followed by a subscripted number. The fundamental is written as F_0, the first formant above it is written as F_1, and so forth.

The positions of F_1 and F_2 on the spectrograph in Figure 4–8 are produced because of the following:

- The low F_1 is due to the large space at the rear of the oral cavity; since it is large, it resonates a low pitch-area of the spectrum.
- The small, high space at the front of the oral cavity causes the high F_2; a smaller space resonates a higher pitch area than a larger one.

Correlate these concepts with the view of the articulator configuration for /i/ shown in Figure 4–9, in which one can clearly see, due to the position of the tongue, the small oral cavity and the large pharyngeal area.

The vowel /a/: A Back Vowel

For the vowel /a/, one lowers the mandible, an action that also drops the tongue because the mandible is the base for the tongue. This action, along with some muscular reshaping of the tongue, results in a large oral cavity and a small pharynx (Figure 4–10).

The spectrogram for this vowel clearly shows a typical pattern for a **back vowel** (Figure 4–11); /a/ has a high F_1 (the highest of any vowel) and a low F_2. The massing of the tongue in the back of the oral cavity results in a small pharyngeal area that produces the high F_1; a large oral cavity in the front accounts for the low F_2. Thus a relatively small shift in anatomy produces a major difference in resonation characteristics between the two vowels. The brain recognizes the acoustical effect of these differences by calculating the

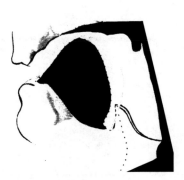

Figure 4–9. Sagittal view of the head showing the resonance configuration for the vowel /i/. (Schematic sagittal view adapted from *The Science of Vocal Pedagogy*, by D. R. Appelman, 1967, p. 299. Bloomington, IN: Indiana University Press. Copyright 1967 by Indiana University Press. Adapted and reprinted with permission.)

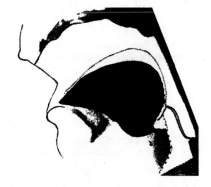

Figure 4–10. Sagittal view of the head showing the resonance configuration for the vowel /a/ showing the small pharyngeal cavity area and the large oral cavity. (Schematic sagittal view adapted from *The Science of Vocal Pedagogy*, by D. R. Appelman, 1967, p. 331. Bloomington, IN: Indiana University Press. Copyright 1967 by Indiana University Press. Adapted and reprinted with permission.)

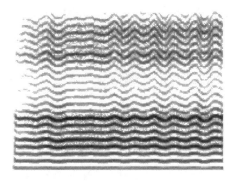

Figure 4–11. Spectrogram of the vowel /a/. 💿

placement and strength of formants. With that information, it is able to recognize the individuality of the two vowel sounds.

Shifting articulator placement produces changes in formants that result in a wide variety of sounds. Languages present a bewildering variety of resonator shapes, which is one reason that the study of speech and song is so fascinating. One can even study subtle differences in pronunciation within a single language. The formants in two accents will be subtly different but similar enough that one should still be able to identify the word as the same when spoken by the two individuals.

The Singer's Formant

There is another vital contribution, critical to fine classical singing, that the ability to produce various formants makes possible. How can a single person sing in front of a 90-piece symphony orchestra and not be acoustically overwhelmed by the sheer mass of orchestral sound? When people attend the opera or an orchestral concert, they think about this phenomenon only when the singer cannot be heard. The audience blames the conductor and the orchestra for the imbalance, but how can the singer be heard at all when competing against such a formidable sound-making machine?

The answer is found in the well-trained singer's ability to produce a formant in a specific area of the spectrum that is considerably different from the resonances produced by the orchestra. Figure 4–12 shows the difference in the formant structure of the vowel /a/ when both spoken and sung. In the upper line that denotes the singing voice, note the peak that begins to build at about 2400 Hz, peaks at 2800 Hz, then falls off at about 3200 Hz. This is the **singer's formant**.

Production of the Singer's Formant

In the well-trained voice, the singer's formant dwells in the neighborhood of 2800 Hz, ± 500 Hz; its center frequency is primarily dependent on the effective length of the vocal tract. The singer's formant is considered to be a clustering of the third, fourth, and fifth formants. As early as the mid-1930s, Bartholomew (1934) observed this formant and suspected that the **epiglottal tube** was its prime source (this is the area between the top of the glottis and the opening into the pharynx at the base of the epiglottis, also called the **epilarynx**). Johan Sundberg (1974) proposed that the formant is produced when the

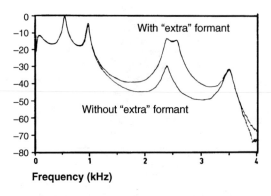

Figure 4–12. Spectrum48

showing the vowel /a/ with and without the singer's formant. (From *The Science of the Singing Voice* by Johan Sundberg, 1987, p. 118. DeKalb, IL: Northern Illinois University Press. Copyright 1987

cross-sectional area of the pharynx immediately above the laryngeal tube opening is approximately six times greater than the area of that opening.

Traditionally, the presence of this desirable formant has been referred to in terms such as "ring" or "point." It is one of the principal distinguishing characteristics of the trained singing voice. (The use of the singer's formant is more prevalent in male singers than in females.)

Importance of a Low Larynx in Singer's Formant Production

It is thought that the production of this critical formant is aided by a low laryngeal position while singing, a position which lengthens and widens the pharynx (Sundberg, 1987). Ingo Titze (1998) offered some interesting insight into this theory by concentrating on pharyngeal widening as an important tonal balance to the brilliance of the singer's formant (as long as the epiglottal tube is kept narrow). He also proposed that the widened pharynx leads to a decoupling of the vocal folds from the changing phonemes above.

Most singers pay particular attention to the development of the singer's formant during their training, as its presence is considered an integral and highly desirable facet of their technique. There are many other beneficial reasons for developing freedom in the laryngeal area beyond the production of the singer's formant.

Figure 4–13 is a graph of data collected by Johan Sundberg (1987) showing two long-term-average spectra (known as **LTAS**). It shows the mean of the spectra of all sounds during a long audio sample correlating the sound of a symphony orchestra with that of speech and singing. The loudest partials in both speech and orchestra fall in the area of 450 Hz. The line denoting speech stays very close to that of the orchestra, but the singer produces a vastly different spectrum with a peak in the area of 3 kHz. It is the singer's formant that permits the voice to be heard over the orchestra. Readers who

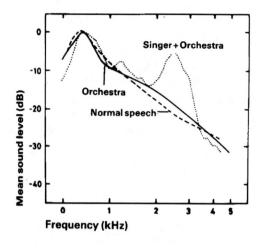

Figure 4–13. Long-term-average spectra for the sound of an orchestra with and without a singing soloist showing the differentiation that the singer achieves by the use of the c. 3000 Hz (the singer's formant). (From *The Science of the Singing Voice* by Johan Sundberg, 1987, p. 123. DeKalb, IL: Northern Illinois University Press. Copyright 1987 by Northern Illinois University Press. Reprinted with permission.)

wish to know more about this crucial aspect of vocal technique should consult Sundberg's excellent discussion of the phenomenon (Sundberg, 1987).

Genetic Inheritance

Of course, there are other factors that determine a vocalist's viability on the large stage. The singer's general ability to produce sounds of significant amplitude is vital. Not all singers are created equal when it comes to the issue of amplitude potential. Most people never have the experience of standing beside an internationally ranked singer during a loud passage. If they could, most would be astounded at the sheer magnificence of the amount and richness of the sound pouring forth. These singers are a part of an extraordinarily select group. Their physical and neuromuscular gifts rank them with the best athletes. A singer possessing such gifts can easily produce a tone with an amplitude range which, if attempted by a smaller voice, would fatigue and perhaps even damage the larynx. With the gifted singer's higher average amplitude comes a higher singer's formant amplitude as well. This amplitude enables the gifted singer to soar above the symphony orchestra with apparent ease.

Consonants

Using the vocal articulators, people are capable of making a wide variety of sounds that are not vowels. These sounds are called **consonants**. As we will see in later chapters that focus on consonants, it is difficult to arrive at a simple, clean definition of the word. It is far easier to create consonant subclasses that can be categorized by the commonality of their physiological production than it is to create one overriding definition.

To understand the complexity of consonants, observe that consonant sounds in English include those produced as:

- bursts of energy, with or without a pitch emanating from the larynx (stops such as /b/ or /p/)
- rushing-air sounds, with or without pitch (fricatives such as /z/ or /s/)
- momentary shutting off of the airflow at the vocal folds (the glottal stop /ʔ/ and **glottal stroke** /ʔ/[2])

- phonation at the vocal folds but with the output directed through the nasal cavity (nasals such as /m/ and /n/)
- rapidly executed semivowels (the glides, /ʲ/ or /ʷ/[2])
- vowels with a partial blockage in the oral cavity (liquids, /l/ or /r/)
- combinations of the above (affricates such as /tʃ/ or /dʒ/).

Most of these consonant types can be produced at various sites in the vocal instrument. In the "burst of energy" category alone, one might use the:

- lips (/p/ and /b/)
- tongue on the **alveolar ridge** (/t/ and /d/)
- tongue on the **velum** (/k/ and /g/)
- occluded vocal folds (the glottal stop, /ʔ/)

SUMMARY

This chapter has presented the basic physics of human vocal production with a concentration on the effects of vocal tract resonation. The myriad of possibilities presented by our malleable resonation system permits the production of the wide variety of phonemes that make language possible, and singing a joy. The heart of this book will be the chapters that explain the use of the spectrograph in the voice studio and how it can provide much usable information about these vocal sounds.

---

[2]The use of the nontraditional superscripted version of these IPA symbols will be explained in later chapters.

5

SINGING VERSUS SPEECH TECHNIQUES

We began the last chapter with a statement that few singers ever pause to truly consider the miracle of song. Many facets of that miracle can be revealed and quantified in the graphics and explanations that will form the heart of this book.

Voice practitioners engaged in the creation of song routinely produce sounds that are *far* from the physiological norms encountered in native speech production. The more one understands the nature of those differences, the easier it is to bridge the gap between speech and fine singing.

HOW WELL DO SINGERS KNOW VOCAL PHYSIOLOGY?

Try an interesting exercise; ask a singer, "How do you make a /d/?" Most of the time, the singer will immediately sing or speak an example of the consonant. Then tell the singer, "No. Imagine that this particular phoneme isn't part of my language, and I haven't the slightest idea how to produce it. Explain what one does to produce it." Often the result will be a frustrated, blank stare because the singer has never paused to explore the physical production of that phoneme. Singers can perform it, perhaps with distinction, in all of its **joins** with the other phonemes that may be required. They may have even risen to the level of the art where production of the consonant varies with the dramatic needs of the moment. Still, they are rendered silent when asked to explain what they do to produce it.

It is a major tenet of the philosophy of this book that whether voice practitioners teach or perform the art of singing, they *must* know the mechanisms by which they produce the constituent parts of language. For both the student and the teacher, this knowledge can only enable a quicker diagnosis and surer grasp of the solutions to vocal problems.

Much of the Work Has Already Been Done

Professionals in the field of vocal pathology have conducted an enormous amount of research on phoneme production. Out of necessity, they have had to develop this knowledge in order to treat their patients. A perusal of research about singing does not reveal comparable research. To remedy the situation, how many voice practitioners ever study the speech literature to see what they can learn? In a very real sense, a voice teacher/coach is a *song pathologist* or a *song therapist*. These practitioners should know every bit as much as their colleagues in the speech field before attempting to teach their first voice student.

Some Translation Is Needed

As the reader will soon see, while there are many similarities between speech and singing, there are also considerable differences, both in a general sense and in the production of individual phonemes. To learn from the speech physiology literature, these differences will require acknowledgement and translation if such a study is to be truly applicable to singing. To enable this translation, this chapter will explore some of the major differences between speech and song.

SINGING AND SPEECH: A TWO TEMPLATE MODEL

An exploration of the differences in the production of speech and song must begin by looking at the two vocal tasks independently as templates for language action.

 ## The Speech Template

Speech is with us throughout most of the waking moments of each day, and, for some people, in the sleeping moments as well. We spend a considerable amount of time executing speech sounds in order to communicate with those around us. Our language-producing technique is a background process that doesn't usually require conscious thought. To understand the concept of this background processing, consider the computer as a model for the speech template by drawing analogies between brain function and the function of the central processing unit of a computer.

When one contemplates speech, one can imagine that the brain houses a neural "database" that contains all of the necessary neuromuscular instructions, not only for the production of each phoneme, but for all possible joins of phonemes that may be needed to express thought. In this imaginary model, the brain calls upon this database for the instructions needed to manipulate the physical structures of the vocal instrument to express thought. This is a gross oversimplification of a remarkable process, but for the purposes of this discussion, this rather simplistic computer analogy will suffice.

When infants make their first pre-speech sounds, their speech database is in the first stages of development. As a child continues to mimic the speech sounds that surround him or her, the raw materials for speech are entered in the database with ever-increasing specificity. As the child learns to speak and express thoughts, the database grows ever stronger with each repetition of the neuromuscular instructions. By the time the individual is a young adult and ready to begin the study of singing, the speech database can present an enormous impediment to the acquisition of proper singing technique.

Once the speech template is developed, it works in the background (subconsciously) much the same as the workings of a computer. When searching a computer database, one does not see the process of the search, only the result. The subconscious nature of speech can be a great problem in the development of good singing habits.

The Singing Template

Voice practitioners must accept a simple truth:

In ways that can be quantified using scientific methods, we must arrive at the conclusion that

well-executed song is NOT speech.

Figure 5–1 shows graphic evidence of the differences. The language sounds used in classical singing are:

- sustained for periods of time far longer than those required for speech
- generally richer (more resonant) than speech
- purer and executed with cleaner joins than those of most speech
- performed with a range of pitch *far* wider than that required for speech
- executed with a rhythmic accuracy determined by the notation of the music

Since the production and use of phonemes in song is unlike speech in so many ways, most singing students must construct a new template for singing separate from their speech template.

Much of the time, as the singing template becomes operational, it will cause corollary changes in the speech template. Usually the singer's speech becomes richer, more resonant, and less dialectally idiomatic. Such subtle shifts often enable one trained singer to recognize another from the singing-modified sounds of their speech alone. This modification of speech patterns is not always a given, however. The author knows more than a few trained singers who, after singing a classically formed "alleluia" of great tone and beauty, turn around and ask, /ɪz ðæt wʌt yal wʌn'?/, employing the strong southern American dialect learned in childhood.

The Shadow of the Speech Template

The speech template represents an awesomely powerful set of behavioral instructions. During a lifetime of speaking, a person's brain executes the phonemic instructions from its speech template "billions and billions" of times (sorry, this tip of the hat to Carl Sagan just had to be made. His voice became imprinted on our minds with his famous line, "billions and billions of stars;" it was his special way of treating the stop consonant, /b/, that made it so memorable). Because this powerful speech processor works in the background of conscious thought, most people do not have to stop, compose a thought, and then *consciously* piece together all of the instructions needed to articulate the thought. Those instructions are compiled in the background, as if by magic.

This subconscious nature of speech may create vexing problems for singers. When beginning students attempt to sing words properly, their brains (working in the background), seem to assume that they are attempting some form of "overdone" speech. It is almost as if the speech template determines, "That's not the way we say that!" and then, without the singer's conscious knowledge, inserts speech instructions, thus sabotaging the attempt to execute the properly sung sound. This phenomenon instantly destroys the effort to sing the desired sound.

The SAS Exercise

Insight into the pervasive influence of speech is gained when a behavioral modification exercise invented by the author, called SAS ("Say it as a Singer"), is employed in the studio. During this exercise, the student is asked to *speak* the sounds of the phrase he or she is attempting to sing utilizing a *full, rich singing technique*. On the first attempt, the student will most often break into laughter, exclaiming, "This

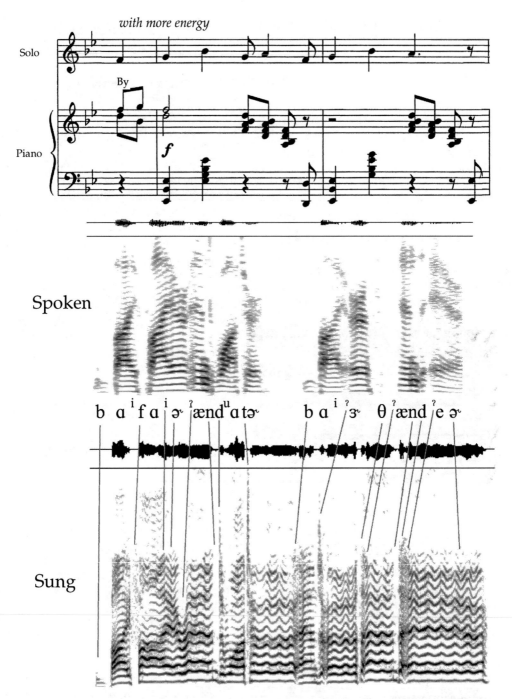

Figure 5–1. Spectrogram of a phrase that is spoken and then sung. (Phrase from *Listen Beloved* by Garyth Nair, poetry by Virginia Nadel. Copyright 1998 by Garyth Nair). 💿

sounds SO stupid!" After it is explained that this judgment is coming from the speech template, the student often seems more willing to consciously attempt to keep that template at bay. When the exercise is successful, the student is well on the way toward the development of the second template, the one needed for song.

Occasionally the student will not be able to perform the SAS exercise until the teacher models it. The best modeling technique for demonstrating SAS is for the teacher to start singing a phrase. Midway through the phrase, switch to speech while preserving the "set" of the song template (as used in this book, the word **set** means the configuration of *all* of the facets of the vocal instrument needed to produce a given phoneme). When the student hears how ludicrous well-sung phonemes sound as speech, they are often more willing to accept the "overblown" sounds of the new template.

Are There Separate Speech and Song Sites in the Brain?

If the tasks of speech and song are separate templates, are they both handled within the Broca's area, the speech center of the brain? Or is there a separate language site in the brain, located away from the speech center, that processes singing instructions exclusively? Only future research will provide the answer. One thing is certain: A shift in the way the singer *perceives the process* appears critical to the development of the different habits necessary for song. If proper song behavior is to be learned and habitualized, on either a conscious or subconscious level, the singer will probably need to accept speech and song as separate entities whether or not those entities are centered in different areas of the brain.

LEARNING FROM SPEECH SCIENCE

It is unfortunate that so few singing practitioners attempt to utilize the gains made in speech science. Those in the singing field seem to assume either that the speech models have no bearing on song or, having attempted to read the literature, do not make the effort to modify the physiological models of speech so they can apply them to song models.

Four Necessary Translations

When voice practitioners do attempt to study speech literature, they usually encounter four critical areas of difference between speech and song that require translation:

- In song, most phonemes (principally the vowels and some consonants) are sustained for much longer periods of time than they are in speech. Thus, there is time for the singer to take far more care in the execution of the **VC** (vowel-to-consonant) and **CV** (consonant-to-vowel) joins. In a well-trained singer, these joins tend to be executed with greater speed than in speech.
- Top-rank singers tend to employ these VC/CV joins, not only with greater speed, but greater *precision* than is typical of speech. The result is a considerable reduction of **coarticulation** (a state where the production of one phoneme influences the production of the phonemes on either side of it, resulting in detrimental effects on the purity of the sounds). In succeeding chapters, more will be said about the use of computer analysis and its efficacy in reducing or eliminating coarticulation in singer's vocal production.
- One of the primary goals of classically trained singers is to employ far more resonance in the formation of all phonemes than is common in speech. Thus, the set of the articulators and the subglottal pressure needed for these sounds may be significantly different, especially in the realm of the consonants.
- With these shifts in speed and precision of articulation, a subtle shift in the use of IPA symbols may be required to more accurately **transliterate** the *sung* sounds of various languages.

If the differences between speech and song are kept in mind, the translation of the knowledge base from speech to song is not difficult and can prove considerably enlightening. Voice practitioners are urged to bridge this gap with serious study. In addition, speech and voice scientists must be persuaded to work together to learn more about the physiological differences between speech and song, especially the differentiation so obvious to the experienced listener when hearing the song production of international-class singers. Such information could be of great benefit in the acquisition of physiological (and psychological) knowledge about the voice, providing an invaluable aid to singers and their teachers.

Much of the knowledge that would be useful to voice practitioners is already in the speech-science field waiting to be read, translated, and applied to song. Later in this book we will work with computer technology as feedback in the learning process, but without an intimate knowledge of vocal physiology, we cannot reap all the benefits of such a strategy.

INFLUENCES ON CLASSICALLY SUNG WESTERN LANGUAGES

The Italianization of Sung Language

Upon careful consideration, most classically trained singers may realize that there is yet another major departure from a speech production that must temper a singer's study of speech science. These singers tend to "Italianize" the languages found in the Western classical repertoire. The author proposes the use of the term **Italianization** to mean the use of production norms of well-sung Italian to enrich and open the sounds of other languages.

The Italianization influence stems from the singing habits developed while learning to master that language. These habits tend to influence the way all other Western languages are sung. This stems from the habitualization of the following classically sung Italian language norms:

- *purity*—meaning devoid of any local dialectal influence.
- *openness*—sung with the mandible down and the mouth more open than is the norm in most speech
- *richly resonant vowels and consonants sung on pitch* and with the *optimal resonance* fostered by the use of a low larynx with its concurrent lengthening of the pharynx
- singing that is imbued with the *singer's formant* (especially in the male voices)

These compelling sounds, so common in well-sung Italian, tend to color the production of all other languages because they are suited to the demands of the concert hall and opera house.

That explains why many classically trained singers sound overblown and stilted when they try to sing a Broadway classic; they utilize their classical singing template. The sounds of Italian have influenced international-rank singing either consciously or unconsciously ever since Italian singers started teaching in foreign cities, and their non-Italian counterparts began to use the language as an elementary starting point in the education of singers.

Why Do so Many of Us Begin Vocal Study With Italian?

For many teachers, Italian has traditionally been a starting point for a student's development. There are two main reasons:

- Italian is a WYSIWYG ("what-you-see-is-what-you-get") language. After some shifting of vowel production away from the norms of the student's native language, the pure vowel sounds found in classical Italian enable the student and teacher to spend most of their time on vocal development instead of dealing with the problems of speech-template interference emanating from the student's native language.

- Because Italian presents so few phoneme-to-phoneme articulative problems, the singer's developmental focus can quickly shift to the avoidance of coarticulation.

For most singers, Italian is probably the first language that they sang well. For all but native-speaking Italians, moving outside one's native language may make it easier to quickly advance to a better, richer sound. After establishing good habits in Italian, it is easier to open up the vocal production of the other languages (Italianize them). In this process, the newly acquired Italian sounds can (and many believe, should) exert a powerful influence on the other sung languages.

For native-born Italians, depending on their region of origin and its local dialect, one could make a case that they have a head start in the development of good tone because their speech template is already much closer to the desired goal than that for most other languages.

Italian-Influenced Vowel Shifts

Italianization has occurred in the realm of the vowels because, in a quest for the best and most consistent tone, many singers tend to discard colors that get in the way of that quest.

Listen to a Spanish-born classical tenor sing in Spanish for example. For the most part, one will not hear the placement of the vowels that is common to spoken Spanish. In speech, Spanish vowels tend to employ a more forward production than those found in Italian. The need to produce rich vowels that thrill audiences and make it easier for the singer to project these sounds into large halls entices the singer to shift the language *toward* a more Italianate production.

English is no exception to this process. Consider how the subtle distinctions be-

tween the first vowels of the spoken words "father" (written as /a/), and "bought" (written as /ɔ/) may be unified into a single vowel /a/ because this vowel is generally perceived as marginally richer than /ɔ/.

Reduction in the Amount of Subtlety

Many of the speech subtleties endemic to native languages, especially those that are the provenance of local dialects, become an impediment to the type of sound required on the international stage. At that level, one usually will not hear the variety of vowel coloration employed in a singer's performance that one would hear in his or her speech.

Most singers, at one time or another, have asked a native-born speaker (non-singer) of a language to coach them in their singing diction. After perhaps hours of laborious work, they find that they must discard most of the subtle colors and linguistic distinctions urged by their native-speaking coach and return to Italian-influenced sounds in order to produce credible vocal output.

During the process of Italianization, the singer learns:

- which sounds must be retained so the language keeps its unique "markers" intact (sounds such as the French nasal vowels)
- how far such markers can be modified toward Italian-like openness and resonance without doing harm to the klang of the language. (*Klang*, short for *Klangfarbe*, is the German synonym for timbre. This shortened form is often used by musicians in preference to the word timbre.)

Of course, there is a great deal to be learned by exploring the speech subtleties of languages. Singers find that in the beginning stages of their training, most of the subtlety must be avoided in the quest for consistently beautiful phonemes. As the singer's experience and skill progress however, more of those minute differences can be worked into the technique without doing harm to the basic vocal fabric.

A Recent Catalyst: The Recording

The proliferation of recordings since World War II has had an enormous influence on the development of a world-standard for singing. The availability of recordings of great singers has offered models for students and helped shape their ideas and technique. With so much great singing available on recordings, singers can continue to learn from the best throughout their career.

Is This "Universalization" a Good Thing?

The answer to this question will vary considerably from teacher to teacher and from singer to singer. When one listens to world-class singers, this universalization is virtually consistent, no matter what the nationality of the singer.

One point of view holds that the development of such universal standards through the use of recordings has not necessarily been a beneficial development. In the process, idiomatic, uniquely nationalistic vocal production is gradually disappearing from world-class stages. This same phenomenon has also occurred in the world of the orchestra. Just 30 years ago, one could easily identify the timbre differences between a French and a Czech orchestra. Today such differences in klang and style are more difficult to find.

Where music students, singers, and instrumentalists once had only local mentors and an occasional touring ensemble to emulate, they now have the greatest international talents to serve as models, whenever and wherever they want. Whether we applaud or decry the development of the recording, it has had an undeniable effect on the standard of singing worldwide. In so doing, it has widened the gulf between speech and song.

Beware of Shifts in the Standard

A caution is in order here; *the norms of this international singing standard are continually shifting.* Within the past 30 years, there have been significant shifts in what constitutes fine singing. A good example is the performance of /r/ in French. French singing diction once demanded that the /r/ be rolled (trilled, /ř/) to avoid giving the diction "great vulgarity" (Bernac 1970). Teachers such as Bernac, held that the use of the so-called "Parisian" /ʁ/ inhibited the production of legato line so necessary to the French style. Today many ranking singers use a more idiomatic Parisian /ʁ/—the very one Bernac rejected—with little or no apparent damage to the sung legato line.

One can also point to the pervasive influence that Dietrich Fischer-Diskau had on an entire generation of singers. In his prime, Diskau was *the* model Lieder singer. His particular technical predilections were the standard for German diction for years and were emulated by countless students worldwide. But during the past 10 to 15 years, there has been a shift toward other norms.

Voice practitioners must constantly attend live performances, as well as listen to recordings of today's internationally ranked singers, to ascertain the direction in which the current is moving. Many voice instructors don't maintain such vigilance and still utilize standards that they learned as students without updating their knowledge. Often the result is students who are inadequately prepared, destined to spend many hours and much money unlearning what they were taught by well-meaning teachers. Given the availability of the greatest singing on recordings, there is no excuse for teaching outdated norms.

RECOMMENDED SHIFTS IN IPA SYMBOLOGY

Books on both speech and singing employ the International Phonetic Alphabet (IPA). **IPA** is a system of symbols that enables us to transliterate language sounds in a way that others can understand and replicate specifics of the pronunciation of a language or dialect (transliterate means to write the sounds of a language in another alphabetical system). The English word "diaphragm," for example, can be written in IPA as, /daɪəfræm/. Non-English-speaking students, utilizing the phonetic standards of the IPA, can avoid many of the mistakes that their phonetic instincts, honed from their own language template, might engender. If properly used, IPA allows voice practitioners to discuss the pronunciation and physiological production of phonemes knowing that, for most phonemes, they are discussing the same sound regardless of one's language background.

At first glance, IPA appears as a rock-solid standard for transliteration and transcription of language. Upon closer inspection, one realizes that an IPA representation of words is dependent on the individual ear of the transliterator—an ear that hears phonemes through its own native language filter. One need only look at the IPA representation for a single word across different sources to see examples of the subtle variations that can creep into the process.

To further complicate the process, the author proposes that differences between speech and song require some small shifts in IPA symbology and use. When considering an IPA chart for singers, few authorities seem to take this differential into account, and the resulting transcriptions, while valid for speech, are not totally valid for song. Thus, some shifts in IPA usage, based both on aural and spectrographic evidence, seem to be in order.

Vowel Shifts

In the realm of vowels, the Italianization factor discussed earlier in this chapter may necessitate reassignment of some vowels in the quest for beautiful singing tone. These reassignments fall in three principal areas:

- reassignment of certain vowels to conform to actual singing practice
- reassignment of both vowel and symbology for offglide vowels in diphthongs
- reassignment of both vowel and symbology for onglide vowels such as /j/ and /w/

To illustrate the potential need for reassessment of vowel symbology, consider the diphthong in the word "my." A study of the current speech and voice literature reveals disparity in the way this diphthong is transliterated (see Table 5–1).

However, based on both aural and spectrographic evidence, the author proposes another way to transliterate this common diphthong. Why not /mʌⁱ/? When spoken, the vowel /ʌ/ is often a fairly shallow sound and would not make a viable singing vowel for the diphthong. However, when sung well in words such as *up, duck, supper,* and so forth, it takes on a resonant life of its own, far removed from speech norms. The power spectrum in Figure 5–2 illustrates the difference between the sung vowels /ʌ/ and /a/ (the vowel called for in the table of IPA transliterations). This spectrum shows the formant pattern for these vowels obtained by using Donald Miller's vocal fry method. The greater intensity shown for the formants in the midsection of the spectrum for /ʌ/ might suggest that it would be a better vowel for use in this diphthong.

Consonant Shifts

The principal divergence from the more traditional IPA classifications offered by our chart will be in the realm of the con-

Table 5–1. Comparison of IPA listings for the diphthong in the word "mine."

Vennard (1968) wrote: Phonetitians differ as to how to transcribe these words (Coffin, Denes and Pinson, Kantner and West, Wise) reflecting different percepts as they listen, and I suspect different concepts as to what the subject "thinks" as he speaks. . . . These questions are more meaningful in speech than in song, since they refer chiefly to the duration of the sounds in speech and duration in singing is a matter of music more than of phonetics. (p. 177)

Source	Symbol	Word	Notes	Book Subject
Sataloff (1998)	A:I	mine, high	Doesn't list primary vowel in vowel list; typo?	Sing/Speech
Sataloff (1998)	A:I	mine, high	Doesn't list primary vowel in vowel list; typo?	Sing/Speech
Moriarty (1975)	A:I	mine, high	/A/	Singing
Moriarty (1975)	A:I	mine, high	/A/	Singing
Vennard (1968)	not listed			Singing
Marshall (1953)	AI	night	See note 1. Never substitute /i/ for the /I/.	Singing
Appelman (1967)	AI	lie	Doesn't use the term, diphthong, but prefers vowel glide.	Singing
Titze (1994)	αI	aisle, sigh	/a/ is listed as "ask, half, past"	Singing
Miller (1990)	AI	nice	Lists /A/ as "father."	Singing
Doscher (1994)	not listed			Singing
McKinney (1982)	αI	buy, night	lottery, I (first sound)	Singing
Edwards (1997)	αI	kind, etc.	Doesn't list primary vowel in vowel list. See note 2	Speech
Kent & Read (1992)	αI	bite	In this dialect, [α] does not occur as a monophthong, but occurs as the nucleus of two diphthongs. See note 3.	Speech
Borden, et al. (1994)	αI	aisle, sigh	/a/ is listed as "ask, half, past"	Speech

Note 1. Some writers list the primary vowel as /α/. Marshall omits this vowel from her list of singer's vowels claiming, "When English is sung, the shadings of /A/ and /α/ are so nearly alike as to be imperceptible to the listener." (p. 163)

Note 2. Edwards includes a Distinctive Feature Analysis (adapted from Chomsky & Halle, 1968). He says, "They also do not include the slightly advanced /α/ as a definable sound used to initiate two of the diphthongs. Therefore, the feature Advanced has been added to show the tendency among speakers of American English to shift /A/ slightly forward for the production of these diphthongs."

Note 3. Northern Midwestern dialect.

One of the authors, Moriarty, lists the secondary vowel /i/ as an option in his IPA listing for singers (Sataloff who adapted his list from Moriarty retains the distinction).

sonants. Well-trained classical singers perform these sounds with much more color and resonance that many consonants edge closer to the vowel classes than their corollary speech phonemes.

The complete IPA chart for this system is given in Appendix A and will be referred to in the coming chapters as we explore the particulars of sung vocal production and the use of computer technology as an aid in acquiring good singing habits.

ARTICULATORS OF THE SINGING INSTRUMENT

Before moving on to a detailed study of vowels and consonants, we must briefly take the time to discuss the mechanisms by which we create all language sounds, sung or spoken. These mechanisms are called **articulators**. We must take note of physiological differences in the use of

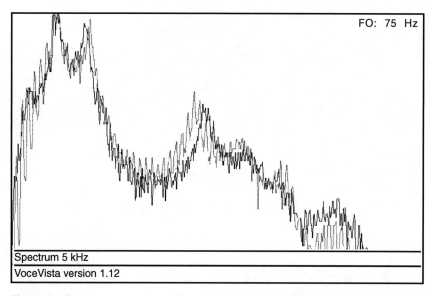

FO: 75 Hz

Spectrum 5 kHz

VoceVista version 1.12

Figure 5–2. A power spectrum showing the formants of the sung vowels /ʌ/ (lighter line) and /ɑ/ (darker line).

the articulators—the movable oral, pharyngeal, and laryngeal structures—that we manipulate to produce phonemes.

Note: The technical norms of vocal production offered in this text are the result of countless hours of close observation of internationally ranked singers. The inclusion of these norms is not meant to preclude other pedagogical norms, but rather to present ideas that illustrate how computer feedback can service those norms, no matter which ones are ultimately chosen by the voice practitioner.

Basic Oral Configuration

A well-trained singer employs articulative motions that are primarily vertical and/or anterior/posterior. In proper singing technique, most articulations that involve side-to-side movement (called **spreading** in most schools of technique) are considered undesirable. When singers use a spread configuration, they most often lose the consistency of beautiful tone across the full length of the phrase.

In contemplating the motion of the articulators, voice practitioners must constantly remind them that all the movable structures of the vocal instrument are interconnected. Any articulative action performed with one anatomical structure will instantly affect many others. This interconnectedness is both a miracle to behold *and* a source of endless problems for the voice practitioner in the quest for verticality in the instrument. It is this verticality that provides much of the increases in resonance so typical of fine singing. Thus, if voice practitioners are to achieve a good singing technique, they must strive for a constant improvement in the vertical plane of their instrument.

The spectrogram in Figure 5–3 will illuminate this important point (refer to both Chapters 4 and 7 for more information on reading spectrograms). It shows a spectrogram of a singer singing the vowel /ɑ/. At the far left, the vowel is the properly sung vowel. As the spectrogram continues, the production is gradually shifted to a spread (horizontal) production and returns to the properly produced vowel by the end of the example. Note the distinctive pattern of the properly sung vowel on the left and

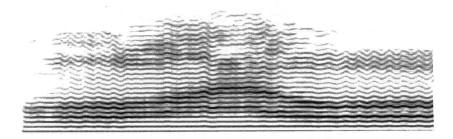

Figure 5–3. The vowel /a/ as a benchmark, spreading and then returning to the benchmark. Note the shift in the formant structure. This singer also has trouble maintaining the "set" of the vowel; tension sets in, and the vibrato disappears for a while as the vowel settles back toward the benchmark. 🔘

use that as an example of a target vocal production (a benchmark) as you compare it with the beginning of the vowel on the right. The vowel that begins on the right is the same vowel but severely spread:

- the formant patterns shift considerably,
- new harmonics appear in the higher regions that give an "edge" to the tone, and
- the vibrato, as evidenced by the waviness of the higher harmonics as they track the fundamental, is unsteady; it only begins to settle back into an acceptable pattern by the end of the example as the spreading ceases.

If one inspects thousands of photos of great singers taken during the act of singing, one will see a virtually universal mouth shape, the vertical oval. Much more will be said later in this text about maintenance of this configuration and the means by which computer-aided feedback can help establish this desirable habit.

The Principal Articulators

Mandible

The Amazing TMJ

The jaw is attached to the skull structure at the temporomandibular joint (known by the acronym TMJ). This universal joint (so

called because it can move on several possible planes) is truly amazing. The TMJ permits the jaw to move:

- as a fulcrum for the mandible (especially useful while chewing. Working in this way, the jaw can exert enormous pressure on the teeth);
- in a forward and backward motion (posterior/anterior);
- in a side-to-side motion (which should not be a consideration in singing technique); and
- as an elevator for the posterior part of the mandible. When the TMJ relaxes, the back of the mandible drops.

Gains From the Use of a Relaxed, Low-Mandible Strategy

In an acoustical system where mere millimeters of shift in the singer's anatomy can have a significant effect on tonal output, the ability to relax the TMJ and thus lower the posterior mandible becomes worthy of attention. Figure 5–5 shows the two principle reasons why. A drop of the mandible by relaxing the TMJ:

- tends to increase the vertical space in the posterior oral cavity as the tongue drops with the mandible, thus increasing oral resonance space; and
- drops the larynx. The larynx and the posterior mandible are connected via ligaments and the hyoid bone. A drop of the mandible consequently allows a

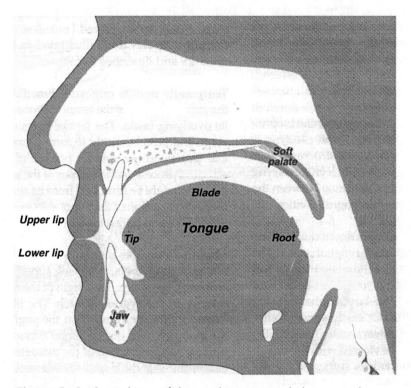

Figure 5–4. Sagittal view of the vocal structures with the principal articulators labeled. (Adapted from *The Speech Sciences* by D. R. Kent, 1997. San Diego, CA: Singular Publishing Group. Copyright 1997 by Singular Publishing Group. Adapted and printed with permission.)

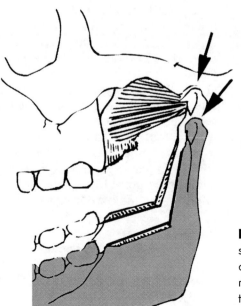

Figure 5–5. Sagittal view of the mandible showing the drop resulting from TMJ relaxation. The upper arrow indicates the normal mandible pivot; the lower indicates the position of the ramus with the relaxed TMJ. Notice the increase in oral space.

corresponding drop of the larynx. This action permits the amount of vertical *and* horizontal resonance space in the pharynx to increase.

The resonance gain accomplished by the drop of the posterior mandible is one of the prime differences between the techniques of speech and song (although classic speech training for the theater also may employ this strategy for the same acoustic benefit). To experience the sensation of posterior mandibular drop, place the fingers of one hand on the back of the jawbone where it makes its vertical turn. With the fingers of the other hand, monitor the protrusion of the thyroid cartilage of the larynx. Now, yawn and experience the coupled action of the anatomical structures from the posterior mandible down to the larynx.

Consequences of a Low Mandible on Tongue Articulation

The dropped-mandible technique has consequences for tongue articulation as will be noted in the following discussion of the tongue. Nonetheless, most singers find that the payoff in increased resonance makes it worth the effort to train the mandible to relax downward as well as employ the greater tongue articulation required by such a strategy.

TMJ Syndrome and Resonance

There are some medical conditions that can affect the proper function of the TMJ, such as TMJ syndrome and certain arthritic conditions. Singers who have such problems should seek medical help, as impaired TMJ function may seriously affect the ability to produce optimal singing resonance.

Tongue

The tongue is the major articulative device in the vocal instrument. As it performs most of the work in the production of language.

It is an astounding collection of muscles that permit it to assume a variety of complex shapes.

One of the principal differences between speech and song is the degree to which the tongue must move to provide the proper phonemes. The previous section explained that many well-trained singers tend to sing with a low mandible position, in which the plane of the tongue is also lowered. Since the tongue, in that position, is farther from the palate, the singer must develop greater agility and extension of the tongue in order to accomplish linguistic tasks. The added effort of retraining the tongue for such maneuvers can be offset by potential gains in oral and pharyngeal resonance. The singer, especially in the early stages of training, must be constantly alert for the influence of the speech template and its tendency to raise the jaw as a means of getting the tongue near the palate. In training the tongue to perform these new extended actions, it might be helpful to continually remind the student that "The jaw should not be an elevator for a lazy tongue." Insight into how much of a change the low-mandible technique makes in the articulation of the tongue can be seen in the Table 5–1.

Many phonemes require contact between the back edges of the tongue and the upper molars. Table 5–1 is a comparison between the palatograms shown in Edwards (1997) and one of the classics of vocal pedagogy literature, Appelman (1967). A **palatogram** is a graphic representation of the degree of tongue-molar contact as viewed from below the jaw.

Note that the data compiled from X-rays of a singer show less tongue-molar contact for sung phonemes than for spoken ones, a possible indication of the use of a lower mandible during singing.

Vowel Drift Due To Involuntary Tongue Movement

Also note tongue drift tendencies in the far right column of the table. While learning the mandible-down strategy, untrained

Table 5–2. Comparison of tongue-molar contact for vowel production in speech versus song.

	Speech—Edwards Number of Teeth/Side	Song—Appelman Number of Teeth/Side	Tongue Drift Tendencey During Singing
Front			
i	4.5	4	
ɪ	5	3	
e	3.5	0	
ɛ	2.5	0	
æ	2.5 to 0	0	↓
Central			
ʌ	2 variable	0	
ə	2.5 variable	Not shown	
ɚ	3	Not shown	↕
ɜ	not shown	0	
ɝ	3.5	0	
a	not shown	0	
Back			
u	2	0	
ʊ	2	0	
o	1.5	0	↑
ɔ	0	0	
ɑ	0	0	

singers may allow the tongue to drift from the more extended positions toward more neutral positions in the center of the oral cavity. This tendency is a particular problem during the performance of a long *melisma* (many notes sung on one syllable of a word, a favorite device of Baroque composers). Many frequently arrive at the end of a melisma producing a different vowel than the one on which they started the passage.

As we move on to the application of computer technology in later chapters, much attention will be paid to this major articulator, the tongue.

Velum

The velum can raise and lower during the articulative process. In singing, the height of the velum is of critical concern. It can substantially effect the amount of oral-resonance space that is available. Furthermore, velum elevation also appears to be a critical factor when a singer must go into the high voice.

Uvula

The uvula is the posterior part of the velum. It is responsible for opening or closing the velo-pharyngeal port (the opening between the oropharynx and nasopharynx). The opening of the velo-pharyngeal port permits the creation of the nasal consonants (such as /m/) and the French nasal vowels (such as the /ã/ as in *sans*).

Lips

For the shaping of some vowels and consonants, the lips are critically important articulators of the resonance system. Some singers also use lip protrusion to lengthen the vocal tract and thus lower the fundamental (F_0).

Laryngeal Elevation

Some mention has been made of the interaction between laryngeal elevation and the TMJ. But laryngeal elevation can change without the involvement of the mandible. Again, for the same reasons as listed previously, the ability of the larynx to change elevation has a significant effect on the posterior oral, pharyngeal, and laryngeal resonance space. It is thought that the relaxed, low larynx plays a pivotal role in the development of the singer's formant (Sundberg, 1987).

Pharyngeal Diameter

This is the area to which teachers refer when using the term "open throat." While increasing pharyngeal diameter does not seem to optimize resonance as effectively as dropping the larynx, the diameter of the pharynx should be of critical concern to the singer. Titze (1998) provides some interesting observations on acoustical gains made with a widened pharynx as long as the epiglottal tube remains narrow.

Glottis

Glottal closure, either momentary or prolonged, can be employed as an articulator for certain vowel initiations.

Epiglottis

The epiglottis seems to occupy somewhat of a backwater in our knowledge of the vocal articulators. A scan of the literature produces some illumination on epiglottal positioning and its effect on resonance shaping in the pharynx. Appelman (1967) shows an intriguing diagram of differences in epiglottal attitude for each of the vowels (p. 79). He claims that the anterior-posterior shifts in epiglottal attitude are the result of movements of the tongue root, stabilized by the thyroepiglottic and aryepiglottic muscles. Other authors such as Estill (1983) and Dmitriev (1979) shed additional light on the subject. When envisioning such epiglottal movements during phonation, one can formulate many questions about the role these movements play in the acoustics of the epiglottal tube.

Neck Position

This often overlooked factor can play a major role in the shape of the pharynx and hence, in the resonance.

SUMMARY

The differences between production norms of song and speech can be quite pronounced. More research is needed to clarify these issues. With that clarification vocal practitioners may be able to make greater use of speech research and perhaps gain a new understanding of the different demands singers must place upon their articulators. Because singers seem to be in a constant battle with speech instincts during their training, it is worthwhile for them to learn as much as possible about the subject. Such acquisition of knowledge of the workings of the articulators may enable them to more easily modify their technique, away from speech norms, toward the sounds of great classical singing.

CHAPTER

6

FEEDBACK IN THE VOICE STUDIO

According to the *Concise Oxford Dictionary* (1976), feedback is the modification or control of a process or system by its results or effects. Such external knowledge of results is absolutely necessary during the process of acquiring the neuromuscular skills needed for fine singing (much more will be said on this subject later in Chapter 14 by Katherine Verdolini and David A. Krebs).

Feedback has been employed extensively in sports to help athletes achieve the fine honing of their motor skills that produces champions. Voice teachers are coaches as well. When vocal practitioners discuss pedagogical methods with athletic coaches, they are often amazed at how much they have in common.

The task facing the voice teacher is, perhaps, more difficult than that faced by an athletic coach because most of a singer's vocal process is internal and cannot be seen. Coupled with that imposing difficul-

ty is the fact that what a singer hears has little or no relationship to the acoustical reality reaching the environment (see Chapters 2 and 14 for more discussion of this problem). Saddled with these two complex inhibitors, voice students need external indications of their success or failure during the course of acquiring good singing habits.

Let us look at feedback as it has been employed in the traditional voice studio and then look forward to some of the ways in which the computer might be utilized to great advantage in the process.

TRADITIONAL FEEDBACK

All voice practitioners use some form of feedback in the voice studio. When used in a constructive way, it is a form of positive-feedback behavioral modification.

Verbal Feedback

Voice teachers offer comments throughout voice lessons to give the student indications of their progress. Such comments include indications about improved production as well as problems in need of correction. Statements such as, "That's great, do it again," "Your jaw is creeping up," and "Good breath management on that phrase," are all examples of verbal feedback. These statements give students an external indication of the status of their progress, and, in the best sense of the word, constitute feedback.

Model/Imitation Technique

Verbal feedback is often combined with the model/imitation technique during which the teacher sings an example of the desired sound and asks the student to replicate the model. During this process, the teacher must ascertain what the student is hearing internally, determine the degree of the perceptive shift that is occurring, and then verbalize a corrective instruction to solve the problem. This commentary may involve precise instructions about necessary anatomical shifts or vague imagery such as, "Make it as soft as moonlight."

Aural Feedback: Mechanical

A common cliché when one envisions singers is the use of the cupped hand as an attempt to channel the sound leaving the mouth directly to the ear. By doing this, singers attempt to obtain a better idea of the actual sound of their production.

Although such a strategy may help the singer overcome the influence of his or her internal hearing, the hand conveys only a part of the acoustical signal to the ear (and certainly modifies it). Now that electronics are more common in voice studios, electrical aural feedback is a far better solution.

Aural Feedback: Electrical

Some studios utilize tape recordings and other forms of electronic aids as feedback devices. Such feedback devices can be utilized in two ways.

Post-Performance Aural Feedback (PPAF)

In this method, the singer's performance is played back after the singing is finished. At this time, both the good and bad points of the student's technique can be discussed. Such feedback helps the student ascertain the acoustical reality of his or her performance.

ARTF (Aural Real-Time Feedback)

ARTF is a closed-loop aural feedback system that allows students to hear their voice as it exists outside their head, in real-time. This method can dramatically aid the shift in the perception between a singer's internal aural sense and the acoustical reality presented to the audience.

To use ARTF, a microphone is placed in front of the student. The electrical signal from the microphone is sent through an amplifier and then back to the student's ears via earphones. By increasing the volume with the amplifier, one can overwhelm the student's "internal" hearing. This method, since it presents the student with the external acoustic reality and not his or her internal perception of it, can rapidly speed up the acquisition of necessary neuromuscular skills.

It is important to note that as soon as the desired skill level has been achieved, the student must be quickly weaned away from ARFT. To do this, the teacher can gradually turn down the headphone volume, allowing the student's internal hearing to take precedence again. This gradual shift continues until the student is hearing without external aid and is able to consistently produce the desired vocal sound.

Setting Up an ARTF System

One can easily set up an ARTF system in a voice studio that is equipped with tape recording equipment. To use the equipment in this mode, place a tape in the recorder, place the recorder on Pause/Record, shut the speakers off, and plug earphones into the earphone port of the amplifier or recorder. The use of the Pause/Record allows the preamplifier in the tape deck to amplify the microphone signal (it is not necessary to have to tape running), pass it on to the amplifier, and then on to the earphones.

After success is achieved, the signal in the earphones is gradually reduced to allow the student to produce the sound without external aids. If the student's technique begins to regress due to the influence of the powerful input of their internal hearing, one can either verbally coach the individual back to the new technique or return to the closed-loop for another modification session.

The purpose of this method is twofold:

• Unencumbered by their own misleading aural input, students can more quickly accomplish the anatomical shifts needed to produce the proper sound and learn how the desired technique *feels*.
• Students can quickly learn to differentiate between what to accept in their internal hearing and what to disregard.

Should the voice practitioner wish a discrete, self-contained ARTF system, Kay Elemetrics Corporation has introduced a device designed by Dr. Daniel R. Boone, called the Facilitator. In addition to ARTF, this small unit can provide looping playback, delayed auditory feedback, speech noise masking, and metronomic pacing.

PPAF Versus ARTF

The choice of aural feedback depends on the needs of the student. Often, during the performance of a passage, the singer's brain is so involved with notes, rhythms, words, and specifics of vocal technique that he or she cannot hear subtle differences in the production. For this type of problem, playing back the taped performance while the teacher comments on it is a valuable method.

Since so many of a singer's problems originate in the differential between his or her internal versus external sense of the voice, the use of ARTF can greatly accelerate the student's shift of vocal production to the external reality.

By using PPAF, one can help improve the acuity of a student's ear. Once the student can hear the subtle differences, ARTF is the next logical step in the pedagogical progression.

Visual Feedback

Visual: Nonelectronic

Many teachers have a mirror in their studio, often full-length. As students sing in front of the mirror, they receive external visual feedback about their technique *in real-time*. One distinct advantage of the use of the mirror is that the students can visually confirm certain aspects of what the teacher tells them.

The mirror can be an enormous help in demonstrating:

• Posture
• Breathing
• The location of visible muscle tension
• Mouth aperture and jaw position
• The degree of success in releasing visible tension
• Various facets of artistic expression

Visual: Electronic

A more "high-tech" form of visual feedback has recently entered the voice studio. With the advent of inexpensive video cameras, some studios have begun to use videotape as feedback. When students sing in front of a mirror, they cannot pay full attention because they must also concentrate on their performance at the same time. By watching a videotape of a sung segment following its performance, singers can more easily concentrate on both the visual and aural aspects of their technique. As is the case with both tape recording and closed-loop feedback, the teacher must decide when to use each mode of electronic feedback based on the student's needs at the moment. As voice teachers gain experience with these methods, they soon develop a sense for which feedback methods are most useful for the correction of specific types of vocal problems. It is important to remember that each student will be unique. A mode of feedback that works for one individual may not work for another.

DIGITAL ANALYSIS: THE NEW FEEDBACK POTENTIAL

With the advent of today's high-speed computers, voice practitioners and their students can now enjoy the benefits of real-time, computer-generated visual feedback, **VRTF**, as an everyday pedagogical tool. Software is now available that can analyze a singer's sound and present it as a full-color visual display.

What Must Voice Practitioners Know To Employ VRTF?

For voice practitioners to utilize VRTF, the following skills are necessary. They must:

- be able to both aurally and visually recognize elements of good and bad vocal production
- know enough anatomy, physiology, and vocal acoustics to understand what they observe in a student's articulator,

breath, or support setup and how these considerations produce the sound in question
- be able to articulate precise instructions that will accomplish desired shifts in technique
- be able to offer exercises to reinforce desired behavior and transform it into good vocal habits.

A New Term: Physioacoustics

The main goal of this book is to teach voice practitioners how to read, interpret, and utilize computer-generated imagery that can be used as feedback in the voice studio.

Chapter 1 stated a case for the creation of a body of terminology on which voice practitioners and scientists can agree. In that spirit, consider a new term: **physioacoustics**, defined as the union of the anatomy and physiology of the singing voice with computer-aided analysis of vocal acoustics. Voice practitioners should know how phonemes are physically produced. They should be able to recognize telltale acoustical features when viewed on the computer monitor.

VRTF

Chapter 1 went into considerable detail on the potential value of computer feedback and its utilization of visual input as a way to guide a singer's hearing, and hence his or her vocal production. A few other points must be considered at this point.

Acceleration of Skill Acquisition

By employing visual input to guide the ear, computer-driven VRTF can greatly *accelerate* the acquisition of vocal skills.

An excellent example of the acceleration that can be accomplished is the case of a student who had spent months attempting to develop a credible Baroque trill without success. When she saw the teacher's model of a properly performed trill on the computer screen, she was able to compare her production with the model, replicate it, and then move on to the execution of wonderful trills. This process, utilizing computer VRTF, took less than 10 minutes.

Objective Communication

Another benefit of its use is that it provides a means for objective communication between student and teacher or coach. What is seen on the computer monitor is something tangible to which both parties can refer.

VRTF in Teaching Anatomy, Physiology, and Physics

VRTF can be a valuable adjunct in the teaching of the anatomy, physiology, and physics of good voice production. As the student sees objective evidence on the monitor, the teacher can utilize the display as a springboard for discussion of the physical causes of the vocal sound analyzed on the monitor. The more students can visualize the physiological processes that produce a given sound, the easier it is for them to alter their own anatomy to achieve the desired goal. It is during this realization process that teachers can most easily reveal technical knowledge about the vocal instrument.

Important Points To Remember About VRTF

VRTF Is a Bridge Technique

It must be stressed that, when properly utilized in vocal pedagogy, computer-generated feedback is a bridge device. It is a way to help the singer see and correct vocal detail and then advance to hearing and feeling the improved vocal production. Once the singer crosses that bridge, he or she should be able to replicate the improved sound without the need of the

feedback. If students are not carefully weaned away from feedback, the resulting benefits can quickly disappear. The goal of the teacher or coach must be that the students must ultimately rely on their own sensory input, both aural and tactile.

VRTF Is Most Helpful in Helping With Micro, not Macro, Events

Figure 6–1 shows a spectrogram of the sung phrase, "O Lord, be my refuge." It is an impressively complex display containing mountains of useful information. As this cascade of information scrolls by the singing student in real-time, it may seem overwhelming due to the wealth of information available. While it can be helpful to sing while watching the analysis of the performance because students may garner general knowledge of their technique, it is in the realm of the micro, not the macro, that VRTF comes into its own as a pedagogical tool. This point cannot be overstressed.

In the studio/lab at Drew University, the VRTF image is running the entire time a student is singing, but it is used only briefly during the session to address specific short-time events. In all other respects, the lesson or coaching goes on as a *traditional* voice lesson.

Most often, a large part of an entire phrase may be compromised as a result of one micro vocal event, the "spreading" of an "m," for example. The utilization of VRTF to solve the production of that one sound and then to learn how it connects with its neighboring sounds is where VRTF becomes an extraordinary adjunct in the process. Once the problem with the micro event is solved, the singer's good singing habits can operate efficiently for the entire phrase.

The problems that singers experience with consonants constitute an excellent example of the need to look at micro events. In singing, vowels are sustained for relatively long periods of time, which allows the brain to concentrate on properly formed singing vowels. Most students

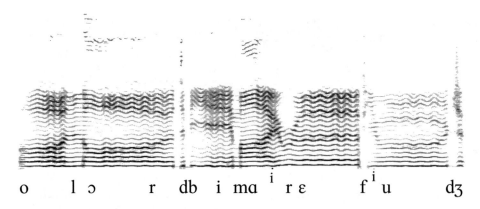

o   l ɔ   r   db i ma ⁱ r ɛ   fⁱ u   dʒ

Figure 6–1. Spectrogram of the sung phrase, "O Lord, be my refuge." 🆑

will very quickly reach a point where their vowel production has improved far beyond the standard of their speech. At that point in a student's progress, work should begin to focus on the production of consonants—both as individual phonemes, as well as in their joins with their neighboring phonemes.

While the singer enjoys the luxury of taking time with the sustained vowels, no such time is available in the production of consonants. Most consonants must still be executed at the same speed in singing as they are in speech. As a consequence, most singers are left with no resort but to turn to their speech templates for the necessary neuromuscular instructions. The result is sung phrases where the singer's technique often oscillates between beautiful vowels and poorly sung consonants. Because the speech consonants being employed are so far from the resonance and openness of the singer's vowels, the constant shift of the articulators may compromise the vowels as well. This leaves students with the frustration of poorly sung phrases that are only slightly superior to their own speech.

Because of the speed of execution in song, CV-VC join problems may be difficult to correct within the context of whole phrases. No matter how hard the student tries to produce the proper sounds, the offending joins may still wreak havoc on the phrase.

When this occurs, one may have to move to a more micro level, working only with individual joins in an effort to correct both the problem of the production of the consonants and the joins with their neighboring vowels. It is at this level, VRTF comes into its own. It permits the student to "see" problems and solutions on the monitor that can guide the ear and brain, greatly reducing the amount of time spent solving those problems.

TECHNIQUE-BUILDING STRATEGIES FOR USE WITH VRTF

Following are some VRTF strategies that have proven successful in the voice teaching studios at Drew University. The reader is urged to explore these strategies and then create his or her own uses that better match the reader's teaching style.

Structured Building: A Macro Strategy

In real life, there is seldom one problem present in the singing of a phrase, especially in the vocal production of beginning students. The teacher is often presented with a small cluster—sometimes galaxy!—of local phonemic problems, all crying for attention. The **structured building** technique can build neuromuscular skills in a hierarchy that, with the use of feedback, can build proper vocal production of the whole phrase, as well as function as a diagnostic tool.

In the structured building strategy, the student is asked to sing the phrase in question using the following hierarchy:

- The student sings the phrase as a vocalize on a single vowel (useful if the problem is breathing or support related).
- The student sings the phrase utilizing only the vowels of the words in the phrase. The phrase "O Lord, be my refuge," would be sung as /o ɔ i aⁱ ɛ ʲu/ (the use of superscripted IPA symbols will be explained in later chapters). This eliminates the potential problems that may stem from production of consonants and permits the inspection and improvement of the phrase vowel line. This method can impart the "feel" of the correctly sung vowel line. As other phonemes are added later, the singer stands a better chance of knowing when a particular vowel has been compromised.
- After the vowel line has been set, the student adds the voiced consonants, those that are sung with pitch. Now, the phrase would be sung as: /o lɔr i maⁱ rɛ ʲu/.
- After the student correctly sings phonemic sequence of vowels plus pitch consonants, he or she adds the rest of the phonemes: /o lɔrd bi maⁱ rɛ fʲu dʒ/.

By using this structured sequence with the aid of VRTF, the building of a beautifully sung phrase can then be considerably accelerated. The skills and habits acquired during this structured sequence can be called on in subsequent phrases.

Local problems encountered in this structured buildup are amenable to correction using the next method, the skill accelerando.

Skill Accelerando

A singer in the voice studio is attempting to master extraordinary sequences of complex neuromuscular instructions. If one ponders the magnitude of the skills necessary for beautiful song, one may come to the conclusion that no one has a genetic right to sing *Pagliacci*. Most great singing skills do not happen naturally because the level of neuromuscular coordination is considerably more complex and demanding than that utilized in everyday speech. Thus, the skills must be attained very slowly and carefully. This necessity leads to the technique of the skill accelerando.

The heart of the **skill accelerando** is slowing down—sometimes drastically—the phoneme-to-phoneme production. Such an approach can permit the student's brain to image sounds at a slow enough pace that he or she can consciously control the vocal process in a way that is close to impossible when the same passage is performed at speed. With the increased likelihood of success, a singer is more likely to quickly learn and *habitualize* the skills needed to sing the phrase properly.

After spending time singing the phonemic sequence correctly in slow motion, the phrase is repeated, each time a little faster, until the student can perform the newly acquired technique at the speed needed for performance.

This strategy takes its cue from the classic method by which singers learn a patter song. This type of song is a very rapidly executed series of syllables that delight us because of the "high-wire" difficulty involved. Gilbert and Sullivan's, *"I am the very model of a modern major general,"* or the central section of the aria, "La vendetta" from Mozart's *Le Nozze di Figaro* are two of the more famous examples. A good coach or teacher generally has the singer slow these songs down to a speed at which the singer can "pre-think" each syllable. Concurrently, the student may also be instructed to overpronounce the phonemes.

When the phrase can be *correctly* performed in *slow* motion, the student then increases the tempo slightly. If the singer stumbles on a syllable, the speed is dropped back to a level where the passage can be correctly performed. The gradual acceleration begins again until the passage can be performed at the desired speed.

This method slows the vocal-language process down so the brain can focus on each sequential shift in musculature. By doing so, the brain can build a memory sequence that contains all of the necessary neuromuscular commands that can be turned on without conscious thought and executed at breakneck speed. Most singers who have learned patter songs in this way find that, with very little practice, they can perform them years later without difficulty; their brains seem to have retained the sequence of neural instructions. What works for the syllabic difficulties in a patter song can work just as well for any phonemic sequence encountered in singing.

The technique doesn't have to be employed for full phrase lengths. It can be used on units as small as a single CV or VC join. The secret of the method's success is to sustain each phoneme (vowel or pitch consonant) for a length of time that enables correct production. When the correct phoneme is acquired, the student is urged to think ahead to the next phoneme in the sequence, imagine getting to it cleanly and accurately, and then shift the articulators to the next phoneme.

In the process of slowing down the phoneme production, it is usually necessary to take the phoneme sequence out of the rhythmic structure demanded by the music. Other situations may call for the more drastic step of requiring the singer to drop the pitches of the melody and intone the passage on a single note. The key to the success of the strategy is to unencumber the brain so the singer can concentrate on building skills.

Utilizing this method, students often learn the skills in a fraction of the time than if they had simply kept repeating the passage within its musical context at speed. When a student repeats the phrase at speed without any attention to skill building of phonemic sequences, the result is usually a badly sung passage that becomes engraved in the student's memory.

Consider a case where skill accelerando would be advantageous. Imagine a phrase in which the Italian word *amore* occurs and the student begins the word with a wonderfully produced /a/, sung with the mandible down. The vowel rings with resonance and "point" (the presence of the singers formant). When the move is made to the /m/, however, the speech template insinuates itself. The jaw is raised, and the lips are tightly pursed in a horizontal configuration. This forces widespread changes in the instrument that singers call spreading. As a consequence, the ending of the initial /a/ collapses as the articulators are moved toward the spread /m/, the production of the consonant suffers and the remainder of the word probably will be compromised.

Once the teacher and student have addressed the problem of the rising jaw, utilization of the skill accelerando to correct the local problem of the /am/ join will most likely improve the production of the remainder of the word. It will also add the proper /am/ muscular sequence to the students singing template, making it available for all future occurrences of that VC join.

Many micro problems begin with an opposite acoustical scenario, the CV join. In those situations, the use of the **benchmark** strategy, an excellent technique-building device at the micro level, is called for.

Benchmark

The benchmark strategy always begins with the utilization of a student's strength when addressing a technical problem. An example is the VC join at the beginning of the word "kindness," /kaɪndnəs/. As in the previous example, a problem might occur if the student tends to raise the jaw for the production of the consonant rather than utilizing the tongue to do the articulative work. If the jaw was left in the relaxed, vowel-like position and the tongue performed the upward extension needed to produce the /k/, the production of the consonant would most likely improve because spreading would be avoided. The singer would then be able to form an easy join between the consonant and the vowel.

Step 1: Establishing the Benchmark

To perform a benchmark exercise, vocal practitioners must initially focus on the first vowel, /a/, to make sure that its proper execution is well ensconced in the student's technique. Using that vowel as a benchmark, the singer is then asked to reverse the two phonemes of the word, first sounding the /a/ and then the /k/. The goal is the use of the articulative set of the vowel to initiate a proper resonance environment for the /k/. When the student can execute the join properly, the next step in the benchmark process can be added.

Step 2: Bracket the Benchmark

The student now brackets the consonant between the two benchmark vowels, /a k a/. In this form, the exercise now becomes a VCV set. The goal is to maintain the sound of the initial vowel, /a/, in its repetition following the consonant. The student should be instructed to take care that the second iteration of the vowel should sound exactly like the first. When this is accomplished, the singer should be instructed to drop the benchmark, the initial /a/. If properly done, the CV join, /ka/, should work satisfactorily. One can then use the skill accelerando to engrave the habit in the student's technique.

This may seem like a great deal of time and effort to spend on a single VC join in one word. But, how many times will that student have to perform the same join, not only in this phrase, but in all instances of that VC join in all the other singing languages? If performed properly, this exercise can embed the technical sequence in the singer's song template making it less likely that he or she will turn to the speech template for a solution.

For this reason, every lesson in the author's studio begins with exercises that train the various CV-VC joins at the micro level. This skill acquisition is approached by having students start on a consonant, then sing five pitches up and down in their middle range on a vowel, completing the exercise with a return to the original cosonant (see the chart given in Appendix B). By following the orderly sequence of the chart, one may take a close look at each join in an attempt to learn proper articulative habits (notice that the various consonants are dealt with in groupings by production class). In this way, good CV-VC join habits are formed simultaneously with the vocal warmup.

Toggle Strategy

Toggling is a way to increase student awareness of the way a well-produced sound *feels,* as well as fostering conscious knowledge of the articulative configuration that produces it. When a phoneme has been modified sufficiently so that it can be deemed "well-sung," it is time to reinforce that learning with the **toggle exercise**. To perform this reinforcement, the teacher asks students to alternate between the good and bad productions without stopping phonation. By doing this, students gain much valuable knowledge by comparing the set of articulators needed for the production of both good and bad sounds. Should they begin to drift back to a speech-influenced sound, they are more likely to recognize the drift as the brain compares the good and bad productions.

Two-Screen Modeling

Whether working at the micro or macro level, the computer can be used in the studio as a high-tech version of the traditional model/imitation technique. By running the spectrogram program twice on the same screen (simultaneously), a static model can be shown in one window while the student utilizes VRTF on the other in an attempt to duplicate the model. The correctly sung model can be recorded by either the teacher or the student. Earlier in this section, an example of a student who learned the proper execution of a Baroque trill by utilizing computer VRTF was presented. With the model in one window and her own voice in real-time on the other, she had no trouble using her eyes as a guide in the attempt to match the image; the correct use of the vocal anatomy followed, and the skill was hers. Once a student has mastered a technical point in this way, we at the Drew University studio/lab quite often save the spectrographic model on a floppy disk to use again,

should it be needed in subsequent work sessions.

SUMMARY

The first chapter spoke of the need to pay careful attention to detail in our acquisition of vocal technique to enable the art to flourish. It is difficult to keep that in mind, as the student understandably wants to enjoy the emotional satisfaction of singing the whole song. Indeed, satisfying that emotional drive should be part of the voice practitioners pedagogical goals. Without that satisfaction, why should the student submit to the long and sometimes wearying process of learning to sing well? Voice practitioners must balance that emotional need with technique building at the micro level. Without such attention to detail, the phrase and song may improve, but not as fast as they might with careful instruction. Do not be afraid to move to the micro level and use RTF as an adjunct, especially **VRTF** that employs the input of the computer.

CHAPTER

7

USING THE SPECTROGRAM IN THE VOICE STUDIO

We have already seen some examples of spectrograms and power spectra in earlier chapters. Those images were produced on a PC using acoustical analysis software called Gram. A complete, fully functional copy of this software is included on the CD that accompanies this book. This program will permit vocal practitioners to immediately start learning how to use the spectrograph, as well as how to apply it as a feedback/research tool in the voice studio. All that one needs to begin using this technology is a PC, Gram, a sound card, and a microphone. With these in hand, a studio will have a working spectrograph capability.

This chapter discusses the basics of spectrograph use. A thorough understanding of the spectrograph and how it works is critical to mastering the feedback applications that will appear in this chapter and later in the book. More detailed discussion of the workings of Gram can be found in Appendix C.

LEARNING TO USE GRAM

Richard S. Horne, an electrical engineer living in Virginia who has had a long interest in the use of desktop computers for audio analysis, wrote the first versions of the spectrographic software included on the CD that accompanies this book. He originally wrote Gram in 1994 for use in studying the audio frequency spectrum of bird song.

Since that time, the program has been improved and expanded many times. Horne posted it on the Internet as freeware and, as people discovered it and began to use it, its use has grown to include many different fields of research far removed from its original purpose. Some of those applications include:

- analysis and identification of biological sounds
- analysis and identification of human speech
- analysis of vocal and instrumental music
- evaluation and tuning of musical instruments
- evaluation and calibration of home audio systems
- ham radio audio reception and tuning

How Gram Works on Your PC

Spectrograms and power spectra are created on a PC by the following means: First, the sound emanating from the singer is converted into an analog electrical signal by the microphone. Then the microphone signal is fed into a device in the PC called a sound card, which converts the analog microphone signal into a digital signal that the computer can understand (much as a modem converts telephone transmissions into the digital language of a computer). This type of signal conversion is called A/D (audio to digital) conversion. The computer, running the spectrographic software, analyzes that digital signal and presents the results as a graphic display on the computer's monitor or printer.

Running Gram

When you run Gram on your computer, the screen shown in Figure 7–1 will appear.

Main Screen

The large blank area in the middle of the display is the window where the acoustical analysis will be displayed. In addition to that window, there are other features on the screen that add greater functionality to Gram.

Waveform

The subdivision at the top of the main window is a waveform display (see Figure 7–2). It will show the amplitude of each audio sample as it is analyzed. It runs simultaneously with the spectrographic display below it. If Gram is configured to a very fine resolution, one is able to see evidence of each full cycle of vocal fold vi-

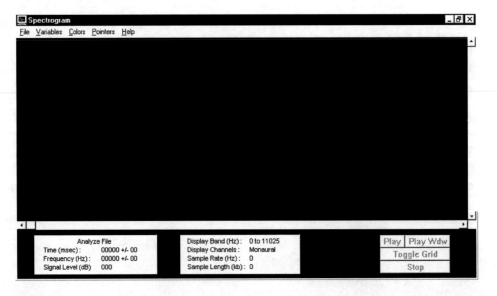

Figure 7–1. Full screen view of Gram as it appears when the program is first run.

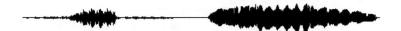

Figure 7–2. A waveform as it appears on the Gram screen.

bration (which appear as vertical stria-tions in the waveform).

Drop-Down Menus

The menus that control the program are found at the top of the screen. They are typical, drop-down menus (when one clicks the mouse on a selecton, menus drop down giving further options under that choice). These drop-down menus present a wide variety of parameters for running the program.

The File menu shown in Figure 7–3 is the main control panel for setting up the various types of analysis. Figure 7–4 shows the result of choosing "Scan Input" on the File menu. This menu gives the user extremely fine control over the way in which Gram will conduct the analysis (details on the various parameters can be found in Appendix C). Once the parameters are properly set, clicking on the OK button, or pressing the Enter key, will run the analysis.

Lower Portion of the Screen

In addition to the spectrograph's three-dimensional analytical display and the waveform on the main screen, there are three small boxes at the bottom of the screen that provide additional information about the analysis in the main window and control the program while in analysis mode.

Center Box: Information About the User-Set Parameters

The three upper lines in the center box show information about how the user has set Gram's parameters during and prior to performing the analysis. If the program is being run in one of the modes that creates a new file or reads a preexisting one, the bottom line of the box will show information about the number of kilobytes the sample has used (and hence, the size of the file being read or saved).

Left Box: Cursor-Derived Information About the Analysis

Once an analysis has been performed and saved, or paused on the screen, the left box becomes a source of valuable information. By moving the cursor to points on the display screen, the user can obtain more precise information on the following parameters:

- Time, in **milliseconds** (thousandths of a second, abbreviated as ms) at the cursor position. Many aspects involving time and vocal production are of interest in the spectrographic display. Information such as relative time spent on phonemes, length of silences between stop consonants (i.e., /p/) and the following vowels, vibrato rate, and so forth, are all readable by moving the cursor and reading the values on this line.
- Frequency: When the cursor is placed on any part of the screen, this function shows the frequency of the harmonics, the formants, or both at the location of the cursor. Depending on the type of analysis, there is a variable in the accuracy of the readout (±).
- Amplitude: The relative amplitude of a harmonic in **dB** (**decibels**) can be obtained at any point on the screen.

Right Box: Control Buttons

More will be said about these right-hand control buttons when Gram's various types of analysis and displays are discussed later in this chapter.

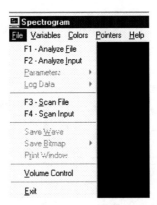

Figure 7–3. A drop-down menu revealed by clicking the File menu option.

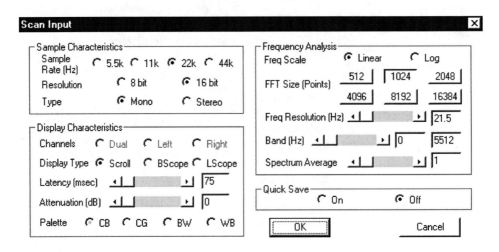

Figure 7–4. Scan Input menu shown after choosing Scan from the drop-down File menu.

GRAM'S ANALYSIS TYPES

Voice practitioners can use Gram to produce the two different types of analysis seen thus far in illustrations given in this book, the spectrograph (scroll) and the power spectrum (scope). The user can choose either of these functions by highlighting the option menu that appears on the screen shown in Figure 7–4. Under the File menu, select Scan Input. Toward the bottom of the screen, note the section called Display Characteristics. At Display Type, the user may select "scroll" or "scope."

Scope: The Power Spectrum

As noted in Chapter 3, a power spectrum graphically represents the harmonics of a sound at a given point in time, a kind of acoustical snapshot, in a real-time amplitude versus frequency plot. The spectrum analysis is useful for certain real-time feedback applications in the voice studio. Donald G. Miller's discussion on the subject of power spectrum use, found later in this book, will go into considerable detail about analytical techniques and utilization of the results.

To review, the power spectrum displays a dual-axis graph:

- X-axis: This information shows the sequence of harmonics reading from left to right. As one scans from left to right, the frequency of the harmonics portrayed gets higher. The numbers that run along the bottom of the display indicate frequency in kilohertz (1000 Hz increments); thus the 8 in the display stands for 8000 Hz, or in shorthand, 8 kHz.
- Y-axis: This axis reveals the amplitude (relative loudness) of the harmonics. The higher the apex of a harmonic, the louder it sounds in the spectrum. In this way, one can see the relative strengths of harmonics in the sonic spectrum. The numbers along this axis indicate amplitude of the signal in dB.

There are two types of power spectrum display in Gram, the B Scope and the L Scope. For an explanation of the difference, see Appendix C.

Scroll: The Spectrograph

Readers first encountered the spectrograph in Chapter 4. It performs the same analysis on the incoming microphone signal as the power spectrum, but displays it very differently.

The spectrographic analysis is displayed as a continuous color ribbon. Each harmonic found and analyzed in the audio signal has its own horizontal line that runs across the screen continuously in real-time. This display is actually a three-dimensional graphic with information encoded as:

- X-axis: representing time moving from left to right, and
- Y-axis: frequency; the higher a harmonic or formant appears on the screen, the higher its frequency.
- Amplitude: the amplitude of the displayed harmonics and formants is rep-

resented by the color and intensity of the color on the display. In black and white, darker shades of gray represent greater amplitude. In color, brighter colors indicate the same effect (a full-color illustration of the vowels /ɔi/ is found on the front cover of this book).

With all of this information readily available in an easy-to-read format, the spectrogram is the analysis display that is at the heart of most of the feedback techniques discussed in this book. Instead of being an aural snapshot of a moment in time like the power spectrum, the spectrograph shows what is happening acoustically at every moment. It is especially useful in the tracking of language events in the vocal signal.

Toggle Grid

While the spectrogram scroll is running, there are no time and frequency indicators on the main screen. While exact information can be obtained by placing the cursor on a spot on the screen and then reading the results in the lower left box, more approximate time and frequency information is available though the Toggle Grid function found at the bottom right of the screen. Pressing this button will cause a grid to overlay the main window that will give frequency and time references during the analysis. It is available in only some of the analysis modes.

DISPLAY DIFFERENCES BETWEEN THE POWER SPECTRUM AND SPECTROGRAM

The difference between the power spectrum and spectrographic displays are illustrated in Figures 7–5 and 7–6, which show the same sung event in the two different types of display. Because a power spectrum shows only a snapshot of time,

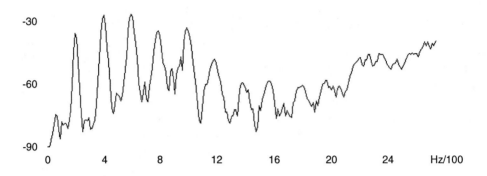

Figure 7–5. A "snapshot" of one moment of a sung phrase analyzed with the power spectrum, Gram's Scope function. 🆑 (Note: Use Gram to analyze the wave file for this figure that can be found on the CD. In this way, by using Scan File/Scope, the reader can view the entire phrase in real-time.)

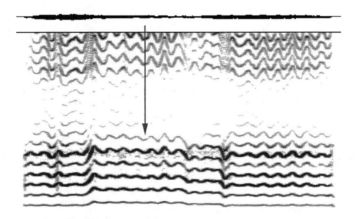

Figure 7–6. Spectrogram of the full sung phrase from which Figure 7-5 was taken. The arrow indicates the moment that the power spectrum "snapshot" shown in Figure 7-5 was captured. 🆑 (Note: Play the wave file for Figure 7-5 using Scan File/Scroll to view this image on the CD.)

it will only show a specific moment of the phrase; the spectrogram shows all that happens during the entirety of the phrase. The arrow on the spectrogram in Figure 7–6 shows the moment in time that was captured in the power spectrum in Figure 7–5. The accompanying CD contains the files that show the complete analysis to enable the reader to be able to view the entire power spectrum sequence and compare it with the spectrogram.

Play!

The very best way to learn how to use these displays is to run the program and sing into the microphone while watching the display. As you manipulate your voice and watch the results on the monitor, you will learn more than any book can teach you. Before going on to some learning exercises, run Gram and PLAY!

DIFFERENCES IN THE DISPLAY BETWEEN MEN AND WOMEN

The author, a bass-baritone, produced most of the spectrograms found in this book. If one looks at a spectrogram of a woman singing in Figure 7–7 (in this case a soprano), the display looks quite different. It does not seem to contain the density of information that is found in the same passage sung by a man.

Why do they appear so different? Why is the density of the information on the right graph so much greater than that shown on the left? The answer is that a spectrographic display converts the result of mathematical calculations into graphic form. All differences in frequency appear as differences in measurable distance on the graph. Since the relativity of the differences between frequencies is graphically represented as distance, the frequency differential between frequencies for middle C and the C below it, 130.8 Hz, will be shown as smaller than the difference between middle C and the C above it, which is 261.6 Hz.

Musicians tend to think of the distance between octaves (a doubling or halving of frequency) as equidistant because they are visually equidistant when viewed on the piano keyboard or in printed music. In those visual references, an octave appears as the same distance no matter where it is in the frequency spectrum.

This differential in distance between harmonics can be seen in the graph in Figure 7–8. As the fundamentals that are being sung go higher, the distance between harmonics becomes greater (a function of the mathematical values). On the spectrogram, one can clearly see this effect in Figure 7–9 in which a singer starts on 140 Hz, moves up the octave to 280 Hz, and then returns to the original pitch. Also notice that the dark lines that represent the formants stay in the same frequency area because they are products of the vocal resonance. On the other hand, the harmonics produced by the vocal folds (the lighter lines) move in lockstep with the F_0.

The Need To Track Higher Frequencies in the Woman's Spectrogram Display

While this display for the woman's voice reveals the information necessary for

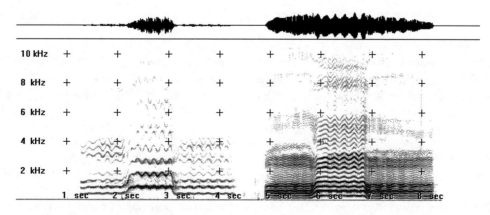

Figure 7–7. Spectrogram of a passage sung by a woman (left) and a man (right). 📀

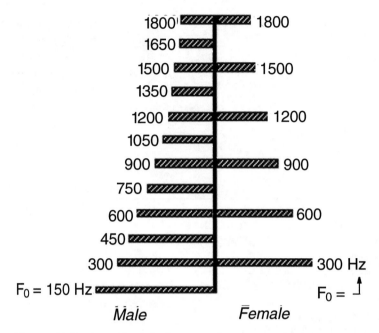

Figure 7-8. A graph of the harmonic frequencies of a bass singing an F_0 or 150 Hz (left), and a soprano singing an F_0 or 300 Hz or one octave higher (right).

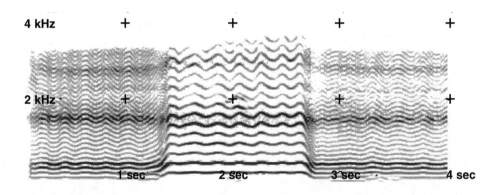

Figure 7-9. An /e/ sung at 140 Hz, up one octave to 280 Hz and then returning. 💿

vowel feedback, it may need to be expanded for the higher frequency resolution needed to work on many of the consonants (i.e., /f/ /ʃ/ or /θ/).

When analyzing the sound of a female singer, if a higher frequency resolution is needed for consonant work, one should change the resolution in the Frequency Analysis portion in the Modify Analysis Parameters menu that appears just before

running an analysis. The user will be changing the FFT size near the top of the right column. The choice will depend on the needs of the moment; generally 1024 FFT points is the preferred resolution for men, and 512 FFT points is useful for women when more upper frequency detail is desired (see Figure 7–10). If you wish to know about FFT points, or any other Gram analysis parameter, consult Appendix C.

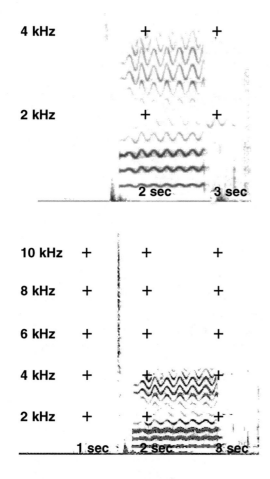

Figure 7–10. Two spectrograms of the word "top" sung by a woman. The upper image was analyzed at 1024 FFT points and the lower at 512 FFT points. The difference in diction detail, especially the stop consonants, are significant. 🔘

Teacher and Student: Same Gender/Different Gender

When the teacher and student are of the same gender, the frequency resolution can remain the same throughout the session. When the gender of the two is not the same, it is advisable to toggle between the two resolutions when the teacher wishes to show the student an example on-screen. Beginners in the field of reading spectrographic VRTF can be confused by the difference in the two displays shown in Figure 7–7. By toggling between the two display resolutions (1024 and 512), the male-female/female-male display differences can be made to almost disappear, making it easier for students to compare their analysis with the teacher's.

LEARNING TO READ GRAM: THE DISPLAY

The following exercises present static images in order to learn the types of physioacoustical information that one can observe. Later in this chapter, there will be a series of hands-on exercises, in real-time, to further the reader's understanding of how the spectrogram works.

Looking at a Single Vowel

Signature Formant Pattern for the Vowel

In the spectrogram shown in Figure 7–11, the brightest lines (shown by the arrows) indicate areas of the frequency spectrum where the formants (supraglottal resonances of the vocal tract) are at work. Remember that each vowel has a characteristic formant "signature." We can recognize the pattern in Figure 7–11 as the classic formant pattern for the vowel /i/; the F_1 (bottom arrow) is low, F_2 appears at about 1.6 kHz. There is also evidence of a strong singer's format (F_3), indicated by the top arrow.

Vibrato Evidence

Notice that the horizontal lines representing the individual harmonics oscillate in a more or less periodic manner. This is evidence of the singer's vibrato. Since each of the harmonics stays in lockstep with the minute frequency changes in the F_0, most of the harmonics will display the same "rolling-hills" pattern during the vibrato cycle.

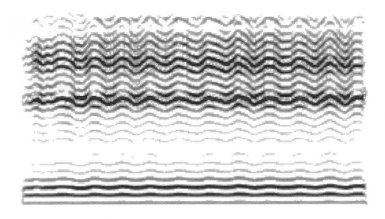

Figure 7–11. Spectrogram of the vowel /i/. 🆑

Onset and Exit Evidence

Readers can also learn some things about the technique of the singer from this example. The beginning of the phonation, called the **onset**, is well executed; the majority of the harmonics constituting the structure of this vowel appear at the same time at the beginning of the display. The only ones that lag are in the 1 kHz area, and they only lag by about 8 ms). This indicates that the singer had virtually all of the articulators set in their proper position in advance of the beginning of phonation. This enabled the voice to produce its full acoustic richness right from the start. There was no "bloom" period as the sound settled.

The *exit* (cessation of phonation) from the vowel is equally well performed; the spectrographic evidence suggests that the singer maintained the proper articulator configuration for this vowel throughout the process of terminating the flow of air at the glottis. Thus the sound remains consistently rich right up to the silence. Such onsets and exits, so well coordinated, are desirable vocal habits in most pedagogies of vocal production.

Possible Evidence of Undesirable Muscle Use

Observe that the vibrato is present throughout the entire period of phonation. This is probably an indication that the singer initiated the air stream with the abdominal musculature instead of over-involving the laryngeal or pharyngeal muscles. Had the pharyngeal and/or laryngeal musculature been overinvolved, the effects may have been seen as one of the following:

• Absence of the vibrato (the harmonic lines would have been straight)
• Unsteady vibrato (the consistency of the waviness would have been compromised)
• Late onset of the vibrato (the vibrato would have set in as the laryngeal and pharyngeal muscles relaxed after phonation had settled)

Two Vowels in Comparison

When phonemes are executed sequentially, the spectrographic evidence of the complexities of physioacoustics become rapidly apparent. The next exercise (Figure 7–12) features two vowels, sung without pause, to enable one to observe the difference in the formant patterns endemic to each vowel (for the remainder of this book, the term **F-pattern** will be used). One can also see the join (the brief period of transition between phonemes) as the singer shifts articulator configuration for the second vowel.

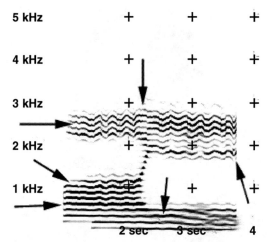

Figure 7–12. Spectrogram of the vowel /ɔ/ moving to /i/. 🔘

Note the difference in the placement and intensity of the harmonics and formants. There is a gap in harmonic generation toward the top of /ɔ/ that shifts downward for the /i/. Also notice that the /i/ is richer in upper harmonics.

In the shift from the /ɔ/ to the /i/:

- F_1 (indicated by the lower left arrow) falls slightly (lower central arrow);
- F_2 shows a considerable migration from its position in /ɔ/ (middle left arrow) to that in the /i/ (right arrow); and
- During the short time that it took the tongue to shift from the /ɔ/ to the /i/, one can clearly see evidence of the shift as F_2 makes a dramatic rise (area shown by the top arrow).

As was the case with the single vowel /i/, shown in Figure 7–11, the area right around 2700 Hz reveals the continual presence of a strong singer's formant throughout the execution of the two vowels.

The physioacoustic factors revealed in the shift of the F-patterns can be seen in the following sagittal view (an imaginary slice down the center of the anatomy as viewed from the side) of the head of a singer as derived from X-rays.

In Figure 7–13, the /ɔ/ shown on the left, the tongue is relatively flat and low, a configuration that creates a large oral cavity

and a small pharyngeal cavity. In the /i/ vowel shown on the right, the tongue has formed a large hump in the middle of the oral cavity. As a result, the oral cavity is small, and the pharynx is large.

Voice practitioners can learn more about formants by combining the information from the spectrograms with that of the X-rays. The /ɔ/ vowel, with its small pharyngeal cavity, tends to produce a relatively high frequency F_1. As the tongue shifts to /i/, the pharyngeal cavity enlarges, and the pitch of F_1 drops correspondingly (larger resonance space = lower frequency).

F_2 is generally susceptible to shifts in the amount of resonance space in the oral cavity. Since that area is large in the /ɔ/, the F_2 is low. As the tongue moves to nearly fill the oral cavity for the /i/, F_2 rises dramatically, an action that gives this frontal vowel much of its considerable brightness.

An Entire Word: /vɔⁱs/ ("Voice")

Let us now add some consonants to the same vowels to form the word "voice." Once the two vowels are executed within the body of the word, they comprise an excellent example of a **diphthong** (more will be said about diphthongs in Chapter 8). A few observations about the nature of diphthongs are in order here.

A diphthong is a sequential pairing of two **monophthongs** featuring a differential in the amount of phonation time between the two. In singing, one vowel is usually sung for more time than the other. The two vowels shown in Figure 7–12 do not constitute a diphthong as there is no differential in performance time between the two vowels; to form a diphthong, there must be a time differential between the pair of vowels.

The /ɔ/ and /i/ vowels shown in Figure 7–14 constitute a diphthong because the /ɔ/ takes up more time of the execution than the /i/. In speech, while moving

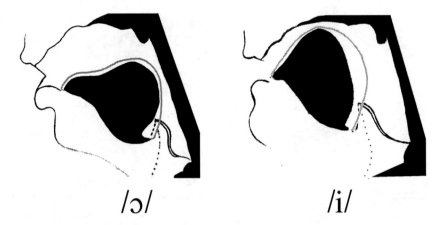

/ɔ/   /i/

Figure 7–13. Sagittal view of the tongue position for the vowels /aɔ/ and /i/. (Schematic sagittal views adapted from *The Science of Vocal Pedagogy* by D. R. Appelman, 1967, pp. 315, 299. Bloomington, IN: Indiana University Press. Copyright 1967 by Indiana University Press. Adapted with permission.)

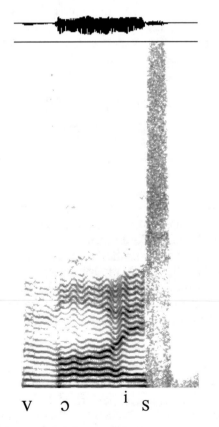

v   ɔ   i   s

Figure 7–14. Spectrogram of the word "voice." 💿

from the longer of the two vowels to the shorter, the tongue often does not get into a proper position, a condition called **tar-**

get undershoot. In singing, target undershoot can result in the impression of sloppy diction. Well-trained singers tend to move the tongue more quickly from one well-executed vowel to another. As a result, target undershoot is generally less of a problem in the production of a singer as compared to that of the average speaker.

In addition, Figure 7–14 shows two new sounds, the consonants /v/ and /s/, that are needed to complete the word. The initial /v/ shows a good amount of vowel-like resonance (although not as much as the coming /ɔ/) because of constriction of the space needed between the lower lip and the upper front teeth for the production of /v/. In Figure 7–14, one can see that the transition of the articulators (the lips and tongue) from the /v/ to the /ɔ/ is rather quick and efficient. The ending /s/ shows the aperiodic pattern of noise (all of that "fuzziness" high in the spectrum). One may also observe that the singer has performed a very clean movement from the /i/ vowel to the /s/, as indicated by the almost vertical wall of harmonics at the end of the vowel.

If the singer had encountered trouble with the execution of any of these phonemes or the joins between them, the problems would have shown up in the spectrogram, ready to be diagnosed and corrected.

LEARNING TO USE GRAM: HANDS-ON

It cannot be stressed enough: Working with one's own voice is the best way to learn to use the spectrogram. Voice practitioners should try to replicate the exercises given in the previous section with their own voices and then move on to the new ones given in the following section.

Running Gram for the Study Exercises

After running Gram by double clicking on the Gram.exe file, left click on the FILE pulldown menu at the top left of the screen and choose SCAN INPUT. This will display the analysis parameter menu. Set the parameters on this screen as you see them represented in Figure 7–4. If you are male, set the FFT size to 1024; if you are female, you may want to set it to 512 to account for the pitch differential in the appearance of the spectrogram, allowing one to see the higher frequency detail needed to track some consonants. Also, make sure that the Display Type is set to SCROLL.

After clicking on OK, the spectrogram will run in real-time, and you can begin to further explore the acoustical properties of your voice.

Stopping the Scroll: The Right Mouse Button

One important feature of Gram is that with the cursor in position in the middle window, the user can temporarily stop the scrolling at any time by pressing the right mouse button. This will pause the spectrograph and permit the user to inspect the display on the screen. Clicking the right mouse button a second time will start the scroll going again (remember to keep the cursor in the main window).

REAL-TIME EXERCISES

Vowel Differentiation

As the reader will remember, each vowel has its own distinctive F-pattern. It is the differences in the F-pattern, from vowel to vowel, that enables the brain to differentiate between the various vowel phonemes that one hears.

In learning to use the spectrograph, one must learn to correlate the visual display with what is happening inside the vocal instrument. Learning to distinguish between vowels is an excellent starting place. This correlation of the distinctive appearance of each vowel's F-pattern with the anatomical shifts that cause the differences allows voice practitioners to employ the spectrograph as real-time feedback.

Sing the vowels /i/, then /u/, giving the two phonemes equal time. You should see a pattern that appears similar to that shown in Figure 7–15. Repeat the slow execution of the two vowels while paying attention to the following:

- Observe the harmonic pattern on the screen and note the shift in the F-patterns.
- If the formants in your performance of the two vowels shift at a slower rate (i.e., the shift occupies a longer section of the

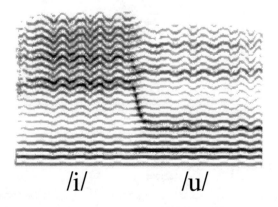

/i/   /u/

Figure 7–15. Spectrogram of the vowel /i/ moving to /u/. ⓒⓓ

screen), it means that your articulators are not repositioning fast enough during the shift. Sing the exercise again and attempt a shift that looks more like the one in Figure 7–15. By using the spectrogram, you should be able to make your shift both more accurate and more rapid, a necessary component in many styles of technique.

- Next, sing the two vowels slowly while looking at the anatomical drawings in Figure 7–16. These drawings illustrate the tongue positions that produce the two vowels. Use your eye to increase your awareness of how the tongue moves in the course of producing the vowels.

- Shut your eyes and sing the two vowels again in order to concentrate more on the positioning and movement of your tongue. With some practice, you will be able to sense where the tongue is for the /i/ (held in a high curve near the hard palate, then dropped in the center for the /u/). Also, you may sense a slight rounding of the lips while sounding the /u/.

- A big difference between the production of the two vowels is the occlusion of the tongue and the back upper teeth

for the /i/. Figure 7–17 is a palatogram, a representation of the occlusion between the tongue and the palate or upper teeth. This type of lingua-dental constriction is performed for some vowels but not others. Singers and speakers are rarely aware that such occlusion is a critical part of the articulative process. If you did not feel this occlusion, shut your eyes and try the exercise again.

This is an excellent illustration of the use of feedback. In this case, your eyes, while looking at both the spectrogram and the anatomical drawings, help guide your brain to a sensory awareness of the tongue positions involved in executing the two phonemes. Many singers never consciously experience this until the visual aids give them a reference point.

Repeat the exercise while looking at the real-time spectrograph. You should become even more aware of the tongue's movement as you watch the formants change on monitor.

Finally, sing the two vowels again, but begin to experiment with little shifts of your articulators, producing sounds that are not representative of your best vocal

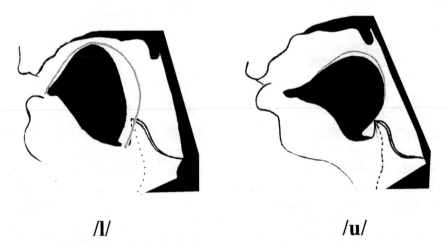

/I/   /u/

Figure 7–16. Sagittal view of the production of /i/ and /u/. (Schematic sagittal views adapted from *The Science of Vocal Pedagogy* by D. R. Appelman, 1967, pp. 299, 321. Bloomington, IN: Indiana University Press. Copyright 1967 by Indiana University Press. Adapted with permission.)

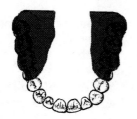

Figure 7–17. Palatogram of the vowel /i/ showing the degree of contact between the tongue and the upper teeth. (From *The Science of Vocal Pedagogy,* by D. R. Appelman, 1967, p. 299. Bloomington, IN: Indiana University Press. Copyright 1967 by Indiana University Press. Printed with permission.)

production. Try to sense the configuration that produces the less than ideal sounds. Then alternate (toggle) between the good and bad sounds to learn the relative positions of your articulators. As you gain experience in sensing the articulative shifts that cause unwanted vocal production, you will be well on your way toward using the computer as feedback in the voice studio.

Following are some experiments that illustrate spectrographic differences during the performance vowels produced with faulty vocal production.

Vocal Production Problems as Seen on the Spectrogram

Try the following exercises employing the vowel /i/ again. This time, we will start with one that looks like the spectrogram on the left in Figure 7–16. We will use this as a benchmark, our point of reference for the well-produced vowel. In this case we want to keep an ideal /i/ vowel in mind as we vary its production to learn the type of things that can go wrong with articulator position during its execution.

Spread Production

Sing the vowel normally until you are pleased with the sound and note the configuration on the display. This will be your benchmark. Now sing the vowel while spreading the production (tense and spread the corners of your mouth).

- What happened to the sound?
- What happened to the set of your articulators? What shifts in the spectrographic display occurred as a result?

Problems in Vertical Configuration

Next, sing the vowel and slowly raise your jaw without concurrently spreading at the mouth. Ask the same questions that were asked during the spreading exercise given above.

Finally, lower your jaw as far as you can (almost to a yawn). In doing this, one of two things may happen:

- Your tongue may drop with the jaw, and the vowel may drift toward another vowel (in the studio, we call this "vowel creep"), or
- You may learn that, by making the tongue work with greater flexibility and extension than you habitually use in speech, you may be able to lower the jaw and achieve a far better vowel.

In fine vowel production, one would be well advised to accept the maxim, "*The jaw is not an elevator for a lazy tongue!*" Most speakers employ their jaw in a high position, allowing the tongue to make only minor adjustments for vowel differentiation. Learning to utilize a more active tongue, while maintaining a relaxed jaw, can greatly increase the resonance space (and hence, an increase in "richness") that we associate with fine singing and speaking. Experiment with jaw elevation during the production of all the vowels and hear the result.

Because your speech template is hard at work trying to "correct" this type of production, executing the vowels with a lowered jaw platform will probably feel strange. If you substitute the word "different" for strange, you will be on your way to some interesting discoveries.

Consonant Production

Let us now explore a few different types of consonants to learn about their physical production and their resulting graphic displays.

Fricatives

The production of **fricatives** involves the noise of **turbulent** air. An excellent example to employ in one's first experiments with the spectrograph is a /ʃ/, the sound at the beginning of the word "should." Since this phoneme is a noise, it will not display any harmonic definition such as seen during our earlier vowel exploration. You may, however, see one or two areas of resonance that are being created by the supraglottal resonance spaces.

/ʃ/ is created when the tongue narrows the space between itself and the palate so that the air stream strikes the front teeth. If there is insufficient constriction of the flowing air, little or no turbulence will result, and a weak consonant will result.

Run Gram in the real-time analysis mode and explore the interaction between your production of this fricative and the spectrographic display utilizing the following exercises:

- Produce the consonant and observe the spectrographic display.
- Experiment with the degree of constriction by moving your tongue and note the changes in the display.
- Sustain the fricative for a second or so and then, without stopping the airflow, initiate phonation at the vocal folds.

You will recognize the sound as the voiced cousin of /ʃ/, the voiced /ʒ/ (as in the word "division"). Toggle between the two phonemes; during each sounding of the /ʒ/, you should see the beginning of a structured harmonic development (emanating from the vocal folds) in the first several harmonics at the bottom of the Gram display. When you stop phonation, these harmonics will disappear, and you will only hear the /ʃ/.

Try toggling between /s/ and /ʃ/ and note the differences on the display. Finally, induce phonation in each of these consonants and you will hear (and see) /s/ /z/ /ʃ/ /ʒ/. If you are unfamiliar with the concept of the toggling exercise, consult Chapter 6 for details.

Nasals

Sing an /m/ while observing the spectrogram in real-time. This consonant requires a full closure of the lips to block all airflow from leaving the front of the oral cavity. As the front of the oral cavity is shut off, the soft palate relaxes (it is normally sealed against the nasopharynx for most vowels). This permits the moving air stream to escape through the nose (hence the designation nasal). You will observe little harmonic structure in the spectrographic display because the trip through all of the absorbent tissue of the nasopharynx and the nose causes the loss of most of the higher harmonics.

An excellent way to learn the feel of the opening of the velopharyngeal port during the production of nasal phonemes is to sing an /m/ and pinch your nostrils shut after phonation has begun. Phonation will cease immediately as the air stream has no way to leave the instrument. Pressure above and below the glottis quickly equalizes, causing the cessation of all air motion. By alternately opening and closing the nose or the mouth, one can learn to sense the opening and closing of the velopharyngeal port.

Stops

Stops are produced by building up air pressure behind a full occlusion of the oral cavity, followed by a precipitous release of the pressure that creates a burst of energy called a **transient**. These transients appear on the spectrographic analysis as "spikes," sharp vertical displays of noise. Perform a /t/ and then a /p/. While watching the spectrogram, you will notice an area of resonance in the pattern of the spike. It will be high for the /t/ because the oral cavity during and after the pressure buildup is small, and lower for the /p/ because the cavity is larger.

SUMMARY

We have just explored the tip of the spectrographic iceberg. As we proceed through the next four chapters, much more detail about vocal production and how it is revealed on spectrograms will be discussed. The research on the use of real-time spectrography as an everyday adjunct in the process of teaching singing has just begun. Vocal practitioners may find that virtually every session with a singer that uses the spectrograph will yield new insights.

Initially, the quickest and most thorough way to learn to use the spectrogram is to use it with one's own voice. As you read the next four chapters, try to replicate each example while observing the results on the real-time spectrogram. As these explorations progress, the user should use the following checklist:

☐ Can you replicate our sample given either in the book or on the CD?

☐ If your production is different, how is it different?

☐ Can you manipulate your voice so that the resulting display is more like the example in the book or on the CD?

☐ If you succeeded in altering your sound successfully, exactly what articulators did you move to accomplish the change?

☐ How much did the articulators move and to what altered position?

☐ If you are not sure of what happened during the shift, do the toggle exercise. Toggle-replicate your first attempt and then, without stopping the voice, shift to the configuration that produces a sound and display more like that in the book. You will begin to feel the changes in your articulators as you toggle back and forth.

Important Reminder

The vocal production techniques espoused in this book and CD may not conform to every vocal practitioners' technical norms. These examples are offered as a way to illustrate a method of analyzing specific technical problems in the hope that they might encourage readers to utilize the technology in service of their own technical norms.

As you explore the world of the spectrogram, consult other books about the acoustics of the voice to deepen your understanding. Correlate what you are observing on the display with what you are sensing in your vocal instrument. Voice and speech literature can help guide the user to gain valuable scientific knowledge about physioacoustics. Users should:

• Learn the proper terminology for the anatomical, physiological, and physical principles.
• Utilize that terminology in the studio everyday for the sake of clarity in communication with students and ultimately other practitioners of the singing art.

CHAPTER

8

VOWELS

DEFINITION AND BASIC PRINCIPLES

Vowels are continuants, phonemes produced by oral configurations during phonation that permit a relatively unrestricted flow of air in the oral cavity. As the articulators (principally the tongue) move during phonation, different resonance patterns are created that the listener perceives as specific vowels are created.

Most books on singing borrow vowel and consonant classifications from the speech literature. As we've noted earlier, however, the differences between speech and song are considerable, making re-ordering of classifications justifiable when discussing the acoustics of singing. Many phonemes that are traditionally classified as consonants, for example, can be thought of as vowels (or at least semivowels) when sung by an accomplished singer because these sounds fit within the vowel definition given above. Attention to the degree of restriction of the oral cavity will be the

deciding factor when these sounds are reclassified into vowels and semivowels later in this chapter and in Chapter 9.

Sagittal X-Ray Imagery of Singers

The **sagittal** images of the vocal tract scattered throughout this book are from a collection of X-rays and palatograms taken from Appelman (1967). This extra-ordinarily valuable collection of images is a result of six years of kinesiologic analysis of phoneme identity in song by the author at Indiana University Medical Center in Indianapolis, Indiana.

In this text, Appelman's original X-ray images have been significantly modified to show only those vocal structures essential to the understanding of physio-acoustical principles under discussion.

The original Appelman images are highly recommended for study by all voice practitioners as they reveal details of the articulator configuration of a singer singing the most common phonemes (as opposed to images of a speaker's vocal configuration on the same phonemes). Furthermore, the Appelman images reveal modifications in articulator position for each of the phonemes that are needed as a result of changes in pitch area across the singer's range. Finally, in addition to showing tongue placement (and tongue groove) details, Appelman also included palatograms of each phoneme (graphics that indicate tongue contact with either the teeth or the palate).

The Dance of the Tongue

While there are some differences in oral and pharyngeal resonance shape created by jaw opening and lip protrusion, the tongue is the prime mediator in the production of vowels. These phonemes are aurally recognizable because each vowel has its own distinctive F-pattern that is produced by a very precise configuration of the tongue.

Figure 8–1 is a vowel quadrilateral that shows the influence of articulative movement (especially the tongue) on the resonating spaces of the oral and pharyngeal cavities. Many texts refer to this type of graphic as a vowel "triangle," an incorrect appellation as the graphic has four corners, not three). Most vowel quadrilaterals reveal only the general placement of the tongue in the mouth. This quadrilateral adds two more elements to help the reader understand the complex interrelationship of the vocal articulators and the causal effect on the acoustical signal:

- sagittal views of the vocal tract to enable the reader to image the articulator positions more precisely, and
- spectrograms of each vowel so the changing F-patterns resulting from the shifts of the tongue in the oral cavity can be observed.

Armed with this visual information, the reader can understand the movements of the tongue in two dimensions, vertical and longitudinal, that create our various vowels.

Especially in the case of the frontal vowels, the changes in the oral/pharyngeal ratio have a dramatic effect on the F-pattern. The shifts in oral configuration and the resulting F-pattern for the back vowels are subtler.

Vertical Tongue Movement in the Oral Cavity

As the tongue moves in the vertical plane, it has a combined effect on both the oral and pharyngeal cavities:

- Higher tongue placement creates a larger pharyngeal cavity as the tongue centralizes its mass while it extends upward.
- Lower tongue placement causes a spreading of the tongue mass and increases the size of the oral cavity while the size of the pharyngeal cavity decreases.

Phoneticians indicate the three areas of production on the vertical plane as:

- Low
- Middle (sometimes called *medial*)
- High

Longitudinal Tongue Movement in the Oral Cavity

In speech terminology, movement along the posterior/anterior axis is called tongue advancement. In voice studios, teachers constantly work with the position of the tongue on this axis, moving some vowels forward and others to the back. Since the term, as utilized in speech science, might imply a motion that is unidirectional (back to front), a substitute term may be more applicable in the voice studio, **longitudinal movement** (meaning move-

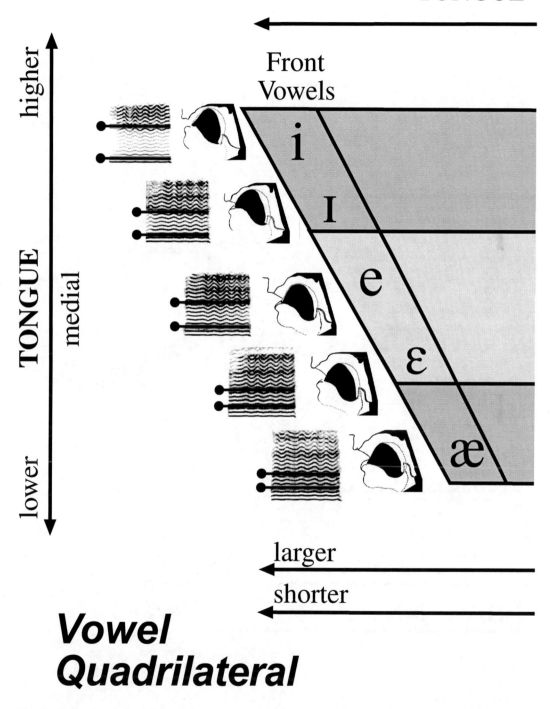

Figure 8–1. Vowel quadrilateral showing placement of the vowels in the mouth, both on the quadrilateral and in schematic sagittal views of the vocal tract. (Schematic sagittal views adapted from *The Science of Vocal Pedagogy* by D. R. Appelman, 1967, pp. 299-325. Bloomington, IN: Indiana University Press. Copyright 1967 by Indiana University Press. Adapted and reprinted with permission.) *(continued)*

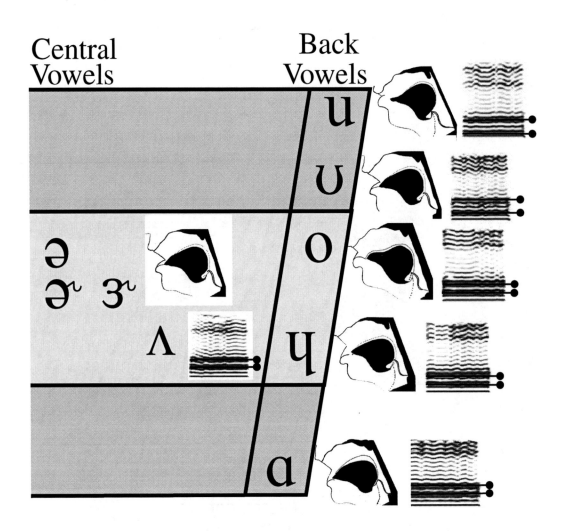

Central Vowels

Back Vowels

FRONT CAVITY   longer

PHARYNX   smaller

●── = formant

Figure 8–1. (continued)

ment along the anterior-posterior axis in either direction).

As in the vertical plane, tongue movement causes shifts in the ratio of aural/pharyngeal resonance:

- Frontal placement along this longitudinal axis creates more pharyngeal space. As this happens, there is a corresponding decrease in oral space.
- As the tongue moves farther back, an increase in oral resonance in experienced with a concurrent reduction of pharyngeal space.

Phoneticians name three areas of the tongue position on this plane:

- Front
- Central
- Back

The Missing Third Dimension

Any tongue configuration features muscular shaping on both planes simultaneously and will form a two-dimensional entity that offers a wide range of shapes and ratios of oro/pharyngeal resonance. The constant reshaping of the tongue dur-

ing the production of language—spoken or sung—is a veritable ballet.

But there is a third dimension in tongue movement that has received surprisingly little attention in the literature. When viewed from the front, the tongue is also capable of executing a variety of compound lateral curved shapes. The outside edges of the tongue can be moved upward, while the area of the midline groove (running on the posterior/anterior axis, called the median sulcus) remains depressed.

As viewed in the X-ray images in Appelman (1967), all vowels employ this groove to a greater or lesser extent; the groove may extend for virtually the entire length of the tongue, from only the middle of the tongue to the back, or from only the middle of the tongue to the tip in the front.

Many of the vowel configurations in speech require these outside raised edges of the tongue to make contact with the upper teeth, occluding an area varying anywhere from the third molar forward to the first premolar. Even if linguadental contact is not required, all vowels feature some degree of this compound curvature.

Figure 8–2 shows the vowel /i/ both in sagittal and palatogram views. The gray line in the sagittal view indicates the out-

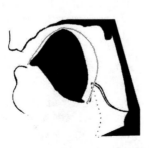
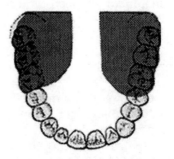

Figure 8–2. Vowel /i/, sagittal view and palatogram showing linguadental occlusion. (Schematic sagittal view and palatogram adapted from *The Science of Vocal Pedagogy* by D. R. Appelman, 1967, p. 299. Bloomington, IN: Indiana University Press. Copyright 1967 by Indiana University Press. Adapted and reprinted with permission.)

side edges of the tongue, including those contacting the teeth in the palatogram, while the black area shows the mass of the tongue at the median sulcus. Since approximate depth and placement of the tongue groove can be ascertained from this information, one can mentally construct a rough three-dimensional image of the configuration.

With the great advances in medical imaging available today, it is time for the creation of a new series of up-to-date images. There is still much to be learned about how great singers manage their vocal systems. Such state-of-the-art images may reveal many important details that will vastly improve our knowledge of vocal production. Such information will become critical as voice practitioners learn to use spectrograms and power spectra in the applied voice studio.

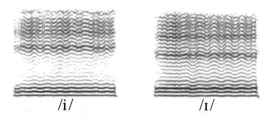

/i/   /ɪ/

Figure 8–3. Spectrograms of /i/ (left) and /ɪ/ (right) showing minor differences in F-pattern between the two vowels. **CD**

VOWELS AND COMPUTER FEEDBACK

Vowel Identity

One of the first things that many voice practitioners envision when they see a vowel spectrogram for the first time is how useful it might be in teaching students about vowel production. Often, because of a differential between singers' internal hearing and the acoustic reality being experienced in the room, they are often convinced that their vowel production is correct, while their teachers or coaches raise objections to the timbre produced. Since each vowel has a distinctive F-pattern signature, minor variations in vowel placement can be visible on spectrograms and power spectra. Thus, the use of computer-generated VRTF may prove to be of great use in the remediation of vowel identity problems.

When improperly formed, vowels often tend to drift toward one of their nearest neighbors (/i/ might drift to /ɪ/, for example). Figure 8–3 shows the spectrograms

and power spectra for these two neighboring vowels.

Figure 8–4 shows a continuously sung vowel slowly moving the tongue from /i/ to /ɪ/ and back to /i/. As one can see, the difference in the F-pattern is not great, but by using a movable cursor to mark a target point on the screen, the spectrograph can be used to help a singer clarify the production of either vowel. This is particularly useful in conjunction with the toggle strategy described in Chapter 6.

Vowel Color

Even if the identity of a specific vowel is correct, small shifts in the longitudinal axis of the tongue may create unwanted colors, or timbre, in its production. If the longitudinal placement of the tongue is too far forward, the vowel may be overly bright; one produced too far back may produce a dull coloration. Evidence of such shifts in the longitudinal axis are observable on the spectrogram. In Figure 8–5, the vowel /i/ is continuously sung and modified slowly from a benchmark production to an extreme anterior production, then to an extreme posterior position and then back to the benchmark. Again, with the use of the movable cursor marking the target F-pattern during spectrographic VRTF, the student should be able to see the results of the tongue-placement experimentation.

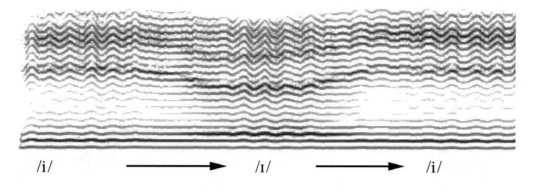

/i/ ⟶ /ɪ/ ⟶ /i/

Figure 8–4. Spectrographic results of slowly shifting the vowel from /i/ to /ɪ/ and then back showing the small movement in the F-pattern. 🖸

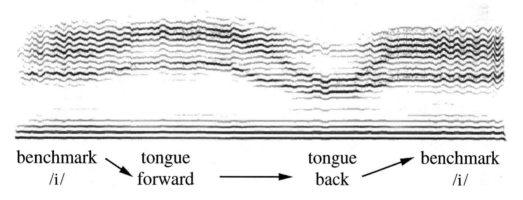

benchmark ↘ tongue ⟶ tongue ↗ benchmark
/i/ forward back /i/

Figure 8–5. F-pattern migration of an /i/ vowel. The migration is obtained by longitudinal movement of the tongue. The vowel starts out as a benchmark, moves too far forward, too far back, and then returns to the benchmark. 🖸

The Power Spectrum Is a Better Tool for Vowel Identity Work

While the differences in both vowel identity and placement are observable in spectrograms, the power spectrum is perhaps a better feedback tool for both uses. In many situations, the manner in which the power spectrum depicts harmonics and formants on the screen may make subtle vowel shifts easier to read than on the spectrogram. In power spectra, harmonics and formants appear as "mountain peaks."

The power spectrum image can, however, easily present voice practitioners with too much information about the harmonic structure of the sung sound because the formants created in the pharynx and oral cavity appear simultaneously with the harmonics being produced by the vocal folds. Even experienced researchers may encounter problems extrapolating those formants out of the total harmonic.

Pioneering work by Donald Miller of the University of Groningen provides an elegant solution in formant imaging. By using the larynx to make a noise (such as "vocal fry"), the harmonics produced by the vocal folds are virtually eliminated from the graphic leaving only format-producing resonances of the vocal tract.

Dual Power Spectrum Images for Benchmark VRTF

Figure 8–6 was made with the commercial program called VoceVista, which has the ability to save an analysis on the screen as a benchmark and then display real-time analysis as an overlay.

Vowel Identity

This saved-benchmark capacity is especially useful in the remediation of vowel-identity problems. If a student has difficulty producing an /i/ vowel, for example, the teacher may guide the student until the proper production of the vowel is achieved, freeze this benchmark image on the screen, and then have the student use the VRTF capability of the program in

an effort to match it (Figure 8–6). This use of a visible benchmark is an excellent example of the use of computer feedback in the voice studio.

Vowel Color

Figure 8–7 shows a more subtle use of the power spectrum. Many times, a singer is able to achieve an articulator configuration that produces an F-pattern easily recognized as the intended vowel, but its coloration (**vowel color**) needs to be corrected. The same technique of overlaying a benchmark display with a VRTF image can be utilized in this situation as well.

Passaggio Strategies

Finally, the benchmark technique is an excellent strategy for shifting vowel production when working with singer's traversal of the **passaggi**. In later chapters,

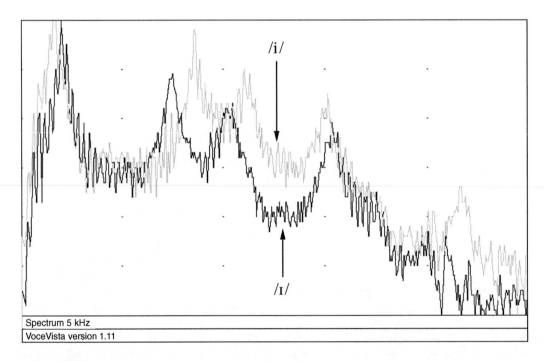

Spectrum 5 kHz
VoceVista version 1.11

Figure 8–6. A power spectrum made with VoceVista showing a benchmark vowel /i/ overlaid with a real-time signal of the vowel /ɪ/. The lighter line is the benchmark.

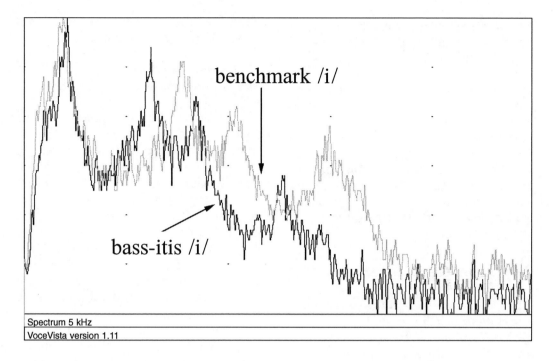

Figure 8–7. A stored benchmark vowel /i/ (lighter line) overlaid with an /i/ that is formed too far back in the oral cavity.

Donald Miller and Harm Schutte will explain these procedures in considerable detail.

Can We Use Gram To Perform These Functions?

While one can perform similar analyses using Gram's power spectrum and movable cursor, the graphics and specialized overlay abilities of a program like VoceVista make it well worth its acquisition when designing a state-of-the-art voice studio.

COMMON VOWEL PROBLEMS: USE OF SPECTROGRAM

Aside from basic questions of vowel identity and color, there are many other matters of traditional concern where the use of VRTF can be a useful adjunct in the voice studio.

Singer's Jaw Elevation: The Major Coarticulative Problem

While any of the coarticulative problems one discovers in a perusal of the speech literature can affect singers, degree of **jaw elevation** stands out as the most problematic. During the singing of a vowel **vocalize**, most singers can produce beautiful, open, and resonant vowels. When those same vowels are interspersed with the consonants required by sung language, the vowel quality drops drastically (except in the case of the best trained singers).

The speech habits of most people include a high jaw position (producing a relatively small oral cavity) during the production of consonants. Of course, many consonants require the mandible to be relatively high to permit the consonant production (/ʃ/ or /f/ for example). Other consonants can be performed with little or no mandible rise (i.e., /k/ or /g/). In many speech habits, the jaw is universally high and the interspersed vowels suffer from a lack of oral resonance. It has already been stated that even if the singer has learned to produce wonderful resonant vowels, the singer will consistently turn to his or her speech template for the neuromuscular instructions for the production of consonants. *This interference of such high-mandible speech habits on the surrounding vowels is one of the major factors mitigating a singer's development of optimal vocal production.*

New Term: Consonant Shadow (CS)

The speech term **coarticulation** refers to the state in which the production of one phoneme influences the production of the phonemes on either side of it resulting in a disturbance of the clarity and/or *timbre* of the surrounding sounds. Coarticulation problems involving jaw elevation and the resulting effects on both consonant and vowel production can be a critical problem for the developing singer. Therefore, a specific term, restricted to consonant production, seems pedagogically desirable. In the studio/lab at Drew University we employ the term **consonant shadow** (CS), a vivid visual image that succinctly sums up the problem for the singer. Consonant shadow, just like shadows caused by objects that interrupt light, can occur in any direction; both CV and VC joins are potential victims of this phenomenon.

CV Shadow (Retentive or Backward Coarticulation)

In a CV join, many singers raise their mandible for the production of the consonant and then leave the jaw parked in this position while moving on to the next phoneme. When this occurs, it will almost surely compromise the quality of the next vowel. Once that vowel collapses, a domino effect often occurs that may seriously affect the production of the next several phonemes; the singer has "painted" him- or herself into an physioacoustical corner.

VC Shadow (Anticipatory or Forward Coarticulation)

In a VC join, consonant shadow can be created when the singer's brain tries to "preset" articulators that are needed for the next consonant (principally the mandible and tongue) during the preceding vowel. In English-speaking singers, this happens most often in the phonemes /r/ and /l/. To a greater or lesser extent, all VC joins can suffer from this problem.

Well-trained singers will produce consistent vowel lines only to the extent that they are successful in mitigating CS problems. Great singers execute consonants with much more resonance than those in speech (see Chapters 9 and 10). A relaxed mandible, centered vocal production, open pharynx, and a relaxed larynx are the principal components of such resonance. This is especially true for notes sung above the speech range.

The spectrograph can be used to help detect vowels compromised by preceding or succeeding consonants. After establishing a benchmark vowel image, the singer can work toward eliminating the consonant's influence from the vowel. This effort will usually engender more resonance in the adjoining consonant as well.

Word-Interior Vowel Blooming

Word-interior vowel **blooming** is characterized by a slow shift of the articulators from the previous phoneme. As the vowel production continues, the articulators continue to move until they are in proper position. Vowel blooms can be both heard as well as seen on the spectrograph as a slow accumulation of the upper acoustical components of the vowel. When properly performed, the harmonic structure of the vowel should be totally complete within a few ms of the initiation of the phoneme. Interior vowels are bloomed either by:

- consonant shadow (forms of coarticulation) or
- problems in delivery of support.

In the latter type, the singer may begin the vowel with insufficient subglottal pressure and then attempt to correct it as the vowel progresses.

Figure 8–8 shows a spectrogram and waveform of a singer blooming word-interior vowels throughout a phrase from the Brahms *Requiem*. The effects of the "support crescendos" are especially visible in the waveform

Spreading

Spreading is one of the few singing terms where there is a near-unanimous agreement regarding its meaning. Vennard (1968, p. 140) says, "The existence of this figurative expression in singers' vocabularies shows that the ear instinctively anticipated what the Sonagraph finally made visi-

ble" [author's note: the Sonagraph was an early commercial spectrogram].

A spread tone is accomplished by increasing the horizontal plane of the instrument at the expense of the vertical. If one spreads the mouth in an extreme example of the production of the word "cheese," he or she can feel some or even all following articulative events:

- Tension builds in the *obicularis oris* muscle that surrounds the mouth. Tension may also amount in the muscles on the side of the cheeks (principally, the *zygomaticus* major and minor, and the *risorius*), which pull the corners of the mouth laterally.
- When this occurs, concomitant tension will probably appear in the muscles in the high cheek and eye areas as well.
- Additionally, there may be increased tension in the anterior and inferior muscles of the chin.
- The larynx will raise.
- Concomitant tension in the musculature surrounding the larynx will occur.
- The velum will tense and drop.
- The tongue will widen and tense.

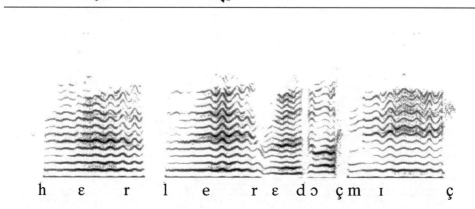

Figure 8–8. Spectrogram and waveform of a singer blooming word-interior vowels throughout a phrase from the Brahms *Requiem*. The effect of the "support crescendos" are especially visible in the waveform. 🔘

Figure 8–9 shows these muscles. It does not take much imagination to see why such spreading is a physioacoustical disaster.

Figure 8–10 shows the spectrogram of a singer gradually shifting the vocal production from a vertical set of the instru-

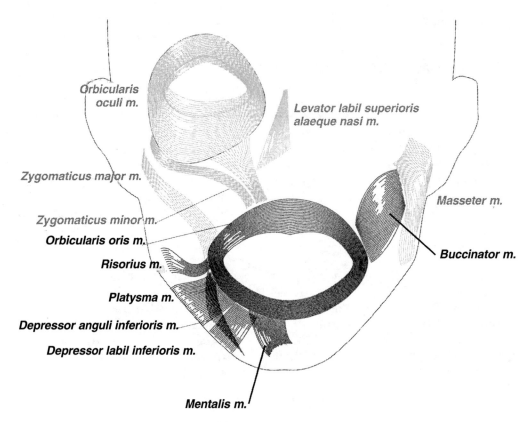

Figure 8–9. A diagram of the facial muscles showing those that play a role in the problem of spreading (darker portions). (Adapted from *The Speech Sciences* by R. D. Kent, 1997, p. 179. San Diego CA: Singular Publishing Group. Copyright 1997 by Singular Publishing Group. Adapted and reprinted with permission.)

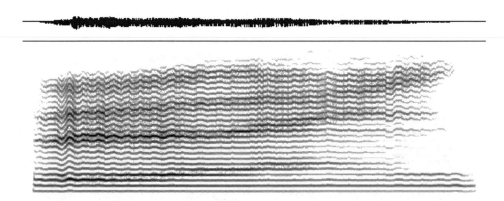

Figure 8–10. Spectrogram of singer's tone gradually evolving from a normal production to a spread production. ⊙

ment to a spread configuration. Notice that as the muscle tension builds, the vibrato ceases. This is likely the result of the tightening of vocal musculature. The shift in the F-pattern causes timbre that is heard by the listener as a blatant, harsh sound. Spectrographic evidence such as this may help the students change their articulative configuration to achieve a more acceptable tone.

Breathiness

Breathiness is another common vowel problem found in the production of the untrained singer. In Figure 8–11, notice the quality of the vibrato. As the singer allows

the tone to become more breathy, the F-pattern looses its structure and finally disappears into wispiness just before the vocal folds lose the ability to maintain phonation. Assuming there are no physical anomalies on the vocal folds, the culprit here is probably an improperly maintained glottal focus (the degree of aperture of the glottis during phonation).

Tight Glottal Aperture ("Pressed Voice")

The opposite of breathiness, which was brought on by a too-relaxed glottal aperture, is the tight glottis, or **pressed voice**. In Figure 8–12, one can clearly see the

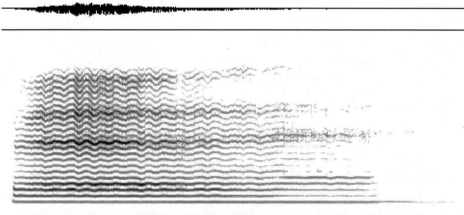

Figure 8–11. Singer's tone shifting from a normal production to a breathy production.

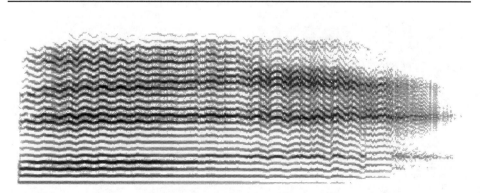

Figure 8–12. Singer's tone proceeding from a normal production to an overtightening of the glottal aperture (pressed voice).

shift in the F-pattern as the glottis gradually overfocuses toward the center line, an act that causes all the energy to focus in one area of the harmonic spectrums.

Tongue Massing ("Bass-itis")

This is a problem that develops in most singers' techniques sometime during the course of their study. It generally occurs when a singer attempts to produce a more resonant tone. In an effort to increase posterior oral resonance by simultaneously raising the velum and dropping the larynx, singers often unwittingly pull the tongue back along the longitudinal plane (sometimes accompanied by a simultaneous inward puckering of the lips called lip covering; see next section). When this lack of muscular independence occurs, the tongue will mass in a vertical mound in the back of the oral cavity. This action effectively cancels the benefits achieved by raising the velum and can artificially depress the larynx as the hyoid bone is forced downward. Figure 8–13 reveals the acoustical effect of this move of the tongue as it progresses from an acceptable tone on the left to one in full "bass-itis" on the right. (This tone quality is

called bass-itis since basses seem to be most prone to its use.)

This can be a particularly difficult technical fault to correct because the singer's internal sense of the sound is very rewarding; to the singer, it feels *huge*. The singer imagines it as a large and beautiful tone. Of course, as the spectrogram shows, it is a tone that looses all of its top luster and carrying power. Simultaneous use of ARTF and VRTF is a viable way of attacking this pervasive problem.

Lip Covering

Lip covering is the use of the upper lip, lower lip, or both to attenuate the upper *harmonics* of a vocal sound (making the sound less "bright"). Such covering may be voluntary or involuntary. There are three variations of this condition:

- **Lip drop**—the upper lip is drawn lower than the bottom edge of the upper front teeth, partially obstructing the opening of the mouth.
- **Lip rise**—the lower lip is drawn above the top edge of the lower teeth, partially obstructing the opening of the mouth.
- **Bilabial covering**—both lips are drawn in an inward "pucker," a state that

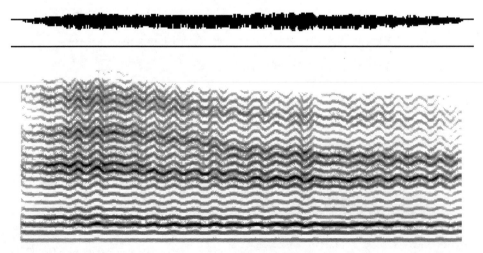

Figure 8–13. Normal tongue position on the vowel progressing toward posterior tongue-massing ("bass-itis"). 🔘

causes severe attenuation (most often a consequence of "bass-itis").

These actions can effectively attenuate the upper frequencies of the sound leaving the oral cavity (especially the bilabial covering).

Lip Drop

When the edge of the upper lip is allowed to drop lower than the bottom edge of the upper front teeth, an unwanted attenuation of the higher frequency components of the sound often occurs. When lip drop is encountered, instructing the singer to execute a slight elevation of the upper lip can produce amazing advances in the upper-harmonic activity that can be observed on the spectrograph (Figure 8–14) and heard by the ear. In this example, a benchmark /i/ is sung, progressing to lip drop, and returning to benchmark. Note the shifts in the waveform at the top of the screen, as well as in the spectrogram.

As mentioned earlier, lip drop can also occur during tongue massing (bass-itis). It occurs because of a lack of muscle independence between the velar and labial areas that occurs when a singer attempts to raise the velum. As was the case with feedback correction of "bass-itis," the use ARTF in conjunction with the VRTF of a mirror or spectrograph can be useful in altering this unfortunate habit.

Lip Rise

Lip rise is less common than lip drop. In this condition, the lower lip is raised to a sufficient height to cause an attenuation of the higher frequencies of the vocal signal. The remedial strategy is the same as that for lip drop.

Bilabial Covering

Bilabial covering is more obvious when seen in a mirror. In its extremes, the subject appears to be imitating a person with no teeth. This problem responds well to the use of simple visual feedback utilizing a mirror for identification of the symptom. Adding spectrographic RTF to show the potential improvement in higher frequency areas, possibly including closed-loop ARTF, can accelerate the correction considerably.

Excessive Lip Rounding

Somes vowels, especially /o/ and /u/, involve some degree of lip-rounding in their production. If one accepts the premise that the lips, when placed in front of the outgoing vocal signal, can attenuate higher frequency sounds, then one must ask how much of that rounding is truly necessary for the intelligible production of a given vowel.

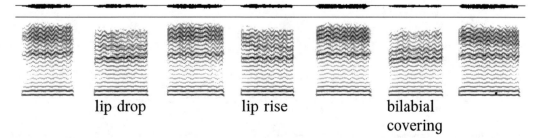

lip drop   lip rise   bilabial
                                    covering

Figure 8–14. Effect of lip drop on the vowel /i/. From left to right, the benchmark /i/, with lip drop, returning to the benchmark, with lip rise, returning to the benchmark, with bilabial covering, and finally back to benchmark. Note the shifts in the spectrogram, as well as the waveform at the top of the screen. 🔘

The answer, based on spectrographic readings (as well as the aural evidence in the room), is far less than most people think. This may be another example of the overlay of speech habits on song.

Consider the phrase, "when the moon comes over the mountain," /ᵘɛn ðʌ mun kʌmz ovə ðʌ mʌᵘntən/ (Figure 8–15). Many singers will produce both the /u/ and the /o/ with considerable lip rounding as is shown on the first image. The second image shows the same passage sung with a more open production on those vowels (not the increase in amplitude on the waveform at the top of the screen).

The spectrograph in Figure 8–16 singles out those same vowels for a clearer view. The first image in each pair is the result of the singer employing less lip rounding and concentrating on maintaining vowel identity with resonance space inside the oral cavity. The second of each pair shows the result of allowing a greater degree of lip rounding. An attenuation of the upper frequencies results in each case.

Consider these two vowels, as represented in the first of each pair, sung within the context of the singing line. Both look and sound like more natural partners instead of the sudden constrictive sound one often encounters.

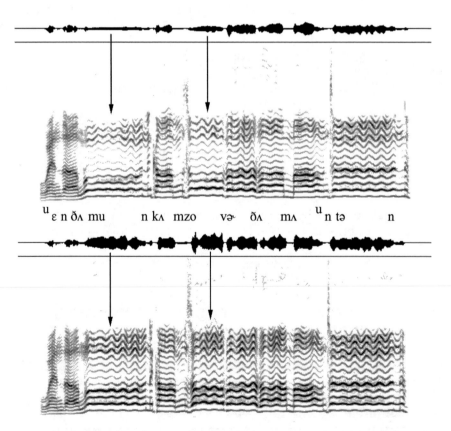

ᵘɛ n ðʌ mu   n kʌ mzo   və ðʌ mʌ ᵘn tə   n

Figure 8–15. The phrase "when the moon comes over the mountain" sung first with closed /u/ and /o/ (top image), and then with a more open production (bottom image). The /u/ and /o/ vowels are marked with the arrows. Notice the significant increase in the strength of the waveform in the bottom (more open) image. 🔘

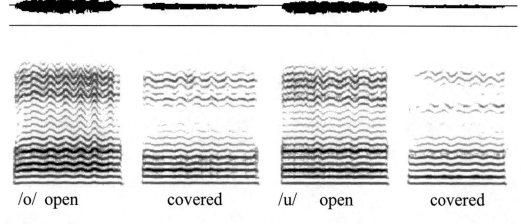

/o/ open   covered   /u/   open   covered

Figure 8–16. Benchmark "open" /o/, followed by excessive lip rounding covering the vowel (left two images); then an "open" /u/, followed by excessive lip rounding covering the vowel (right two images). Note the differences in intensity shown in the waveforms at the top of the image. **CD**

Onset

Onset is the initiation of a sung vowel sound after silence without a preceding consonant to help (or hinder) the set of the instrument. A more common term, used by innumerable voice practitioners, has been "attack." But words that have pejorative meanings, such as "tense," "hit," and "attack," are probably best used when trying to describe unwanted technical practices. To use these words to describe desirable technical attributes may lead to confusion. (Unfortunately, the literal meaning of onset is "acute attack," but most dictionaries list a second definition as "beginning" or "acute beginning." Perhaps the common usage of the word favors this second meaning, making it less objectionable than the word attack.)

The presentation of the spectrographic image makes it ideal for the diagnosis and remediation of problems involving difficulty with onset.

Articulators-Set/Abdominally Initiated (ASAI)

In Figure 8–17, the left-hand image shows an onset in which all articulators were set prior to the initiation of abdominally initiated subglottal pressure and resulting phonation (**ASAI**). The acoustic signal shows a full harmonic/F-pattern development virtually at the instant of initiation. This vertical "wall" of harmonic activity is the visual hallmark of a well-initiated onset. Note that the vibrato is also present from the first evidence of sound, most likely indicating that the laryngeal and pharyngeal musculature was not tensed for the onset.

Support

It is useful to pause here briefly and discuss the word support, another of the words commonly used by voice practitioners that can yield a plethora of opposing definitions. When the word support is used in this book, it means subglottal pressure created and maintained by the muscles of the abdominal wall. As the abdominal musculature contracts, it displaces the abdominal viscera upward, which then exerts pressure under the diaphragm. Control of the delivery of this pressure for use in the vocal instrument is accomplished by the simultaneous contraction of the diaphragm operating as an antagonistic muscle (opposing or downward pressure).

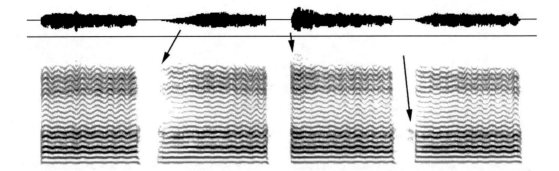

Figure 8–17. Four types of vowel onset on the vowel /o/. From left to right: articulators-set/abdominally initiated, bloomed, glottal attack, aspirate. 🆑

When many practitioners wish to invoke the idea of support they utilize the word diaphragm, as in, "use your diaphragm when going for that note." Unfortunately, the diaphragm cannot produce the needed increase in subglottal pressure because when it contracts, it flexes downward and away from the direction of needed force. This motion is used primarily for the act of inhalation. Urging the singer to contract the diaphragm (except when speaking of it as an antagonistic muscle) can lead to a counterproductive situation, possibly producing a locking of both the intercostals of the rib cage and the abdominals (in our studio/lab at Drew University we call this "hour-glassing").

When properly executed, the use of the co-contracting abdominal versus diaphragmatic musculature can supply pressure to the air stream. Its use permits relative freedom from the temptation to employ the internal intercostal muscles surrounding the rib cage, as well as counterproductive musculature in the larynx and pharynx farther up in the instrument.

Training ASAI

A classic vocal exercise used by teachers to achieve this type of onset has been a series of abdominally initiated staccato onsets. If the articulators remain set, the sound on each staccato utterance will be virtually fully formed from the beginning to the end of its brief existence (Figure 8–18). The spectrograph is an invaluable tool in the teaching of the proper execution of this exercise because the singer can clearly see when the desired coordination is missing and, using the feedback, quickly correct the problem.

Blooming

This problematic onset is characterized by the initiation of airflow in the glottis be-

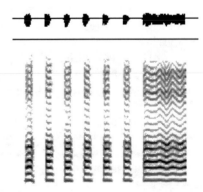

Figure 8–18. Series of staccati ASAI onsets showing the full development of the harmonic components of the sound from the beginning to the end of each staccato tone. 🆑

fore the articulators are completely set to form the desired vowel. The visual marker on the spectrographic image for this type of onset is the slow accumulation of the upper acoustical components of the vowel as seen in Figure 8–19. When properly performed, the harmonic structure of the vowel should be totally complete within a few milliseconds (ms) of the initiation of vocal-fold vibration. In this example, it took 384 ms until the full acoustical structure of the vowel was set, and another 408 ms until the onset of the vibrato. It took a full .79 seconds for the desired sound to appear after the beginning of the onset for a vowel that only lasted 1.73 seconds. In other words, it took 46% of the duration of the vowel before it had its full singing resonance.

Blooming can be caused by:

- lack of coordination between the completion of the articulative set and the initiation of the airflow at the glottis,
- insufficient support (another way of saying insufficient subglottal pressure), which is corrected after the vowel is initiated, and
- a combination of the above.

Blooming can also occur in word-interior vowels, a problem that was discussed earlier in this chapter.

Singers who have not yet developed the habit of ASAI onsets, and who bloom ini-tial vowels, generally try to "correct" the problem with one of the last two ill-advised onsets shown to the right in Figure 8–17.

Glottal-Stop Onset

In Figure 8–20, all of the articulators have been properly configured prior to phona-tion with one exception. The singer has locked the vocal folds together, built up subglottal pressure, and then released the pressure as a strong plosive. The spectro-graphic marker for this type of onset is the dark vertical area seen in the first mil-liseconds of phonation. This dark band is representative of chaotic vocal fold vibra-tion that continues until the larynx can settle into the desired vibrational mode. Notice also that the vibrato, in both the rate and extent parameters, is not stable because of the shock of the plosive onset. More will be said about vibrato, glottal stops, and strokes in Chapter 11.

Aspirate Onset

Figure 8–21 shows an aspirate onset. In this example, with the exception of the glottis, all articulators are properly set prior to the initiation of phonation. The glottal aperture is a little too wide, which instead of inducing phonation produces an aspirate /h/. This image begins with

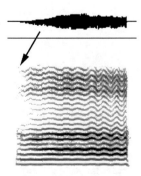

Figure 8–19. Bloomed onset.

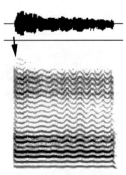

Figure 8–20. Glottal-stop onset. CD

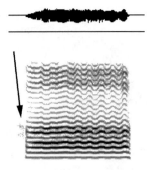

Figure 8–21. Aspirate onset. 💿

the noise pattern of the aspirate /h/ that lasts for 36 ms. During this period, the glottis is narrowed so phonation can begin. After initiation of phonation, it takes another 204 ms before the frequency (F_0) is stable, and another 696 ms until the system is stable enough for the vibrato to appear. A full 53% of the duration of the vowel was spent in developing the singer's acoustical goal. In some vocal pedagogies, this onset technique is taught as standard. In others, it is used as a way station in the process of correcting glottal-stop onset problems.

Voice practitioners can readily recognize the telltale signatures of these four onset types and utilize the spectrographic imagery to guide the singer toward a more desirable vocal production.

Exit

Most vowel **exit** problems are the reverse of the onset types. The spectrograph can present evidence of various modes of exit as well (Figure 8–22).

Articulator/Support-Maintained Exit (ASME)

In the image on the far left, the virtually simultaneous cessation of harmonics (the "vertical wall") indicates that the singer maintained proper articulation and support for the vowel until after phonation had ceased. Had there been any premature lessening of support or shift of the articulators, the next image to the right in Figure 8–22 would result.

Resonance Collapse

This image shows the gradual disintegration of the tone from the top harmonics downward and exemplifies the meaning of our term, *resonance collapse* (RC). It may be the most common of the exit problems heard in the voice studio.

As was also the case in the bloomed onset, the absence or degraded quality of the vibrato might be viewed as an early

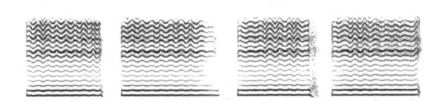

Figure 8–22. Four types of vowel exit on the vowel /i/. From left to right: articulator/support-maintained release, resonance collapse, aspirate release, and glottal grabbing. 💿

warning of a possible increase in laryngeal tension that often occurs as the support and articulators leave their proper set before the cessation of phonation.

There are two principal causes of resonance collapse:

- The articulators shift prematurely before the vocal folds have stopped phonation.

  Usually, this articulative shift is a movement away from song and toward speech norms. These unwanted anatomical shifts may include:

  movement of the velum

  movement of the tongue toward a more central vowel configuration

  raising of the mandible

  raising of the larynx

- Premature release of support, which may cause a drop in air pressure needed for the maintenance of the vowel. As the subglottal pressure drops, the singer may unconsciously attempt to correct for the loss by changing the set of the articulators.
- A combination of the above.

Toggling between two spectrographic images of proper and improper performance can greatly accelerate the student's progress in correcting this coordinative deficiency.

Aspirate Exits

Figure 8–23 shows the result of a shift in the aperture of the glottis as it widens from proper phonating position *before* the application of subglottal pressure has ceased. In this scenario, the spectrographic imagery generally shows two markers in sequence as the vocal folds move away from the centerline:

- The vibrato is compromised as the vocal set weakens when the widening of the glottis begins.

- When the vocal folds can no longer maintain phonation, there is evidence of a rushing-air noise at the end of the display as the remaining subglottal pressure is released as an aspirate /h/.

Glottal-Grab

Figure 8–24 shows a singer's attempt to correct an exit problem by bringing the vocal folds to the centerline and sealing off the flow of air, thereby choking off the sound. Notice the disturbance of the vibrato as laryngeal muscles begin to narrow the glottis, followed by a telltale vertical line of noise as the vocal-fold valve is abruptly shut to terminate phonation.

The examples in both Figures 8–23 and 8–24 show non-ASAI onsets. One can easily spot the slow development of the upper

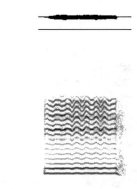

Figure 8–23. Aspirate exit. 🆑

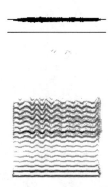

Figure 8–24. "Glottal grab" exit. 🆑

harmonics accompanied by a vibrato that does not settle right away. Had the laryngeal or pharyngeal musculature been improperly deployed prior to the onset, the vibrato probably would have been present from the beginning. (Figure 8–22 shows all four types of exit; compare the onsets shown in the two left-hand examples with the two on the right.)

DIPHTHONGS

In speech, a diphthong is the succession of two monophthongs (single vowel phonemes) that involve a *gradual* shift in F-pattern from one vowel to the other.

Kent and Read (1992) define a diphthong as:

dynamic sounds in which the articulatory shape (and hence formant pattern) slowly changes during the sound's production. . . . most phonetic descriptions specify the starting (or *onglide*) and final (or *offglide*) positions of the diphthong. Some phoneticians use the term *nucleus* to refer to the onglide portion. The symbols in the International Phonetic Alphabet reflect this description. For example, the diphthong in the word *I* (or *eye*) is represented by a digraph /ɑɪ/, where the first symbol /ɑ/ represents the onglide and the second symbol /ɪ/ represents the offglide. (pp. 102–103)

In Figure 8–25, both the spectrograms and extracted F_1–F_2 patterns for the spoken words *bye*, *boy*, and *bough*, show that the F-patterns for the vowels listed in the IPA digraphs never stabilize but are constantly shifting and evolving during the execution of the diphthong.

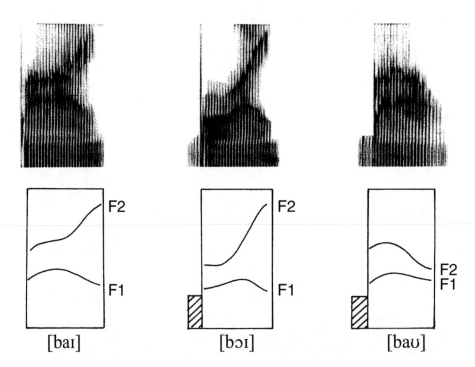

Figure 8–25. Spectrograms of spoken diphthongs and extracted F_1-F_2 patterns for the words bye, boy, and bough. (From *The Acoustic Analysis of Speech* by R. D. Kent and C. R. Read, 1992, p. 102. San Diego, CA: Singular Publishing Group. Copyright 1992 by Singular Publishing Group. Reprinted with permission.)

Monophthong Duration in Diphthongs

Peterson and Lehiste (1961) studied the duration of diphthongs in speech and found that shorter diphthongs, /oᵘ/ and /eᴵ/, tend to change slowly and with an even rate of change from one monophthong to the other. The longer diphthongs that they listed, /aᴵ/, /aᵘ/, and /ɔᴵ/, tended to have a longer first vowel than second, along with a longer transition and a shorter offglide at the end.

The Singer's Diphthong Is Not a Speaker's Diphthong

In singing, when the musical notation forces the diphthong to be performed at the speed of speech, diphthongs are performed very close to speech norms. Once the musical notation requires a diphthong to be performed for a longer duration than those of speech (the vast majority of instances), several critically important dif-

ferences between the speech and singing production can be identified.

- In the performance of a sustained diphthong, the differential in monophthong durations (as noted by Peterson and Lehiste, 1961) tends to disappear. All diphthongs tend to become two monophthongs, one executed with longer duration than the other.
- Since these diphthongs are performed over a longer period of time than those found in speech, the well-trained singer has the luxury of singing purer vowels than those found in speech diphthongs.
- The continually evolving F-patterns of speech diphthongs tend to disappear, and the monophthong of greater duration tends to become a stable vowel (see Figure 8–26).

Changes Needed in the Way We Regard Sung Diphthongs

Considering these differences, the author proposes two changes in how voice prac-

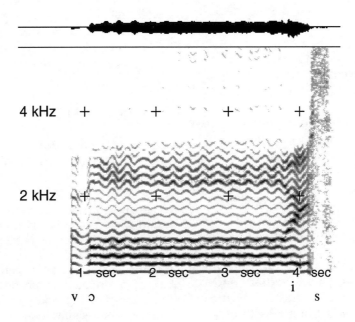

Figure 8–26. Spectrogram of the sung word "voice" lasting c. 4 seconds. Ⓒⅅ

titioners regard sung diphthongs. Because sung diphthongs tend to have a stable F-pattern on the vowel of longer duration, the use of the usual speech terminology (which suggests an unstable F-pattern) could create confusion. Instead of the terms onglide and offglide, consider the use of the terms, *primary and secondary vowels*.

If a singer needs to sustain the word "voice" across a four-second-long note, for example, the monophthong /ɔ/ will be sung for the majority of that time; this monophthong would be called the **primary vowel**. The brief appearance of the other monophthong, because of the shortness of its duration, would be called the **secondary vowel** (see Figure 8–26).

A Special IPA Diphthong Notation for Singers

In speech-based IPA tables, diphthongs are usually written as a digraph showing two equal vowels: (i.e., the word, "say" might be written as /sei/). Speech notation uses the symbol /ː/ to indicate an elongation of the phoneme preceding it and thus can be used to denote the differential in duration between a diphthong's two monophthongs. Using this notation the word "say" would be notated as /seːi/. (Note that the colon is now an acceptable subsititue in IPA for the older length mark, /ː/.)

Because most sung diphthongs have such a marked distinction between primary and a secondary vowel durations, it is useful to differentiate between them by super-scripting the secondary vowel (Kent and Read [1992] use this convention in their IPA appendix but not in the body of the text). That same word now becomes /seⁱ/. Written in this way, singers may more easily understand the pure-vowel distinction between the primary and secondary vowels, as well as obtain a clear idea of the differential in length between the two monophthongs.

Definition in Production of the Secondary Vowel

Most singers naturally achieve the correct apportioning of the length of the monophthongs in a sung diphthong. Still, many singers experience diphthong problems occurring in the quality of and clear differentiation between the primary and secondary vowels. Because the secondary vowel is usually sung at a speed similar to that found in the singer's speech, the singer may inadvertently employ his or her speech template in its execution. This may lead to a secondary vowel that does not match the primary in resonance (providing the primary vowel is properly sung). This often means that the secondary may be difficult for a listener to perceive.

Use of /i/ Instead of /ɪ/ as the Secondary Vowel of /ɔⁱ/

The author has used the vowel /i/ to denote the sung secondary vowel and not the /ɪ/ preferred by the speech community. While a singer may not totally achieve the classic F-pattern for an /i/ during the brief time it is sung, the singer's F-pattern is often closer to that of the /i/ than it is to /ɪ/. For pedagogical reasons, it may be beneficial to have the singer aim for the brighter /i/ for the sake of clarity.

Coarticulation of Diphthong Vowels

The reader will recall the concept of coarticulation which Kent and Read (1992) defined as:

The phenomenon in speech in which the attributes of successive speech units overlap in articulatory or acoustic patterns. That is, one feature of a speech unit may be anticipated during production of an earlier unit in the string (anticipatory or forward coarticulation) or retained during production of the unit that comes later (retentive or backward coarticulation). (p. 228)

Another problem, a frequent occurrence with speakers of American English, is the "homogenization" of the two monophthongs. This form of coarticulation, common in singers, occurs during the production of diphthongs where, although the singer may exhibit proper differentiation in monophthong lengths, the production of both the primary and secondary vowels is allowed to drift toward more central vowels. When this happens, a sort of homogenization occurs in which both vowels become less distinct, and listeners may have trouble understanding the word containing the diphthong (Figure 8–27). An example of such homogenization could occur in the sung production of the word "voice;" it may be sung as /vʌːˈs/ instead of the desired, /vɔːⁱs/.

The feedback strategy for this problem is to diagnose the problem, deciding if it is:

- vowel confusion (substituting a vowel for the one that is required) or
- vowel placement (where the vowel is basically correct, but the production is too far forward or backward).

After a diagnosis has been established, use either the power spectrum or the spectrogram to help solve the problem. When utilizing either technique, use the software's movable cursor to indicate a better target F-pattern for the vowel in question. By trying to match that target, the student can learn the feel and sound of the correct production and learn to sing primary and secondary monophthongs that will then

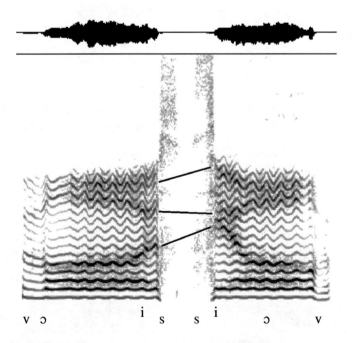

Figure 8–27. The word "voice" sung with insufficient care given to the identity of the primary and secondary vowels (left). Compare the arrival points of the formants on this image with the same points in the right image, a reversed image of the word properly sung. 🆑

match the vowel line surrounding the diphthongs.

Avoiding "Long" Vowel English Diphthongs in Other Languages

Many of the long vowels in the English language are actually pronounced as diphthongs. Thus, the long "y" of the word "my" becomes /aⁱ/, and the long "a" of the word "May" becomes /eⁱ/. In Italian, German, and French, such diphthongization of long vowels is undesirable because such additional monophthongs are not idiomatic to those languages. The following examples will suffice:

- Italian—"vero" should be /vero/, not /veⁱro/.
- German—"Tot" should be /tot/, not /toᵘt/.
- French—"parlé" should be /parle/, not /parleⁱ/.

To illustrate this tendency, see Figure 8–28, a pair of spectrograms of the French word parlé. The one on the left is the word sung properly with the final vowel being sung without an English diphthong. The one on the right is incorrect; one can observe the F-pattern shift to an /i/, thus creating an unwanted diphthong. This is evidence of a strong battle between the singing and speech templates that must be hard-fought in the case of most native English speakers.

The use of spectrographic VRTF is particularly helpful in dealing with this problem because diphthongs appear unmistakably as sudden, swift sweeps of the F-pattern. After the singer learns to spot these telltale shifts, vowel production without unwanted diphthongs can follow very quickly. Remember, after students have begun to master this improved production, they must be weaned away from the computer screen to enable them to translate that gain into the feel and sound of the proper phonemes.

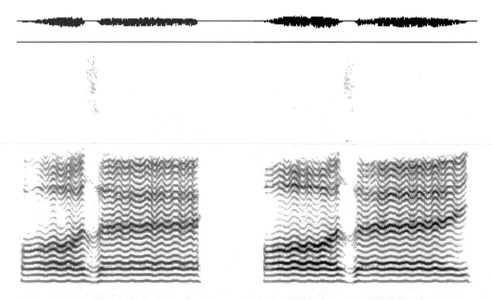

Figure 8-28. Spectrograms of the French word poser. The image on the left represents the proper execution without an ending with an English diphthong. The one on the right is incorrect since the F-pattern shifts to an /i/ on the final vowel. 🆑

SCHWAS

Stressed and Unstressed Vowels in Speech

Many languages, especially German and English, feature considerable stressing and unstressing of word syllables. Two centrally produced vowels, /ʌ/ and /ə/ (along with /ɪ/) are the principal agents of the unstressing, (a central vowel is one that is produced at the center of the oral cavity on both the longitudinal and vertical axes of the tongue). Phoneticists make a distinction between the stressed **schwa** /ʌ/, and the **unstressed schwa** /ə/.

Is the Stressed/Unstressed Nomenclature Needed in Singing?

The case for rethinking some of the phonetic nomenclature when it is applied to singing has already been made. The differentiation between the two types of schwa, stressed and unstressed, may be unnecessary in the voice studio when one considers singing practice.

The stressed schwa of speech is at the core of such words as "cut," "other," "said," "does," "country," and that favorite of the operatic plot, "blood." In English, /ʌ/ occurs in both the initial and middle positions in words (but does not normally appear as an unstressed ending syllable). This sound can be sung with considerable resonance and most singers readily accept /ʌ/ as a vowel that can be classed with all the other sustainable vowels.

On the other hand, it is common for singers to encounter considerable difficulty in mastering the schwa /ə/. Unlike the other vowels analyzed in the lab, there are only minute spectrographic differences between its spoken and sung production. Many beginning students do not even realize that the sound exists in their own speech, even though they speak countless schwas everyday. Even if they are aware of its existence, it is so transitory in speech that singers have great problems producing the sound on command, let alone sustaining it to meet the demands placed on them by composers' musical notation.

Pedagogically, because the schwa /ə/ can be such a problem for the singer (not only in English, but for French and German as well), the author proposes that the /ʌ/ be simply called a **central vowel**, dropping the "stressed schwa" terminology.

That would leave the word *schwa* (without the adjective unstressed) available to act as a unique marker for /ə/. In this way, when voice practitioners use the word schwa in the singing studio they would refer only to the /ə/.

The Nature of the Sung Schwa

The /ə/ sound is a also a central vowel that is required in the production of three of the principal singing languages, English, German, and French. It is related to the central vowel /ʌ/ but is produced with less tongue-root tension.

The schwa /ə/ is the most used vowel monophthong in English. Edwards (1997) reports that it accounts for 20.12% of the vowel frequency in the language. The second-place vowel is /ɪ/, with only 14.44% (in German, the schwa usage percentages are comparable, with French running a distant third). In English, a total of 43 possible spellings have been listed as requiring this sound (Dewey, 1971). It has been called "the dumping ground for all of the variations caused by unstressing" by Kantner and West (1960).

Given the importance of this phoneme in sung language, one would expect that great care would be expended on the sound in the voice studio. Sadly, that is often not the case in the studios of English-speaking teachers and coaches.

The Sung Schwa in an Interior or Final Unaccented Syllable

The schwa is used in English as the phoneme of choice for many unaccented interior and final syllables, as in "frequency" (/frikwənsi/) or "neutral" (/nⁱutrəl/). Poorly performed schwas are the cause of much unfortunate diction among singers who have never properly learned the sound and its uses. Part of the difficulty stems from the fact that in speech, as an unaccented syllable, it shares very little of the total production time in a word. Say the word "neutral" (/nⁱutrəl/) and hear how briefly the schwa sounds. In some dictionaries, the word is listed as, /nⁱutr'l/ in order to account for this brevity of execution.

In song, these unaccented syllables (because they must follow rhythmic indications provided by the composer) may have to be sung for a far greater length of time than in speech. Even more troublesome, they may be placed on a strong musical accent, making the rendering of the secondary nature of the syllable a very difficult task.

If singers are not trained in schwa production, they will invariably substitute a non-neutral vowel. In the word "neutral," one might hear /nⁱutræl/, /nⁱutɪl/, or /nⁱutrʌl/. Once the non-neutral vowel is substituted, the syllable tends to sound accented and of equal weight with the first accented syllable. A famous television advertisement that was on the air for years featured a singer intoning, "That's entertainment" as /ðæts ɛntɛˑteⁱnmɛnt/. Since the last syllable fell on the strong last note of the jingle, the resulting accent was considerable (and to those with "schwa-awareness," laughable).

Using the Spectrograph To Learn Schwa Production

Since there is not much acoustical or physiological difference between /ə/ and other nearby vowels, there is plenty of room for error in the execution of the schwa. The spectrograms of /ʌ/ and /ə/ are shown in Figure 8–29. The biggest difference is in the 1100–2000 Hz area where

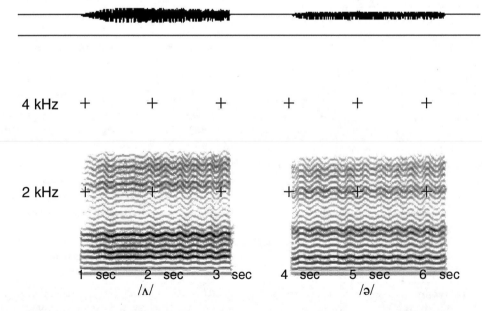

Figure 8–29. Spectrogram of /ʌ/ (left) and /ə/ (right) showing the minor F-pattern differences between the two. ⓒⒹ

the schwa presents less harmonic activity that the /ʌ/. Not as noticeable to the untrained eye is a slight drop in the area of F₃. The difference in F-pattern shows up more clearly in Figure 8–30, a power spectrum showing the difference in placement of F₃.

Spectrographic VRTF can successfully be used to help a student master the schwa by tracking the harmonic activity in the 1100 –2000 Hz area. If one begins with a benchmark /ʌ/ and then shifts to the schwa, the lessening of the middle-area harmonics in that area becomes obvious.

A Case Needing Special Attention: The English Initial Unaccented Syllable

The English words "deliver," "remark," and "believe" all begin with an unaccented syllable. IPA transliterations of these words in dictionaries show great inconsistency in how these syllables should be pro-

nounced. Some list the vowel /ɪ/ as the preferred sound in speech (/dɪlɪvɚ/, /rɪmark/, and /bɪliv/), and others call for the schwa (/dəlɪvɚ/, /rəmark/, and /bəliv/). When spoken, either solution is capable of producing the words with the stress falling on the second syllable.

When these words are sung for longer durations than is normal for speech, however, the use of the /ɪ/ can result in a vowel strong enough to impart equal stress to both syllables. Even worse, singers often substitute the brighter /i/ so the words become transformed into /dilɪvɚ/, /rimark/, and /biliv/ (examples of "schwa atrocities").

A possible solution is the production of a **colored schwa** that can be notated as /əᵢ/. This use of the subscripted IPA symbol indicates the production of the schwa with just a hint of /i/. With a little hard work, students can (and must) master this sound; it is a critical phoneme needed in their English diction if this wonderful language is to sound natural to the audience. One of the most effective ways to lead a

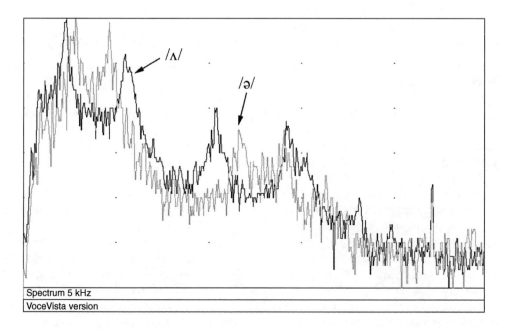

Spectrum 5 kHz

VoceVista version

Figure 8–30. Power spectrum of /ʌ/ (light line) and /ə/ (dark line).

student away from the substitution of pure vowels for schwas is to point out that word meaning can be radically changed as a result. The phrase "O Lord, deliver me," for example, might be understood as a request, not for divine deliverance, but for a fatal operation, /dilɪvɜ-/.

German

The same final-syllable accentuation problem is encountered in German as well. The uninformed singer, substituting a non-neutral vowel in a final weak syllable, experiences an unwanted accent. Thus, the word *Geben* (which should be pronounced /gebən/) becomes either /geb ɛ n/ or /geb ɪ n/.

In addition, the language utilizes the schwa in weak prefixes such as *ge,* as in Gesetz (/gəzɛts/) and *be,* as in Befehl (/bəfel/). Proper execution of the schwa is a requirement for the production of idiomatic, sung German.

French

The schwa gives non-French singers trouble when encountering words like *le* and *premier*, which should be pronounced /lə/ and /pʁəmⁱe/.

Training the Schwa

Many singers may have already mastered this sound for their singing of French but never realize that the same phoneme is useful in their German and English diction as well. Quite often, all that it takes to convince a singer to utilize the schwa in those two languages is for the teacher or coach to point out the problem and remind the singer that they already possess the neuromusculature model for the sound. A combination of raising the singer's awareness concerning the way English and German can be rendered instantly non-idiomatic by avoiding the use of the schwa, coupled with borrowing the sound from the French, is often enough to cure the problem rapidly.

NON-ENGLISH VOWELS ON THE SPECTROGRAM

It is not within the scope of this book to go into detail concerning the non-English vowel sounds of the principal sung European languages. Vowels, such as the German umlauts and the French nasals, can profit from both spectrographic and power spectrum analysis with the same gains in understanding seen thus far with the common English vowels.

IMPROVING VOWEL RESONANCE

At various points in this chapter, differences between singing and speaking resonances have been discussed. Voice practitioners should consider some of the principal ways in which singers can optimize their resonance configurations.

Resonance Creation Checklist

☐ **Low Mandible**

Techniques for achieving this include a:

• Relaxed TMJ area
• Properly opened mouth

Remember that the entire jaw must be considered as a platform; the jaw is not just a lever that is hinged at the TMJ and capable of being opened at the front. When the posterior mandible is dropped by the relaxation of the area around the TMJ, the entire jaw drops. This action can produce a considerable increase in oral and pharyngeal resonance space.

☐ Proper Tongue Configuration

The section on CV/VC joins discussed the concept of consonant shadow (coarticulation), a problem created when the singer does not fully complete a CV or VC join utilizing pure phonemes. As a result, areas of the tongue may still be configured for the consonant that preceded the vowel, or the production of the next vowel may be "looking forward" to the anatomical requirements of the succeeding consonant. In either case, the tongue cannot form the desired configuration for the given vowel. Attention given to the eradication of consonant shadow in singing can gain great advances in vowel production at the phoneme-to-phoneme level.

☐ Proper Set of the Lips

One must be constantly conscious of the degree to which the lips are being used to shape vowel sounds. Several potential problems are:

• Lip covering (lip drop, lip rise, and bilabial covering)
• Excessive lip rounding.

All of these habits can cause an unwanted reduction in both the harmonic richness and the acoustical impact of the vowel in the hall. These are often problems of subtlety, but they must receive the attention they deserve if the sung line is to live in fullness.

☐ Raised Velum

In addition to the resonance space created by the lowering of the mandible, singers must take care to create additional vertical space in the oral cavity by raising the velum. There is insufficient space to fully discuss this complex issue in this text. Suffice it to say that the amount of velar elevation can vary according to vocal register, especially as one nears and enters the top voice. A reasonable concentration on velar elevation usually pays great divdends in the total resonance strategy of a singer.

☐ Pharynx Open and Relaxed

There has been considerable controversy about this concept in the vocal pedagogy and voice science literature. Disparities between authors often center on the use of terminology and not the basic need for and open an relaxed pharynx.

The Potential Role of Pharyngeal Musculature in the Creation of Supraglottal Pressure

It is critical, when considering the areas of the pharynx (especially the laryngo- and oropharynx) to pay careful attention to how the singer creates the air pressure needed to produce certain consonants.

Observations in the lab seem to suggest that in speech, pharyngeal constriction may supply most or, at least, some of the pressurization of the air column needed for the creation of consonants. If this observation is proven correct during future experimentation, it might indicate that the narrowing of the singer's pharynx during such pressurization reduces much-needed resonance space.

Furthermore, upon the release of the consonant, the pharyngeal space many tend to narrow even further, as the vectors of the constricting musculature are all pointing inward. This can have dire consequences for the overall resonance of the instrument, but particularly in the area of the singer's formant (see Chapter 4).

If singers are prone this problem, a practice that may stem from speech habits, great advances in vocal stability and tone may be achieved by training the abdominal area to supply *all* the necessary pressure for the production of consonants. When abdominal support is invoked in the production of these sounds, the pharyngeal muscles can then be largely isolated from the process, resulting in an increase in the pharyngeal diameter. This in turn can produce an increase in the resonance of the consonants themselves as well as their neighboring vowels. See the next two chapters for more information on CR (consonant resonance).

☐ Low Laryngeal Elevation

Many authorities on the singing voice have joined the chorus advocating a low larynx during singing. Chapter 5 cited an interesting passage by Johan Sundberg, who gives a clear rationale for the employment of a lowered larynx (Sundberg, 1987).

There seem to be two principal factors in the determination of laryngeal elevation during singing:

- the degree of tension in the musculature surrounding the larynx and
- the elevation of the posterior part of the mandible. As mentioned before, this may be principally governed by the degree of tension in the TMJ. If this area is relaxed, the posterior mandible can be dropped. With that action, both the hyoid bone and larynx drop as well. The resulting lengthening of the pharyngeal tube increases the amount of space available and potentially has significant resonance consequences for the singer.

Exploring Vowel-Like Consonants

As indicated at the beginning of this chapter, as well as in Chapter 5, the method by which a fine singer performs many of the consonants blurs the distinction between vowels and consonants. This is especially so in singers who favor a mandible-down production. Such a method produces many consonants that offer considerably less resistance to the air stream and can thus be classified as vowels (such as /r/ /j/ and /w/). Others are produced with so much vowel-like resonance behind the point of restriction that they can be truly called semivowels (such as the nasals /m/, /n/, the liquid /l/, and voiced fricatives such as /v/ /z/). The common denominator between these sounds is that they are sustainable on pitch. These reclassifications will be discussed at length in the next chapter.

SUMMARY: ALL OF THE RESONANCE AREAS WORKING IN CONCERT

It is only by paying proper attention to all of these areas of potential resonance that a singer can truly optimize the resonance potential of the vowel (and consonant!) phonemes. Such optimization of resonance is, perhaps, *the* major marker that distinguishes well-produced song from speech.

CHAPTER

9

WHEN CONSONANTS BECOME "VOWELS"

When listening to great singers, one usually focuses first on their vowel production because that is where the beauty and richness of the human voice is most easily heard. At some point, discerning listeners may also become aware of many consonants that are performed with such resonance that they might be considered coequal with the singer's vowels.

How many voice practitioners pay as much attention to the production of consonants as they do to vowels? How do the great singers produce consonants in such a way that their diction is rich, meaningful, and vibrantly alive? How do those same singers manage to have a consonant production that never seems to disturb the beauty and consistency of the vowel line? In the production of consonants, how many singers are able to dispel the unconscious assumptions that stem from their speech templates?

Either by intuition or excellent training, great singers seem to endow their *entire* vocal production—not just their vowels—with a resonance that is far removed from everyday speech norms. In doing so, they have solved a conundrum that pervades the technique of singers of more modest attainment: while it is relatively easy to persuade a singer to produce richer sung vowels, getting the consonants to balance those vowels is often a promethean struggle. It is as if the speech template has "decided" that a properly produced sung consonant feels ludicrously overdone and the singer's consonant production reverts to inadequate speech norms.

THE CONSONANT STRUGGLE

The reason for this ages-old struggle is very simple; most of the vowels that a singer executes are sustained for periods of time that far exceed the vowel-time allotments of speech. There is time, therefore, for the singer to concentrate on improving the resonance of the vowels. But one look at the spectrogram in Figure 9–1 shows that, whether spoken or sung, consonants in singing are performed at the same speed as those in speech. So it is only natural that the speech template maintains control over these phonemes while we are singing. The result is that most singers sing with considerably improved

vowels interspersed with ineffective (speech) consonants: an unacceptable compromise in the quest for fine singing.

OBJECTIVELY EVALUATING CONSONANTS

This chapter proposes that voice practitioners reexamine consonant production by utilizing spectrographic evidence. By utilizing this evidence, one can consider

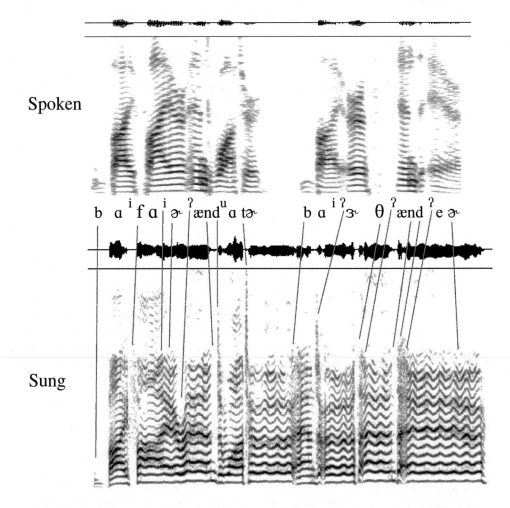

Figure 9–1. A spectrogram of a phrase that is spoken and then sung. (Phrase from *Listen Beloved* by Garyth Nair, poetry by Virginia Nadel. Copyright 1998 by Garyth Nair.) 💿 (Play waves files for Figure 5-1.)

these phonemes as they are actually *performed* when well sung and not simply derive the consonant classifications and techniques of production from the way languages are printed or spoken.

In this text, consonants are divided into:

- pitch (those that involve phonation at the vocal folds), and
- nonpitch (those that have no phonational element).

To the nonsinger, such a division may seem trifling, but to a singer, this shift of paradigm—the consideration of pitch consonants as a separate *vowel-like class*—yields both psychological and physiological benefits.

Rethinking the Production of Pitch Consonants

Based on spectrographic analysis, approximately half of the sounds traditionally classified as consonants can be thought of as vowel-like. These are the *pitch*, or *voiced*, consonants, phonemes that can be sustained on pitch as long as the singer can maintain subglottal pressure. Thus, singers are capable of singing a melody on /v/, /z/, /ð/, /m/, or /r/ just as successfully as if they had vocalized one of the traditional vowels, /a/, /ʌ/, /ɪ/, or /u/.

The pitch consonants include eight continuants and three nasals (phonemes in which the oral cavity is completely shut, forcing the moving air stream through the nasal cavity). Additionally, four more consonants not included with the pitch consonants possess a strong pitch component (/b/, /d/, /g/, and /dʒ/).

When the speech template is the model for a pitch consonant, the resulting spectrograms reveal minimal resonance when compared to the same sounds in a fine

singer's technique. The spectrograms of the pitch consonants of ranking singers show a different story; their spectrograms show considerably more resonance and amplitude in the pitch.

While all consonants require some degree of full or partial constriction in the vocal instrument, such constriction occurs mostly in the anterior half of the oral cavity. When performed by a fine singer, the resonance cavity—the posterior space from the point of constriction back and down to the glottis—can be kept functioning at or close to the level that normally characterizes sung vowel production. Put another way, this text proposes that the resonance areas posterior to the point of constriction (both oral *and* pharyngeal space) be regarded as vowel-like.

New Term: Consonant Resonance (CR)

When speaking of vowel-like resonance and the shift in how voice practitioners regard consonants as sung phonemes, it will be beneficial to have a new term specific to the concept: **consonant resonance (CR)**. The use of this term serves to remind the singer to continually regard the potential gain in resonance for the production of all consonants. CR then becomes a primary issue in the training of vocal technique in which the subject of resonance for all non-vowels is a coequal concept with the resonance of the vowels.

Why Is CR So Critical?

Consonant resonance is a critical consideration for two principal reasons:

- CV balance and diction: singers are trained to produce vowels that are far richer than those in speech. By extension, their consonant production should have greater amplitude and richness to enable intelligible, *balanced* diction.

- Easier CV/VC joins: once the singer has obtained an optimal level of resonance for all consonants, less shifting of articulative structures from phoneme-to-phoneme is required. This results in a more consistently beautiful sound that is also easier to execute. Furthermore, the openness of the instrument seems to foster a lack of strain in the vocal production with a concurrent chance for better vocal health.

Assuming an open vocal production, we can maintain that openness by paying attention to optimal CR. When done well, there is no loss in the clarity of diction.

A Useful Term for the Voice Studio: Consovowel

Some consonants are so vowel-like that they are almost indistinguishable from vowels when viewed in spectrographic images. Henderson (1940) coined the term **consovowel** for /m/, /n/, /ŋ/, /l/, and /r/ (p. 356). Why not apply this wonderful term to all pitch consonants? When used in the voice studio, the term suggests the potential richness that can be achieved when these phonemes are treated as semivowels.

These consonants should be of critical concern to the singer for, when approached in this manner, the entire vocal line, vowels and pitch consonants, can become substantially richer and more easily understood. The IPA table in Appendix A groups all pitch consonants together (instead of intermingling pitch and nonpitch consonants, as is the case with most IPA tables in books about singing). This chapter will discuss the pitch consonants; the nonpitch consonants will be covered in Chapter 10.

TOWARD TREATING PITCH CONSONANTS AS VOWEL-LIKE

Attempts to assimilate a more vowel-like strategy for pitch consonants can gain validation from the spectrographic evidence. In Figure 9–2, the left image is an

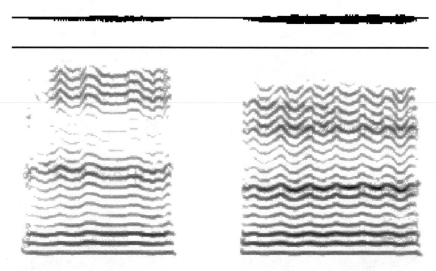

Figure 9–2. Spectrograms of /l/. The left image is sung in a typical speech configuration; the right image is a sung production in which the mandible is down, the tip and the blade of the tongue are vertical. 🆑

/l/ performed with resonance typical of speech; the image on the right is an analysis of the same employing vowel-like resonance behind the point of constriction. This is accomplished by utilizing the tip and blade of the tongue in a more acute vertical configuration than is usually the norm in speech. With the consonantal constriction occurring only near the tip of the tongue, the remainder of the oral cavity can be left more open, resulting in increased resonance space, both in the oral cavity and the pharynx. One can easily see that the sound on the right not only has a far more intense harmonic and formant structure, but it also has far more amplitude due to the increase in the resonance space. The amplitude increase is seen in the waveform at the top of the graphic. This same type of resonance gain is possible on all pitch consonants.

Principal Problems Encountered in Pitch Consonants

There are several factors to consider when training pitch consonants to achieve optimal CR.

Spreading: Perhaps the Principal Anti-CR Problem

If a singer's oral cavity is "spread" during the production of consonants, these sounds will lack the richness and amplitude needed to coexist with richly sung vowels. Figure 9–3 shows photographs of a singer in spread and normal oral configurations. Any or all of the following conditions may be present during the act of spreading:

- Mandible up
- High larynx
- Tongue spread horizontally
- Mouth spread horizontally
- Velum tensed and low

Consult the Jaw Elevation Table at the end of this chapter for information on how to improve CR.

Scooping: Potential for Pitch Undershoot in the Production of Pitch Consonants

In addition to addressing the need for optimal resonance in producing pitch consonants, voice practitioners must also be aware that all of the pitch consonants are highly susceptible to a technical fault called scooping. This problem occurs when a singer begins the pitch consonant slightly below the pitch of the following vowel and gradually corrects the pitch as the vowel is reached. Scooping may occur for one of two reasons: a problem in pitch coordination or as a result of the singer's attempts to bring more emotion to the vocal product. Minor scooping may involve the interval of a minor or major second. Extreme scooping will involve the singer beginning on a pitch in his or her

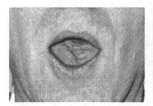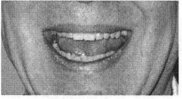

Figure 9–3. Photograph of a normal, vertical mouth configuration (left) and a production in which the lips are drawn tight and spread by means of the facial muscles (right).

normal speech range and then scooping up to the required pitch.

Theory About Flatting of Pitch Consonants (Lack of Pitch Coordination)

Singers often arrive at the studio lacking either the ability to hear the differences of pitch involved in the production of scoops, or lacking the ability to do the rapid laryngeal micro adjustments to avoid them.

Here the author presents a theory that this tendency to scoop is a result of an acoustical phenomenon that is familiar to organ tuners. The open resonator of an organ pipe is a fairly good acoustical corollary for the resonance of the vocal tract. If organ tuners use their hands to directly tune a pipe, the mass of their hand near either the pipe's open resonator or the mouth of the pipe will cause it to flat. When the hand is removed, the "in-tune" pipe goes sharp and is still out of tune. (For this reason, tuners use metal rods to manipulate the top of the pipes in the tuning process because the metal rod has far less interfering mass than a hand. Also, the heat of the tuner's hand tends to heat the walls of the pipe, causing the walls to expand and further alter the pitch.)

When scooping in the voice occurs, this same phenomenon may be at work. A full or partial restriction in the anterior oral cavity, similar to the interaction between the tuner's hand and the organ pipe, is necessary for the production of pitch consonants. The mass of the tongue constricting the front of the resonance cavity probably causes the pitch to flatten slightly.

During the production of pitch consonants, this same phenomenon may be at work. The necessary full or partial constriction of the anterior oral cavity may have the same flatting effect as that seen in the effect of the organ tuner's hand in a pipe's resonance aura.

If this flatting occurs as the occlusion is created, the brain might have to attempt to correct for this minor pitch variation by slightly sharping the pitch with a minute adjustment of the cricothyroid. As the singer relaxes the constriction while proceeding to the next vowel, the cricothyroid muscle would then have to be relaxed slightly to flat the pitch so it would sound constant as the constriction eases.

If the singer does not perform this minute correction, the pitch variation can become quite pronounced. If severe enough, the listener hears it as a *slide* or *scoop*, a riding up to the pitch that isn't notated in the music.

The 10 Hz drop-in pitch shown in the spectrogram in Figure 9–4 occurs as the singer performs the lip closure from the open vowel /a/ to the nasal pitch consonant /m/. If this VC join is reversed (as a CV), the same phenomenon would appear as a rise in pitch because the consonant closure is opened toward the vowel (again, 10 Hz or more).

Emoting

Certain vocal styles encourage scooping as a way to impart emotion to the text (*verissmo* opera, for example). Singers who correctly employ scooping within such a style are often tempted to employ this device in other styles. In those styles in which scooping is not a recommended performance practice, the use of scooping can rapidly become an annoying affectation. Such scooping may become habitual: for the singer, it often *feels* very emotional and thus, very personally satisfying. When scooping becomes habitual, the singer is no longer consciously aware of the extent to which the device is being employed. When encountered at this level, scooping can be a particularly difficult problem to solve.

Fortunately, scoops can be plainly seen on the spectrograph. In Figure 9–5, the first spectrographic image is that of a scooped /m/. Observe the harmonics rising as they track the rising fundamental. Also notice that the misalignment of pitch continues on into the primary vowel of the diphthong /a/. The second image shows how this join should look when the cricothyroid is adjusted to permit a more stable F_0 during the VC join. Even though the singer takes great care to maintain the pitch throughout the join, there is a ± 200 ms

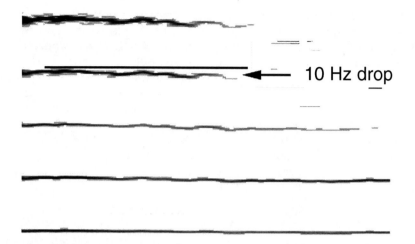

Figure 9–4. Spectrogram of a singer purposely avoiding correction of the flatting tendency of a nasal. As the singer moves from the /a/ to the nasal /m/, one can clearly see a drop of approximately 10 Hz as the closure to the /m/ is finalized. ⊕

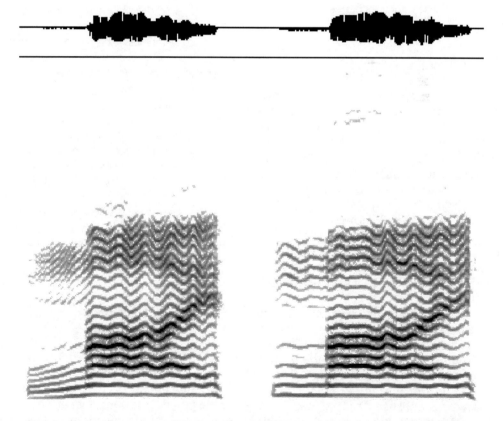

Figure 9–5. Spectrogram of the word "my" showing a full-blown scoop of the nasal /m/ (left) and a properly performed /m/ (right) in which the F_0 of /m/ is stable and on pitch. ⊕

period of adjustment at the very beginning of the /m/. This might suggest that the brain is comparing the actual pitch against the target and is performing the necessary adjustments during that period. As the singer's lips part to reveal the vowel, there is another brief moment of instability that may indicate the presence of a second crosscheck of the pitch. When performed correctly, the listener cannot perceive these brief adjustments, so there is no discernible shift in pitch between CV/VC joins.

Techniques for Correcting Pitch Consonant Problems

The strategies for dealing with pitch consonant problems utilize the feedback techniques of toggling, skill accelerando, structured building, and benchmarking. If review of these concepts is needed, consult Chapter 6.

Spreading

By using VRTF spectrography, singers can quickly learn to ascertain the difference between spread and normal vocal production. Such observations can be augmented by the addition of a biofeedback technique in which the singer places two fingers of one hand at the corners of the mouth while singing. When spreading occurs, the lateral movement of the mouth can be felt and its effects can be simultaneously seen on the spectrogram. The VRTF provided by a mirror can be another successful feedback strategy in our arsenal.

No matter which combination of RTF is utilized, the toggle exercise is of great value in the drive to habitualize the desired sound. By toggling between the spread and unspread sounds while sustaining phonation, the feel of the proper production is quickly accomplished.

The structured building technique is also very useful for the problem of spreading. For example, if the student is spreading the /l/ in the phrase "My Lord, what a

morning," the /l/ should be dropped so the phrase would be sung as /maⁱ ɔrd ᵘʌt ʌ morniŋ/. Once the proper resonance on the vowels /aⁱ ɔ/ is achieved, the offending /l/ can be replaced in the line and the student is instructed to not relinquish the vowel feeling during the production of the /l/.

Benchmarking the CV join /lɔ/ as /ɔlɔ/ in slow, carefully sung exercises is also very effective in the prevention of conso-vowel spreading.

Scooping

The first step to solving a scooping problem is to train the singer's ear to recognize it. While spectrographic VRTF will only indicate the scoop after it has happened, the singer should be trained to stop and re-sing the phrase while correcting the problem.

Once the student is conscious of both the sound and feel of the scoop, one can employ two exercises with great effect. When coupled with the use of the spectrogram, both the benchmark and skill accelerando techniques can rapidly attack the problem of scooping.

Quite often voice practitioners discover that certain pitch consonants are more likely to be scooped than others. If this is the case, begin each lesson with a warm up consisting of exercises in which the offending consovowel is inserted in slowly sung VCV sequences (the benchmark exercise). This enables the singer to retrain the pitch coordination of these consonants, and habits built in this way will quickly find their way into his or her technique.

THREE VOWEL–LIKE SUBCLASSES OF PITCH CONSONANTS

Three subclasses can be established within the pitch consonant class by cataloging the acoustical ramifications of the *degree* of oral constriction used during the sung vocal production of these phonemes. The pitch-consonant classes are as follows.

Class I: The Most Vowel-Like Consonants

A consonant may be considered as Class I if:

- It is sustainable on pitch.
- It presents vowel-like resonance in its F-pattern as seen in spectrograms or power spectra. To be included, the phoneme must possess a clearly definable F_2 and possibly even F_3 or higher.
- The upper harmonic development shows little or no difference between consonants and vowels.

When well sung, the following consonants can be considered as Class I:

- LIQUIDS

  r when it is sounded as /ɚ/ or /ɝ/

  the hard American r /ɹ/.

- GLIDES

  /j/ and /w/

Consider the question posed in the caption of Figure 9–6. When seen on the spectrogram, all four phonemes (from left to right, /i/, /ɪ/, /ɚ/, and /e/), appear to have roughly the same intensity of harmonic development and look like vowels. But, the third image from the left is the consonant /ɚ/ as it might be sung to end the word "father." Most voice practitioners would think of /ɚ/ more as a consonant than as a vowel.

Class II: Less Vowel-Like

These phonemes involve greater constriction in the oral cavity that those in Class I. One may also encounter either a noise component or, when the noise component is absent, sounds that are sufficiently restrictive as to present F-patterns that are only partially developed in comparison to vowels.

A consonant may be considered as Class II if:

- It is sustainable on pitch.
- Its F-pattern shows a vowel-like resonance on spectrograms or power spectra and contains at least F_1 and possibly F_2.
- Formants or harmonic structure above F_1 and/or F_2 may be very weak or non-existent.
- Noise (aperiodic vibration) may be a component.

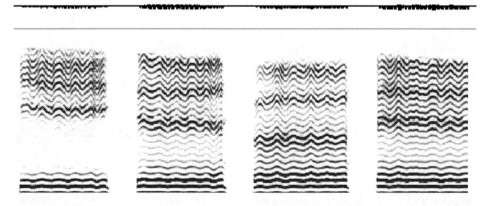

Figure 9–6. Series of vowels including an r form (/ɚ/). Can you determine which one is the consonant? CD

Figure 9–7 shows how properly sung consonants of this class can match surrounding vowels. The lack of upper formant and harmonic structure is due to the attenuation of higher frequencies caused by the higher degree of oral constriction needed for the production of these phonemes.

Under these guidelines, the following consonants can be considered Class II consonants when sung:

- LIQUIDS

  /l/

  foreign forms of r, /ř/, /ɾ/, and /ʁ/—the use of these IPA symbols for /r/ will be explained later in this chapter

- GLIDES

  /ʍ/

The phoneme /ʍ/ is difficult to classify because it begins with a fricative and ends with a vowel. It is placed here because the production of the frontal fricative restricts the /u/ phoneme more than the normal production of that vowel. (See the special section in Chapter 10 for a complete discussion.)

Class III: Least Vowel-Like Consonants

A consonant may be considered as Class III if:

- It is sustainable on pitch.
- Its F-pattern shows a vowel-like resonance on spectrograms or power spectra and contains at least F_1 and, rarely, F_2.
- Formants or harmonic structure above F_1 and/or F_2 may be very weak or non-existent.
- Noise (aperiodic vibration) may be a component.

Although these phonemes (shown in Figure 9–8) do not carry as much upper-harmonic development as Class II consonants, they can also blend well with vowels.

Utilizing these parameters, the class III consonants include:

- NASALS

  /m/, /n/, /ŋ/, and /ɲ/

- VOICED FRICATIVES

  /ð/, /v/, /z/, and /ʒ/

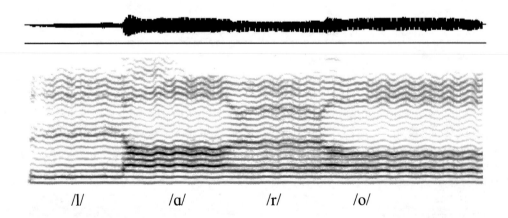

Figure 9–7. /l/ /a/ /r/ /o/: Notice how easily these phonemes blend with the vowels when sung with the singer's resonance. 🆑

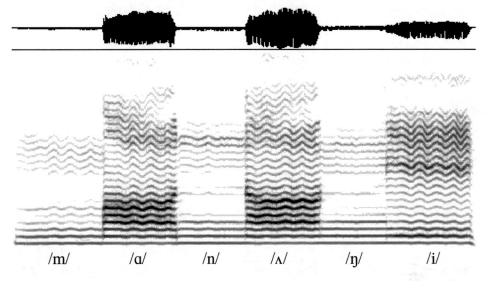

Figure 9–8. /m/ /a/ /n/ /ʌ/ /ŋ/ /i/: These phonemes also blend well with the vowels but do not carry as much upper-harmonic development as Class II consonants.

The Nonpitch Consonants

After all the pitch consonants are separated according to these classes, the remaining consonants are those that cannot be sustained on pitch and that include a strong noise component. These include:

- Stop consonants

    Prevoiced stops: /b/, /d/, and /g/

    Pure stops: /p/, /t/, and /k/

- Unvoiced fricative consonants

    /θ/, /f/, /s/, /ʃ/, forms of /ç/, /x/, and /h/

- Affricate consonant

    /tʃ/

- Prevoiced affricate consonant

    /dʒ/

The prevoiced portion of the consonants /b/, /d/, /g/, and /dʒ/ does contain a brief initial moment of pitch, but because that pitch cannot be sustained for more than a brief moment, the prevoiced fricatives must be classified as nonpitch consonants.

As we will discover in Chapter 10, the nonpitch consonants require as much care and concern in the production of their resonance component as the pitch consonants.

Let us now explore each of the classes of pitch consonant in more detail.

CLASS I PITCH CONSONANTS

These consonants are the most vowel-like and, when well sung, are the least constrictive of the three subclasses of pitch consonants. Glides and liquids are both considered Class I consonants.

Class I Glides

In speech, glides are defined as momentary, muted vowel sounds that swiftly evolve into a primary vowel of longer duration. A good example is the word "yes" (written as /jɛs/ in IPA). Speech texts indicate that the glide /j/ in this word is a sound that begins with the vowel /ɪ/ and quickly evolves into the vowel /ɛ/.

Table 9-1. Glide "vowels."

Written	Traditional IPA	Singer's Vowel	Example
y	i	ⁱ or ᶦ	you [ⁱu]
w	w	ᵘ	win [ᵘɪn]

In singing, however, the spectrographic evidence suggests that a singer may treat glides somewhat differently. A singer's need for longer phonation time on individual phonemes often necessitates a production in which glides become more like "reversed diphthongs," or "diphthongs" that start with a more clearly defined secondary vowel and then rapidly shift to the primary. Throughout the execution of the glide, veteran singers seem to maintain a full vowel-like resonance, making them richer and far easier to join with the primary vowels that follow.

In Figure 9–9, compare the ending diphthong in the word on the left ("my"), with the opening two phonemes of the word on the right ("yes"). One can clearly see that the /i/of the diphthong that ends the first word has the same F-pattern as the glide

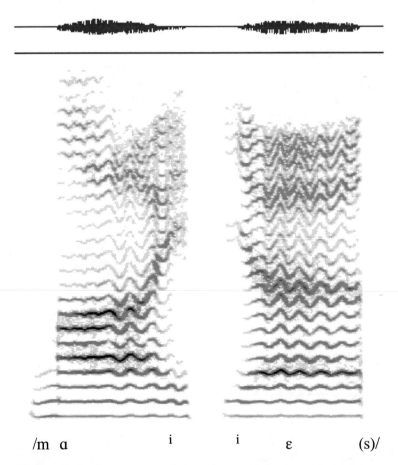

/m ɑ   ⁱ   ⁱ   ɛ   (s)/

Figure 9-9. Spectrogram of the sung words "my" and "yes" (left to right). 🄲🄳

at the beginning of the word, "yes" (/i/). Both utilize /i/ as a secondary vowel and both shift the F-pattern at approximately the same rate of speed.

In certain dramatic situations, singers may linger even longer on the initial sound of the glide to gain greater dramatic intensity. In an emphatic declaration of the word "yes," for example, a singer might perform the secondary vowel as a pure /i/ of such length (far longer than they would ever employ in speech) that the IPA would have to be rendered as /iɛs/ instead of /ⁱɛs/. (Note on the superscripting of /ⁱ/: As was the case for the secondary diphthongs in Chapter 8, the author advocates the superscripted IPA vowels to designate the secondary vowel when it serves as a glide.)

Based on the spectrographic evidence, voice practitioners can recognize that sung glides may be enhanced, according them an appropriate optimal vowel resonance. Approaching these consonants in this manner may be a sound pedagogical strategy. When sung in this way, glides have the potential to match the rich vowels that surround them. In the production of many singers:

- /j/ becomes /i/ or /ɪ/
- /w/ becomes /u/

The Glide /j/

A professional singer produced the spectrograms in Figure 9–10. Starting on the left, there are two benchmark vowels, /i/ and /ɪ/, the word "yes" is then spoken and sung. The characteristic F-pattern for /i/ can be clearly seen at the beginning of both the spoken and sung word (compare it with the F-pattern of the /ɪ/ vowel on the left). Chapter 5 discussed trained singers in terms of the development of separate speech and song templates. In the spoken example, the presence of a strong initial /i/ vowel (rather than the /ɪ/ that one would expect from descriptions in speech texts) may, in part, be due to the performer's singing habits encroaching on the speech template.

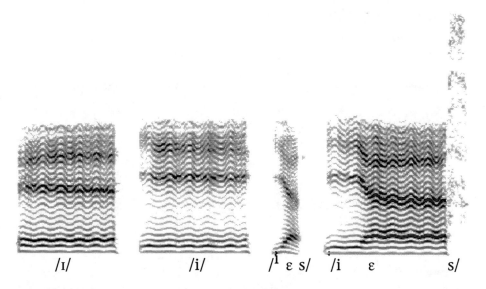

/ɪ/   /i/   /ⁱ ɛ s/   /i   ɛ   s/

Figure 9–10. Spectrograms of the vowels /ɪ/ (far left), /i/ (second from left), the spoken word "yes" (third from left), and the sung word "yes" (far right). 🔵

Spreading of the Glide /j/

Perhaps the most common problem encountered with the glide /j/ is **spreading** (see Chapter 8 for a full discussion of spreading). When spread, the singer may initiate the glide in a jaw-up, "horizontal" vocal production that is very difficult to convert into the succeeding primary vowel. When encountering the spreading of the onglide, several of the feedback strategies discussed in Chapter 6 many help effect the desired physiological shifts.

Vowel Undershoot and the Glide /j/

The opposite problem may occur when (in an attempt to produce this phoneme in the mandible-down, vertical configuration) the singer may not produce enough F-pattern differentiation between the opening vowel of the glide and the primary vowel. At that point, one might work to accomplish greater flexibility and independence of the tongue (helpful information may be found in the section on diphthong problems in Chapter 8).

The Glide /w/

As was the case with the glide /j/, many singers shift production of the /w/ toward a more open /u/. Many speech and singing sources talk about the need for lip protrusion during the production of /w/. Such a practice in the production of this phoneme may produce undesirable results in a singer's diction, both in terms of timbre and unwanted accentuation.

Unwanted Accentuation Problems With the Glide /w/

Figure 9–11 shows paired spectrographs of two words ("woe" on the left and "flower" on the right). In the first image of each pair, the lips are extended and the mandible is relatively high. This use of lip protrusion can cause a considerable rise of the jaw, which, when suddenly released for the next vowel, will probably produce an unintentional accent on the next syllable. This is especially so for a word-interior /w/, as in "flower." The second image of each pair shows the result of the /w/ treated as a more open singer's /u/, a production that involves a low mandible coupled with minimal lip protrusion. The result is a smooth, resonant transition from one phoneme to the other involving no concomitant loss of intelligibility for the listener. For more information on the use of the spectrogram in modifying the production of the /u/

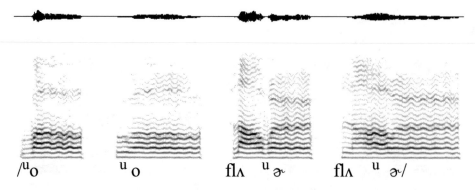

Figure 9–11. Two word pairs, "woe" (left) and "flower" (right). The first image in each pair features a production that is lip-protruded and mandible-up. The second image of each pair shows the results of the use of minimal lip protrusion with the mandible down. 🔘

vowel, see the section on *excessive lip rounding* in Chapter 8.

Class I Liquids: The Open English Central-Vowel /r/ Phonemes

In many texts, liquid r forms are already considered as either full members of the vowel class, or at least as semivowels. As a tenet of singing practice, many voice practitioners prefer to think of these phonemes as full vowels. They are included here among the consonants to make them easier to find when this text is used as a reference.

The /r/ in English

Controversy

Few points of contention receive more attention in the literature and practice of vocal pedagogy than the proper production of the English phoneme /r/. In English, /r/ can occur anywhere in a word in any of its forms. It is the fifth most common phoneme in the English language; only /t/, /ə/, /n/, and /ɪ/ rank ahead of it (Edwards, 1997). There are 11 different ways to spell the sound (consider "l" in *colonel*). Voice practitioners must pay

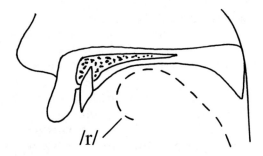

Figure 9–12. Schematic drawing of the articulator position for a spoken /r/. (From *The Speech Sciences* by R. D. Kent, 1997, p. 66. San Diego CA: Singular Publishing Group. Copyright 1997 by Singular Publishing Group. Adapted and reprinted with permission.)

great attention to the production of this phoneme in the voice studio.

Well-Formed /r/ Vowels in English

Goals for the /r/ in English might be stated as follows:

- The sound should coexist easily within the vowel line.
- The sound should not suggest a regional dialect, but be a universal phoneme that all listeners can easily recognize.

Two phonemes are ideally suited for the production of the English r, /ɚ/ and /ɝ/. When both of these phonemes are sung in a mandible-down position, they present

Table 9–2. Liquids as vowels.

Written	IPA	Example and Notes
r (schwa-based)	ɚ and ɝ	Preferred r usage in sung English
r	ɪ	Retroflex or Midwestern "hard" r as in the word, "hurt." In its extreme dialectal usage, the word might sound as /hɪt/. Should not be used in classical sung English.

spectrographic F-patterns that are virtually indistinguishable from those of vowels.

/ɚ/ (The Rhoticized Schwa or Schwar)

This vowel is produced by inducing a little r-color (tongue tension) while singing a schwa. This is known as a **rhoticized** schwa (also known as a **schwar** or unstressed vocalic r). Its IPA symbol /ɚ/ is, in fact, a schwa /ə/ written with the addition of the "wing" /˞/ to the character r (this sign is called the rhoticity sign in IPA nomenclature).

Refer again to Figure 9–6 in which readers were challenged to locate the "consonant" /ɚ/ amid the images of three vowels. There is little difference in the visual display of these four phonemes other than the expected differences in F-pattern. This is an excellent example of the need to rethink how voice practitioners classify consonants in song. If teachers and coaches train singers to think of this /ɚ/ phoneme as a vowel instead of a consonant, then it can achieve virtual parity with the surrounding vowels. VC/CV join problems will be greatly reduced, and the clarity of the singer's diction will improve.

This consonant is preferred for use on unaccented syllables in English. According to Edwards (1997, p. 266), it occurs most frequently in the spellings:

- er, as in lather—72%
- or, as in color—12%
- ar, as in burglar—8%
- The remaining 8% is spread among ir, our, re, ure, and yr

When properly produced, the tongue sits slightly above the neutral schwa position, creating some degree of contact between the edges of the tongue and the upper back teeth. The tip is usually at the lower front teeth. There can be great variation in the way the /r/ is produced, and many students require considerable coaching on its production. This is especially true for singers coming from dialec-

tal traditions in which the retroflex, or hard /ɹ/, is the speech norm. In those cases, work must focus on a gradual relaxation of the tongue from the tensed, retroflex position.

/ɝ/ (Stressed schwar)

For accented syllables in English, one can employ a phoneme that involves a slightly more tense tongue, the /ɝ/. It is called either the stressed schwar, the reversed hooked epsilon, or the stressed vocalic /r/. Edwards (1997, p. 260) lists the following as the most common spellings:

- er, as in herd—40%
- ur, as in urge—36%
- ir, as in firm—13%
- The remaining 11% involve alternative spellings such as ear, or, and our

When this phoneme is properly produced, the tongue is slightly more elevated above the neutral position than is the case in the production of the schwar. While many voice practitioners do not like the use of negative words such as "tense," the word is well used in this case. Compared with the schwar, the tongue position for this phoneme is slightly more tense and retroflexed, creating a more solid contact between the edges of the tongue and the upper molars. The tip of the tongue is usually just in back of the lower front teeth.

As with the schwar, there can be great variations in the production of this phoneme, and many students require considerable coaching in its production.

/ɹ/ (The Retroflex or "Hard" r)

The retroflex /ɹ/ can be considerably constrictive, yet still appear vowel-like on spectrograms. The potentially harsh timbre of this vowel can disturb the vowel line of well-sung English and is best avoided. Singers coming from dialect traditions in which the retroflex, or hard /ɹ/, is the speech norm can require considerable attention as, in its most extreme manifestations, their oral cavities can be so constricted that problems with CV and VC joins will almost always appear. The retroflex /ɹ/ should probably be used by trained singers only if the characterization of a role demands the dialectal use of the phoneme.

Substitution of /ɜ/
for /ɝ/ and /ə/ for /ɚ/

Some pedagogical traditions attempt to avoid the imagined problems of teaching /ɝ/ and /ɚ/ by substituting the un-rhoticized vowels /ɜ/ and /ə/. In these traditions the word "bird" lacks all r-coloration and sounds like /bɜd/ or, even worse, /bʌd/. While such usage does mitigate the retroflex /ɹ/ problem, it substitutes one nonidiomatic production for another, and, as such, should be avoided.

Use of Foreign Phonemes as an
Aid in Learning /ɚ/ and /ɝ/

Far too many English-speaking singers work to master the foreign languages of classical singing, while neglecting their native tongue. Thus, when sung by a native speaker, English may sound like the "foreign" tongue, a considerable irony. When a singer first begins intensive work on English following the mastery of

German, French, and Italian, there are two vowels, probably already mastered, that can be of considerable assistance in the search for the proper English r-vowels:

- O-umlaut in German (written as ö, IPA = /œ/)
- "œ" in French (written as œ, IPA =/œ/)

Other methods of producing the foreign r-sounds and their use in the singing of English will be dealt with in a special section under Class II pitch consonants.

CLASS II PITCH CONSONANTS

This class of pitch consonants is somewhat more constrictive than the consonants mentioned thus far. This greater constriction attenuates the upper spectral structure, but activity in the F_1/F_2 area is still strong. The same resonance strategy presented for the consonants in Class I also applies to those in Class II; optimization of resonance in the instrument from the point of constriction or occlusion throughout the remaining supraglottal spaces must be a primary goal.

Liquid /l/

Refer back to Figure 9–2; the /l/ at the left was sung in a speech configuration, while

Table 9–3. Class II liquids.

Written	Traditional IPA	Singer's Vowel Equivalent	Example or Note
l	l	l	line
ly	ʎ	gl (in Italian)	gli Combination of liquid + glide

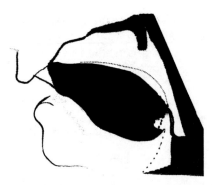

Figure 9–13. Sagittal view of a sung /l/. (Adapted from *The Science of Vocal Pedagogy* by D. R. Appleman, 1967, p. 342. Bloomington, IN: Indiana University Press. Copyright 1967 by Indiana University Press. Adapted and reprinted with permission.)

the one at the right was sung with mandible down and with the tip and blade of the tongue in a more vertical manner than the normal, gradually sloped tongue of speech production. Both /l/ forms have a defined harmonic structure and a clear F-pattern. The one on the right, however, is especially rich in tone and thus can virtually match the color and intensity of the vowels produced by this singer.

By adopting the strategy of using the tip and blade of the tongue in a more vertical position, combined with a lowered mandible, the oral resonance and pharyngeal resonance space can be increased to vowel-like levels.

Class II Foreign Forms of /r/

Few of the world's languages have an /r/ sound such as that found in English, a fact that becomes a two-edged linguistic sword. This phoneme creates difficulties for native speakers of other languages who must learn to replicate the sound in English. On the other hand, English speech habits concerning the production of /r/ can color attempts of native English speakers to produce the phoneme in any of its foreign variants.

IPA Symbols for the /r/ Phonemes

IPA uses the symbol /r/ for the rolled (or trilled) /r/. In this text, some reassignment of the symbology seems to be in order. The author recommends the /ˇ/ symbol (called a wedge) added to the /r/ so it appears as /řr/ (please note that this IPA symbol is generally used to indicate a rising tone, not the trilled /r/). One of the main tenets of this book involves the use of visual clues to invoke proper vocal performance. In that light, the symbols given in Table 9–4 seem more visually appropriate for a singer, as they may convey a visual "feel" of what is happening physiologically:

- The hard, retroflex /r/, when written as /ɹ/, has a "feel" of the tongue pulled back and hardened in the oral cavity.

Table 9–4. Foreign /r/ forms.

Written	IPA	Example and Notes
r (rolled)	ř	Should not be used in American English. Belongs in foreign class.
r (flipped)	ɾ	Should not be used in American English. Belongs in foreign class.
r (Parisian)	ʁ	Interaction of the uvula and pharynx. Oral cavity is set as a vowel.

- The rolled /ř/, with its added "wedge" symbol over the basic phoneme, seems to convey the energetic action of the tongue.
- The flipped /ɾ/ is a very quick tongue action. This symbol, an incomplete /r/, suits it well.
- The symbol for the Parisian /ʁ/ is appropriate as the phoneme is made in the back of the oral cavity (not in front, thus constituting a reversal well symbolized by the backward, upside-down /ʁ/).

The Italian Rolled /ř/

The rolled Italian /ř/ is so vowel-like that one is tempted to place it in the Class I column. But, unlike the rhoticized schwa, the rolled /ř/ combines phonation on pitch with a noise created by the constant strik-

ing of the tip of the tongue against alveolar ridge. This sound is possible when most of the outer edges of the tongue mass are sealed against the upper teeth. This seal results in a very narrow channel at the same location where /d/ is made.

It is possible that this narrow channel allows for the development of a strong Bernoulli effect at that point. When properly configured and performed (with a sufficient increase in subglottal pressure created by abdominal support), the tip of the tongue oscillates between the upward pull produced by the Bernoulli during which it strikes the alveolar ridge, and the return to its original position caused by its own myoelasticity and air pressure.

With the application of a sufficiently high-pressure air stream through the channel, this oscillation can be maintained for as long as the singer can sustain sufficient pressure. In Figure 9–14,

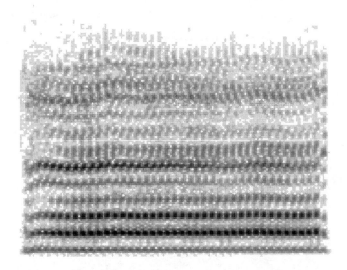

Figure 9–14. Spectrogram of the Italian rolled /ř/. Note the vertical striations in the signal created by the noise of the tongue striking the alveolar ridge. 🔵

one can see evidence of the periodic impact of the tongue hitting the alveolar ridge; the resulting noise appears as faint, vertical striations in the acoustical signal.

The Flipped /ɾ/

The so-called flipped /ɾ/ is executed like an Italian /r̃/ in which the tongue only contacts the alveolar ridge once or twice. In every other respect, its physiological production seems to be the same as that for the Italian rolled /r̃/. It is a sound that should be associated with certain British accents, especially on an interior /r/, such as the one in the word, "very."

If improperly performed, the /ɾ/ can sound like /d/, resulting in the word sounding as /vɛdi/ instead of /vɛɾi/). Most often, a slight increase in air pressure is all that is needed to turn /d/ into /ɾ/.

The Parisian "r" (ʁ)

Likewise, a Bernoulli may be a component of the /ʁ/. This r form, called the Parisian "r," is a few "flaps" of the velum produced in essentially the same way as the phoneme /x/ but with the added elements of phonation on pitch and an increase in pressure and rate of air flow.

To execute a Parisian /ʁ/, as seen in Figure 9–15, the singer must essentially execute an /x/ at the passage between the velum and the posterior mass of the tongue by moving the tongue into posterior oral cavity where its mass can create the constriction with the velum. As in the case of the Italian rolled /r̃/, if a sufficiently high-pressure air stream is passed through the constriction, the velum and mass of the tongue may be pulled together (by a Bernoulli effect) until contact is made. The myoelasticity of the velum and the pressure of the airflow then returns the structures to their normal position. Once this motion is induced, the singer can replicate the resulting oscillation a sufficient number of times resulting in the classic Parisian /ʁ/. The distinctive sonic signature of this phoneme sometimes may be enhanced by the presence of saliva in the area that can contribute noise and thus additional character to the radiated result.

Should These Foreign /r/ Forms Be Employed in Sung English?

The phonemes /r̃/ and /ɾ/ (excluding the /ʁ/ for obvious reasons) may have little or

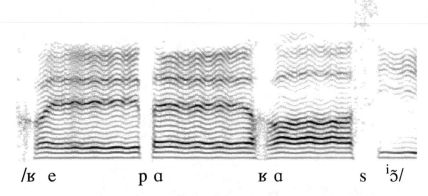

Figure 9–15. A spectrogram of the French word "préperation" (/pʁepaʁasiɔ̃/) showing the appearance of the Parisian /ʁ/. 🆗

no place in properly executed, modern sung English when judged by today's communal standards of diction.

To many listeners, singers who roll the "r" in sung English tend to sound stilted or stuffy. Some teachers and coaches may permit a few exceptions, such as lightly rolling the /ř/ in the word "rejoice" in Handel's aria, "Rejoice greatly" (from *The Messiah*), where such a technique might impart a more festive lilt to the word. The use of the rolled /ř/ on a word-interior /r/ ("arrange")—or even worse, in a word-ending /r/ ("gather")—may seem a bit old fashioned for today's standard English diction.

The flipped /ɾ/ falls prey to the same objection. Some singers have been taught its use as a means to avoid the "problem" of singing the proper phoneme (/ɚ/ or /ɝ/) when encountering an initial or internal /r/. This consonant probably should not be employed in the normal execution of sung English unless the singer is required, by the role being performed, to create a distinctive type of idiomatic British accent.

CLASS III PITCH CONSONANTS

The last set of consonants for reconceptualization involve those phonemes that still feature sustainable pitch but are produced with considerably more oral cavity constriction than either Class I or II. As a result, the spectrographic imagery shows minimal F-pattern development. When sung, however, the resonance required for the proper production of these consonants is no less critical than for those in the prior two classes.

These phonemes may also include an overlay of noise as part of their acoustical signature, a fact that may cause singers to balk at considering them vowel-like. But upon closer inspection, when one considers the spectrographic evidence, they are just as worthy of increased resonance as their Class I and II cousins.

Class III Nasal Consonants

The nasals are produced by simultaneously creating a full closure of the oral cavity at a location in the oral cavity and dropping the velum and uvula to allow the naso-pharyngeal port to open. With this revalving, the airflow and sound radiation are prevented from leaving the oral cavity through the mouth and must pass through the nose instead.

As one can observe in the spectrograms in Figure 9–16, there is significant attenuation of the higher frequency harmonics due to the damping effect of the nose during the production of /m/ /n/ and /ŋ/.

In studies that rank the relative acoustic power of all phonemes, the nasals rank near the bottom of the list; the only pitch consonants that rank lower in relative acoustic power are /ʒ/, /ð/, /z/, and /v/ (Edwards, 1997). With that in mind, particular attention must be paid to maximizing supraglottal resonance space during the singing production of these phonemes, a task for which spectrographic VRTF is particularly wellsuited.

The resonance of all nasals can be greatly enhanced by encouraging a low-mandible production. This technique requires some readjustment at the point of occlusion (see Figure 9–17), as most speech habits require that these sounds be produced with a relatively high mandible to permit an easy occlusion between the lips, or the tongue and the palate. These readjustment techniques will be discussed both in the text that follows and in the

Table 9–5. Class III nasals.

Written	IPA	Example and Notes
m	m	<u>M</u>oment
n	n	<u>N</u>i<u>n</u>ety
ng	ŋ	Beginni<u>ng</u>
n(y)	ɲ	O<u>n</u>ion—see notes below

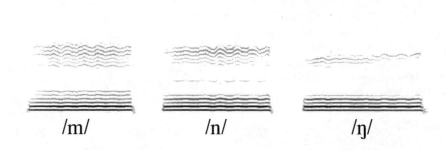

/m/   /n/   /ŋ/

Figure 9–16. Spectrograms of /m/, /n/, and /ŋ/ (left to right). 🔵

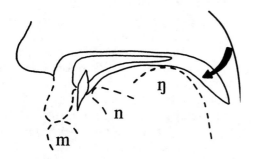

Figure 9–17. Points of oral cavity occlusion required for the production of nasals. Note the drop of the uvula that opens the velo-pharyngeal port to the nose. (From *The Speech Sciences*, by R. D. Kent, 1997, p. 64. San Diego, CA: Singular Publishing Group. Copyright 1997 by Singular Publishing Group. Adapted and reprinted with permission.)

Jaw Elevation Table given at the end of this chapter.

Nasal /m/

The nasal /m/ is the only nasal consonant in which the occlusion is created with the lips; for that reason, it is called a bilabial. At the end of the chapter, considerable attention will be paid to refocusing this phoneme in an attempt to increase its resonance space (see the preface to the Jaw Elevation Table).

The /m/ employs the same articulative configuration as the phoneme /b/. When several phonemes are articulated at the same point in the vocal instrument, they are deemed **homorganic**; thus the pitch consonant /m/, the pure stop /p/, and the prevoiced stop /b/ are said to be homorganic. This principal will become critical in the next chapter on nonpitch consonants. Gains in the quality of phonemes such as /p/ and /b/ can be engendered by encouraging the same type of improved resonance space enjoyed on the /m/ throughout this consonant class. These improvements can be heard as well as quantified on the spectrogram.

Nasal /ŋ/

The nasal pitch consonant /n/ is produced by using the tongue to occlude the oral cavity by establishing a seal at the alveolar ridge. This phoneme is homorganic with /t/ and /d/.

Proper attention paid to centering (instead of spreading) the tongue at the alveolar ridge during the production of the /n/ can yield considerable resonance gains (see the Jaw Elevation Table for more information on centering). By centering the tongue in the oral cavity, the mandible can drop, and increased resonance space can be enjoyed in the remainder of the oral cavity.

Nasal /ŋ/

The /ŋ/ is created with an occlusion of the oral cavity created by the tongue and the velum at the same site as the homorganic consonants, /k/ and /g/(as well as the German "ch" /ç/). As was the case with /n/, care should be taken to center the tongue at the velum during the production of this phoneme.

Many singers go through a stage where it is difficult for them to avoid releasing this consonant as a hard /g/ ("beginning" becomes /bɪgɪnɪŋg/). Most of the time, the same singer may be able to faultlessly execute the /ŋ/ when it is in a word-interior position (n English, consider the words "handkerchief" /hæŋkɜtʃif/and "think" /θiŋk/). Correct interior-/ŋ/ production can be employed as a benchmark while using VRTF to teach the student the proper production of a word-ending /ŋ/. Since the release of the /ŋ/ as a hard /g/ clearly shows up on the spectrogram, it can be most helpful in correcting this problem.

It must also be mentioned here that some American English dialects do pronounce word-final /ŋ/ as /ng/. Because of the pervasive influence of the speech habit in singers with such dialects, the solution to this word-ending /ŋ/ may be more difficult. The corrective technique remains the same; voice practitioners should use the word interior /ŋ/ as a benchmark and drill repeatedly.

Nasal /ɲ/

/ɲ/ is a special case; it begins with the nasal /n/ but is then modified into a glide (/ʲ/). Slowly say or sing the English word "onion" to feel and hear the dual action of this phoneme. A properly centered, initial /n/ should help the singer produce the proper glide vowel and then move on to the succeeding principal vowel, the schwa (/ə/).

Class III Voiced-Fricatives

All fricatives, whether pitch or nonpitch, have the commonality of the sound of turbulent air. There are two types of fricative:

- voiced—sound of turbulent air coupled with phonation on specific pitches
- unvoiced—featuring only the sound of turbulent air

The turbulence needed for fricative production in English is created by a delivery of a high-pressure air stream through a small restriction of the oral cavity located at one of four sites as noted in Table 9–6. In this table, the unvoiced fricatives are shown in the shaded column to establish their homorganic status with the voiced consonants.

As the air stream moves through the narrow constriction, it cannot maintain the integrity of its laminar flow as it leaves the oral cavity. Part of the airflow separates producing turbulence, the source of the high-frequency, aperiodic sounds (noise). When sound produced in this manner is combined with phonation, a lively and interesting mix of timbre is produced.

All admonitions about the centering of the vocal production to permit a lowered mandible apply to this class of consonants with equal validity.

Table 9–6.

Type	Site of Turbulence	IPA Symbol Unvoiced	IPA Symbol Voiced
Interdental	tip of tongue—upper and lower teeth	θ	ð
Labio-dental	lower lip—upper teeth	f	v
Lingua-alveolar	tongue tip-blade and alveolar ridge	s	z
Lingua-palatal	high, grooved tongue and the palate	ʃ	ʒ

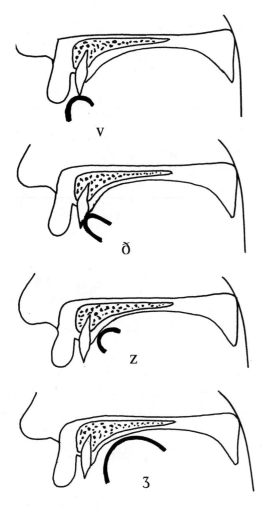

Figure 9-18. Points of oral cavity constriction required for the production of fricatives. (From *The Speech Sciences*, by R. D. Kent, 1997, p. 65. San Diego, CA: Singular Publishing Group. Copyright 1997 by Singular Publishing Group. Reprinted with permission.)

CHECKLIST FOR OPTIMAL RESONANCE IN PITCH CONSONANTS

The same checklist for resonance production that applied to vowels in the previous chapter is equally valid for all pitch consonants (details on technique can be found at the end of Chapter 8).

Resonance Creation Checklist

☐ Low mandible (for more information on technique, see the Target Jaw Elevation Table that concludes this chapter)

☐ Proper tongue configuration

☐ Raised velum

☐ Pharynx open and relaxed

☐ Larynx relaxed and low in the throat

TARGET JAW ELEVATION TABLE

In the attempt to achieve consonant resonance space and avoid consonant shadow (see Chapter 8), critical attention should be paid to the elevation of *both* the anterior and posterior parts of the mandible. Most problematic consonants that appear in the voice studio involve a high-mandible position. This may be due to the influence of the singer's speech habits. These consonants may create problems in adjoining vowel production (on both sides of the consonant), as well as poor resonance during the production of the consonants themselves.

The following table is a compilation of suggested mandible elevation goals that may aid in the singer's quest for well-sung consonants. Many singers who attempt each of the suggested targets find that the target elevation feels considerably lower than those to which they are accustomed. The principal reason that singers resist relearning the set of these phonemes is a common response, "It doesn't feel right." Most of the time, this is another way of saying, "It feels different from the configuration that I use in my speech." This will be especially true for those consonants that are performed above the speech pitch range of the subject.

To accomplish these low-mandible goals, the singer's tongue must be more active in the creation of the sounds. It must be capable of greater extension, and the coordination of the musculature must be more precise.

By utilizing both VRTF and ARTF, the possible benefits of such a resonance strategy become clear, and singers seem more willing to accommodate the suggested target elevations.

Elevation Targets Used in the Table

The symbols used for target jaw elevation are:

L = low—when in this position, the mandible approaches a level similar to that used in the production of a well-sung /ɑ/ vowel.

M = medium—in this position, the jaw is somewhat higher than in the low position but is still much lower than most speech production would suggest.

H = high—this position is necessary when there must be a partial or full occlusion between anterior articulators such as the tongue or lips. Note that this high position should *not* connote a closed jaw.

Pedagogical Strategies

There are two principal strategies for allowing a lower jaw position during the production of all consonants. The following symbols indicate their suggested use:

⊕ Centering

As indicated earlier, when common speech configurations are employed, the mandible is usually higher, and the focus of the sound in the oral cavity is wider (spread) than one would like for the production of fine singing sound.

When the centering symbol is used, it indicates that the jaw should drop and the configuration of the tongue should be brought more toward the mid-sagittal line of the oral cavity than is the norm in a typical singer's speech.

▲ Labial Focus

Three phonemes require the use of lip occlusion (m, p, and b). Care must be exercised to make sure that in an effort to occlude the lips, there is no concomitant spreading and overtightening of the musculature surrounding the mouth. When such spreading occurs muscles in the mouth region are tightened causing the jaw to rise. This tensing can also involve considerable concomitant tension under the chin and in the neck. Most pedagogical traditions consider such use of this musculature to be counterproductive to good singing.

A possible pedagogical strategy for correcting this problem is to train the student to relax the *risorius* muscles. Once this is accomplished the jaw should be relaxed permitting a gentle closing of the lips using the *obicularis oris* muscle. It helps if the student thinks of the labial occlusion as occurring in the central triangle of the mouth (Figure 9–19).

The three-pointed labial focus symbol used for this pedagogical goal seems to convey a visual image to students that helps them grasp the concept.

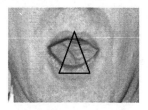

Figure 9–19. Photograph of the normal, vertical mouth configuration with a centering triangle superimposed to help visualize the jaw-down oral configuration.

Table 9–7. Jaw Elevation Table.

Written	IPA	Ideal Jaw Elevation	Strategy		Notes
Liquids					
l	l	L	⊕		
ly	ʎ	L(M)	⊕		
r	r	L	⊕		American English
r	ɹ	M	⊕		Retroflex American r, (mid-west hard r) by definition, cannot be centered
r	ʀ	M	⊕		Parisian (uvular)
r	ř	M	⊕		Rolled Italian r
r	ɾ	H	⊕		Single flip of tongue tip r, as in British "very"
Nasals					
m	m	L	⊕	▲	Both strategies are needed
n	n	L	⊕		
ng	ŋ	L	⊕		
ny	ɲ	M	⊕		
Glides					
y	j–i	L	⊕		
w	w–u	L	⊕	▲	Both strategies are needed
wh	ʍ	M	⊕	▲	Both strategies are needed
Fricatives, Pure and Voiced					
th–th	θ–ð	H	⊕		
s–z	s–z	H	⊕		
sh–(s)si	ʃ–ʒ	H	⊕	▲	Both strategies are needed
f–v	f–v	M	⊕		
h	ç	L	⊕		As in "hue"
ch	ç	L	⊕		
ch	x	L	⊕		

(continued)

Table 9–7. (continued)

Written	IPA	Ideal Jaw Elevation	Strategy		Notes
Prevoiced and Pure Plosives					
b-p	b-p	L	⊕	▲	Both strategies are needed
d-t	d-t	M	⊕		
g-k	g-k	L	⊕		
Affricates					
ch	tʃ	H	⊕		
j	dʒ	H	⊕		
Aspirate					
h	h		⊕		Made at the glottis

SUMMARY

The major goal of this chapter has been to encourage the quest for greater resonance in the production of pitch consonants. Production norms of these phonemes utilized in most singer's speech are generally too shallow and constrained to permit the optimal resonance needed for clarity of diction, fullness of sound in the singing line, and easier CV/VC joins. The simple acts of separating the pitch consonants from the nonpitch varieties, utilizing the term consovowel when referring to them in the voice studio, and employing spectrographic imagery can facilitate a change in the student's approach to the sounds. By thinking of them—not as restrictive speech consonants—but as virtual vowels, the phonemic production of the speech template will soon seem insufficient for the production of these phonemes in a well-trained, singing technique. When these sounds truly approach vowel resonance status, many vowel and join problems tend to disappear.

CHAPTER

10

THE NONPITCH CONSONANTS

Among the nonpitch consonants there are two commonalties:

- None of the nonpitch consonants involve *sustainable* phonation on pitch.
- All are produced with acoustical elements that fall within the definition of noise.

There is a minor pitch component that precedes some forms of stop consonants (prevoiced), but it is not sustainable, making those phonemes inappropriate for inclusion in the pitch-class consonants discussed in the previous chapter.

NONPITCH CONSONANT RESONANCE (CR)

As difficult as it is for some voice practitioners to accept the concept of consonant resonance (CR) during the production of pitch consonants, it seems to be an even more foreign idea when discussing the nonpitch consonants. These consonants seem to be transitory events that do not employ vocal fold vibration and its attendant "feel" of the resonance in the vocal tract. Therefore, most singers find the subject of CR more difficult to accept when considering these consonants.

CR must be considered for the nonpitch consonants to the same degree as that for vowels and pitch consonants if the singing line is to have the richness of both tone and diction that we enjoy when listening to a ranking singer. Figure 10–1 shows an /s/ performed with resonance typical of speech on the left and with full singing resonance on the right.

After reviewing the spectrographic evidence, it is difficult to imagine why the issue of CR—for both pitch and nonpitch

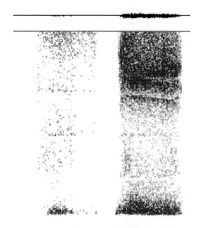

Figure 10–1. /s/ performed with lesser (left) and greater resonance space (right). 💿

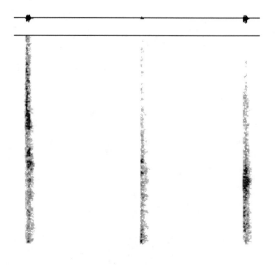

Figure 10–2. Spectrogram transients for /t/, /p/, and /k/. 💿

consonants—is virtually ignored both in the voice studio and in the literature of voice science.

Spectrographic Evidence

Examine some typical nonpitch consonants on the spectrograph for evidence of their potential resonance. In Figure 10–2, notice that there is a "spectral envelope" (an area of resonance in the **transient**) that is distinctive for each of these sounds:

- High frequency for the /t/ as the tongue must rise to the velum, a position that favors high resonance
- Low frequency for the /p/ as the tongue is low in the oral cavity, thus freeing the oral space for resonance
- Mid-frequency for the /k/ as the tongue must move back for the closure, an act that creates a fair amount of resonance space in the front of the oral cavity

The Need for CR in Nonpitch Consonants

As mentioned throughout the last chapter, CR is a critical consideration in singing for two reasons:

- CV balance and diction—singers are trained to produce vowels that are far richer than those in speech. How much conscious, direct attention is given to developing the richness of their consonant production? If they are to enjoy a balanced, intelligible diction, all consonants must enjoy greater amplitude and richness than those commonly found in speech.
- Easier CV/VC joins—once the singer has obtained an optimal level of resonance for all consonants, less shifting of articulative structures is required between CV/VC joins. This results in a more consistently beautiful sound that is easier to execute.

It is simply a matter of mechanics: With the maintenance of optimal CR behind the point of constriction or occlusion needed for the production of the consonant, less articulative movement is required in the progression of phoneme to phoneme. When done well, there is no loss of the clarity of diction, and one achieves a concomitant increase in the overall resonance of the vocal production.

Two Problems Mitigating the Development of CR

Spreading

Remember that, if the singer's oral cavity is "spread" during the production of nonpitch consonants, the resulting phonemes will lack the richness and impact needed for coexistence with richly sung vowels and pitch consonants. Consult Chapters 8 and 9 for a more thorough discussion of spreading. Also, remember to consult the Jaw Elevation Table (Table 9–7) at the end of the previous chapter for information on how to improve CR for all consonants.

Theory: Origins of Consonant Pressurization—Two Scenarios

Is there any evidence that in speech, nonpitch consonant pressurization is accomplished primarily through the use of the musculature in the area of the larynx and pharynx? Spectrographic evidence, gathered during several years of observation in the Drew University lab, suggests that this may be the case.

Could it be that the use of these muscles mitigates the development of optimal resonance and makes the shifting of phoneme-to-phoneme resonance a problem for the singer? When singers minimize the use of the musculature in the area of the larynx and pharynx and substitute abdominal support instead, there is a marked increase in the power and richness of these phonemes.

Figure 10–3 shows three pairs of nonpitch consonants (/t/, /g/, and /tʃ/) and reveals the difference between those pressurized by the musculature in the area of the larynx and pharynx (left of each pair) and those pressurized by the abdominal mus-

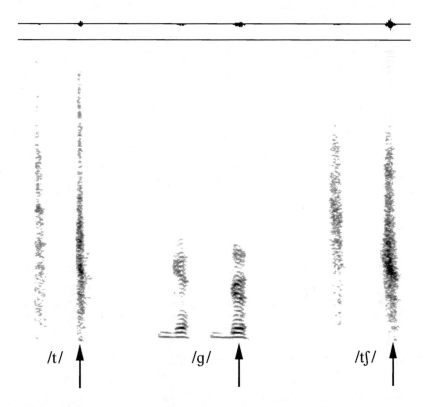

/t/   /g/   /tʃ/

Figure 10–3. Pairs of nonpitch consonants: /t/, /g/, and /tʃ/ (left to right). The arrows indicate those consonants produced with adequate abdominal support. ⓒ

culature (right of each pair). In the first pair of consonants on the left, the first /t/ was pressurized with the musculature in the area of the larynx and pharynx, the second with the abdominal musculature. With the use of the abdominals, the laryngeal and pharyngeal muscles can assume their more vowel-like set, and the difference is clearly visible on the spectrogram:

- There is a drop in the resonance area of the spike of c. 2 kHz.
- The waveform at the top of the screen indicates an increase in the amplitude of the consonant.

Because insufficient amplitude of non-pitch consonants is one of the singer's worst diction problems, this increase in amplitude could be very beneficial to the audience's understanding of the sung text.

In the second set of consonants, the /g/, differences similar to those encountered in the /t/ pair also are evident. In addition, the prevoicing of the /g/ consonant (to be dealt with later in this chapter) is far stronger in the second iteration. Also, observe the difference in the waveform amplitude.

The last pair to the right, /tʃ/, also shows the lowering of the area of resonance and the increase of amplitude as shown on the waveform. The waveform reveals one other critical difference: there is a dramatic increase in the acuteness at the initiation of the consonant. The sound in the concert hall will have a much "sharper" impact within the overall diction of the sung line.

STOPS IN GENERAL

Stops are consonants that require the buildup of air pressure behind a total occlusion (stoppage) of the oral cavity or vocal folds. When the desired degree of pressure is achieved, the pressure is suddenly released, resulting in a spike of energy that is transferred through the atmosphere to the listener. The stop can be executed with or without a pitch component; the author calls a stop that has no pitch component a **simple stop**, and one in which a brief preliminary vocalization is present a **prevoiced stop**.

Both types of stop are illustrated in Figure 10–4 with the word "tag" (/tæg/); it contains both a simple stop /t/ and a prevoiced stop /g/. Note the acoustical signature of the prevoicing just as the /g/ begins.

It is important to remember that all sung stop consonants must be articulated with considerably more energy than those in speech in order to maintain balance with the surrounding vowels. As stated previously, abdominal support plays a crucial role in the proper production of these consonants. For a full definition of support, consult Chapter 8.

Table 10–1.

Simple Stops			Prevoiced Stops		
Written	IPA	Example	Written	IPA	Example
p	p	Pop	b	b	bobby
t	t	Tame	d	d	dame
k	k	Kick	g	g	game
–	ʔ	uh-oh!	–	–	–
–	ʔ	Glottal stroke	–	–	–

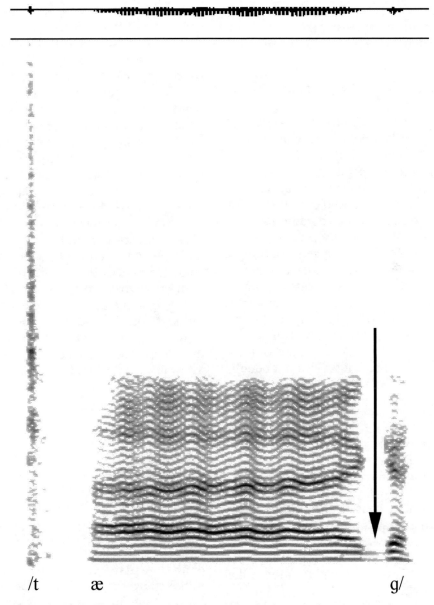

/t   æ   g/

Figure 10–4. The word "tag" (/tæg/) contains both a simple stop /t/ and a pre-voiced stop /g/; the arrow points to the faint signal of the prevoicing for the /g/. Also note the F-pattern evidence of the shift of the tongue as it moves toward the set of the /g/. 💿

Simple Stops

Simple stops are articulated without pitch and are observed on a spectrogram as a spike, or transient (see Figure 10–2).

Stop Onset

At the beginning of simple stops, there is a short time, called a **stop gap**, during which vocalization is interrupted while pressure is built up prior to release. It appears on the spectrograph as a *visual gap* during the scrolling of the spectrographic analysis.

Attaining Stop Onset Coordination

If singers experience problems coordinating support during the stop initiation, they can use a variation of the vowel onset, staccato repetition exercise, ASAI (see Chapter 8 for a definition of ASAI).

Choose any vowel and sing a series of ASAI onsets to feel the coordination and see the resulting evidence on the spectrograph. Then, substitute a stop consonant for the vowel; do not release the consonant but feel how the pressure builds behind the occlusion. After holding the pressure for a short while, the consonant should be released normally. This simple exercise can train the use and coordination of the support musculature (abdominal) and lead the singer away from the use of the neck musculature.

Release of Simple Stops

Simple Stops and VOT

An important consideration when dealing with simple stops is the concept of VOT, <u>V</u>oice <u>O</u>nset <u>T</u>ime. VOT is the time interval between the release of a simple stop and the onset of the phonation of the next vowel.

Syllable-Initial Simple Stops

A well-trained singer often employs a significant amount of essentially silent VOT on syllable-initial simple stops. Spectrographic evidence from singers in the lab reveals VOTs averaging about 35 milliseconds. In those dramatic situations where a particularly strong syllable-initial stop is required, the VOT can be longer.

If a singer attempts to eliminate VOT, the CV join will usually result in a following vowel that may be unstable or too constricted. When this occurs, it may be that there is too much instability in the oral cavity environment following a strong stop release, and time is needed to permit that environment to settle to a point where the onset of the vowel can occur in the stable atmosphere.

It is interesting to experiment with how much VOT gap a listener will accept before they become aware of it. When singers in training first attempt the creation of VOT following an initial simple stop consonant, they may voice considerable resistance to its use, as it seems like an intolerable silence. Once they begin to enjoy the predictable stability of the onset of the next vowel, the use of VOT following a syllable-initial simple stop will quickly become habitual. Figure 10–5 shows a spectrograph of the word "top" and clearly shows the gap of the VOT following the initial stop.

Word-Interior Simple Stops

Most singers tend to employ far less simple-stop force in word-interior situations. Their goal seems to be to continue the flow of phonated sound almost through the stop (a physical impossibility but a psychologically beneficial goal). Whereas VOT may be necessary to settle the oral environment following an acute release of pressure in the performance of syllable-initial stops, the lower stop pressures utilized in the interior of words may not require the use of VOT. As viewed on spectrograms, there appears to be little or no VOT in evidence following the execution of word-interior simple stops.

Word-Final Simple Stops

One of the most intense battles that novice singers have to fight is trying to avoid the propensity to collapse phrase endings before taking a subsequent breath. As discussed in Chapter 8, this collapse

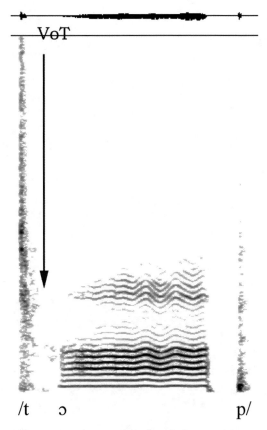

/t   ɔ   p/

Figure 10–5. Spectrogram of the word "top." The arrow denotes the silent space of the VOT following the release of the /t/.

can result from allowing the set of the articulators to drift, or it can be manifested as a weakening—or even a cessation—of support. Either way, this collapse of the production of the instrument is very noticeable, even to inexperienced listeners.

The spectrograph can be a powerful tool in this seemingly eternal battle, a struggle that takes place in virtually every voice studio. A properly performed final simple stop shows up on the spectrographic image as a sharp spike. If singers attempt stop pressurization levels borrowed from their speech templates, such spikes will be minimal or nonexistent. After very little coaching in front of the spectrograph, most singers are able to quickly develop the habit of applying sufficient power to their word-ending, simple stops.

Release Burst

A simple stop is a brief event lasting only c. 35 ms. In most instances in singing, there should be little or no noise emanating from the escaping breath following the release of the stop. When it occurs in speech, this aspirate release is called a **release burst**. Unless it is employed for dramatic reasons, the release burst should not occur in fine singing. One can easily see the difference between a coordinated and an uncoordinated release in Figure 10–6. The first /t/transient lasts 35 ms; the second lasts 60 ms. Furthermore, the /t/ performed with the uncoordinated release does not have the rich spectral development that the more focused execution possesses.

In singing, an unintentional release burst may be a sign of one or both of the following deficiencies of articulative coordination:

- The support that created the high supraglottal pressure necessary prior to the release continues after the stop has been released. As seen in spectrographic evidence, a correctly performed stop will feature the cessation of high supraglottal pressure delivery within approximately 35 ms of release (not the 60 ms seen in Figure 10–6).
- The open, optimally resonant structures of the oral cavities, pharyngeal cavities, or both have partially collapsed with the release of the pressure, causing the out-flowing air stream to dissipate laterally.

If the singer experiences a post-release collapse of the oral and/or pharyngeal cavities, one might correct it by imagining that the pitch component from the previous vowel or pitch consonant can be maintained through the stop and into the next vowel or pitch consonant. If the proper resonance set is not maintained between the production of phonemes and pitch components, proper CR and stop release may be virtually impossible.

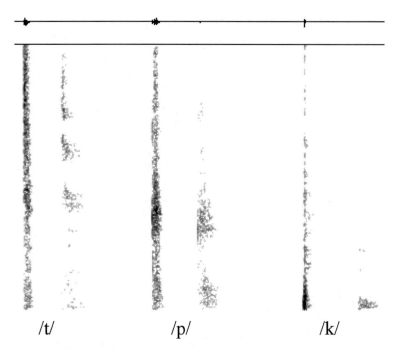

/t/   /p/   /k/

Figure 10–6. Pairs of /t /, /p /, and /k/, each performed as a sharp, focused burst and then as an uncoordinated release burst (left to right). 🔘

Prevoiced Stops

Each simple stop is homorganic with a pre-voiced stop:

- p/b = pursed lips (bilabial)
- t/d = tip of tongue against the alveolar ridge (lingua-alveolar)
- k/g = the posterior part of the tongue against the velum at the back (lingua-velor)

Each pair of sounds is made at the same location in the oral cavity.

Especially on syllable-initial prevoiced stops, a prevoicing of insufficient strength can often be misperceived and heard as a simple stop instead. While listeners may be able to mentally correct the phoneme by contextual means, it is far better not to confront them with the problem in the first place.

Consider the following example: "the boy sang a song." Without the prevoicing, the /b/ in boy may sound like a /p/. A listener may then perceive the phrase as /ðʌ pɔⁱ sæⁱŋ εⁱ saŋ/. The listener must then recompute what was heard in order to understand the phrase as /ðʌ bɔⁱ sæⁱŋ εⁱ saŋ/.

Voice Bars

In the performance of prevoiced stops, the silence that one experiences during the buildup of supraglottal pressure for simple stops is absent; the brief, muffled vocalization that constitutes a prevoicing takes its place. These prevoicings are called **voice bars** and are comprised of only a few lower harmonics. Because voice bars can be clearly seen on the spectrograph, VRTF can be employed to help the singer define the amount of prevoicing that is necessary to make these consonants audible.

On the spectrograph, the singer can easily recognize insufficiently executed prevoicings. They appear as single spikes, with little or no evidence of the prevoicing. Figure 10–7 shows the word "boy" performed with insufficient prevoicing on the left and proper prevoicing on the right.

The Nature of Prevoicing

In a consonant-initial position, a prevoiced stop is performed exactly like the pure stop except, during the buildup of pressure behind the oral occlusion, sound is created by the vocal folds. Since the oral *and* nasal cavities are totally occluded during this pressure buildup, the time in which phonation can be maintained is severely limited. It does not take long to attain equalization of sub- and supraglottal pressure. When that equilibrium is attained, phonation ceases.

At the last moment before phonation stops, the singer releases the pent-up pressure. Since the prevoicing that precedes the release is sung on pitch, that pitch will resonate in the oral cavity during the release of the plosive.

Problems with Prevoicings

There are two crucial considerations to keep in mind when dealing with prevoicings:

- Correct Pitch: The prevoicing must be executed on the same pitch as the vowel that follows it. If the word "daddy" (/dædi/) were to be performed

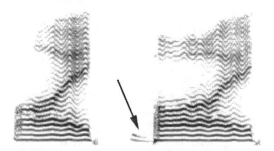

Figure 10–7. The word "boy" performed with and without prevoicing on the left and with a proper prevoicing on the right. 💿

on a single pitch, for example, all the phonemes of the word would have to be intoned on that pitch, including the prevoicings. If the second syllable were notated on a lower pitch than the first, however, the prevoicing of the second /d/ phoneme would have to be executed on the new pitch of the second syllable.

Failure to sing the proper pitch on the prevoicing preceding the release of the stop can be perceived as "scooping." (A speech therapist might use the term "target undershoot" [TUS] to denote the same problem.) As was the case for scooping during the production of all pitch-consonant phonemes, scooping can stem from a misguided attempt to impart emotion to the text—or worse, inattention to pitch stability within a sung line. While scooping can be a desirable ornament in some styles of operatic singing (principally, Italian *verissmo*), it should be avoided in most styles of classical singing. Most often, singers are not consciously aware of the presence of scooping in their vocal production, a fact that makes this a difficult technical flaw to correct.

Spectrograph is an ideal way to deal with the problem. Since most singers who habitually scoop are not aurally aware of the fault, it is an unconscious act. Often, when a teacher or coach points out the fault, the singer will deny having done it.

On the spectrogram, the evidence of scooping is unmistakable. Because the harmonics above F_0 track in lockstep with the fundamental's pitch, the harmonics of any scoop will appear in an up-sweeping pattern that moves rapidly toward the correct pitch required for the vowel. This evidence is easily recognized in Figure 10–8.

Once the singer learns to recognize this telltale visual clue, he or she should begin to hear it as well and be well on the way toward a solution.

Substitution of Liquids for Prevoicings

Another prevoicing problem that shows up with some regularity is an unconscious

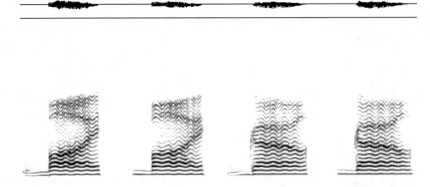

Figure 10–8. Paired spectrograms of the words boy (left) and girl (right). In each pair, the prevoicing is scooped (rise in the F_0) and then performed correctly as the F_0 of the prevoicing is stable and matches the F_0 of the initial vowel. ⏺

habit of singing a nasal pitch consonant as a substitute for the prevoiced sound.

The following substitutions can be encountered:

- /m/ replaces the prevoicing for /b/
- /n / may be employed before the /d/
- /ŋ/ may be used before a /g/

The difference between a properly performed prevoicing and an improper substitution can clearly be seen in the series of spectrograms in Figure 10–9. If the student cannot hear or feel the difference, the spectrograph can provide visual help to aid in solving the problem. When properly performed, a prevoicing will present a small voice band at the bottom of the harmonic spectrum; improperly substituted nasals will appear fully formed and almost vowel-like, making the difference easy to spot on the monitor.

Prevoiced Stops and VOT

The short vocalization that is characteristic of prevoicings seems to eliminate the need for VOT in both syllable-initial and word-interior prevoiced stops. It could be that the pharyngeal resonance needed for the prevoicing, when properly produced, ensures that the pharynx remains open

up to and through the release of the pressure. Thus, the CV problems encountered in the production of the simple stops are most likely eliminated in the case of prevoiced stops.

GLOTTAL STOP AND STROKE

The glottal stop and glottal stroke could be included among the simple stop consonants because, with the sole exception being that they are produced at the glottis and not in the oral cavity, they possess all of the qualities of simple stops. Because they are not traditionally listed as consonants, discussion of these stops will be found in Chapter 10 to make it easier to find for the reader using this book as a reference.

UNVOICED FRICATIVES

A **fricative** is produced by creating turbulence in the air stream as it passes through the oral cavity. This turbulence is produced when pressurized moving air is passed through a point of narrow constriction formed by the proximity of oral

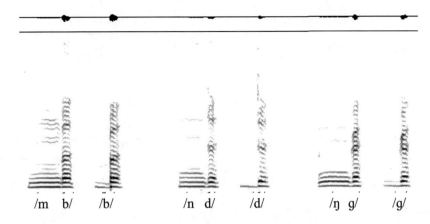

Figure 10-9. Pairs of prevoiced consonants, /b/, /d/, and /g/. The left image in each pair shows the improper substitution of a nasal consonant for the prevoicing; the right image is performed with the true prevoicing (improper substitutions are /mb/, /nd/, and /ŋg/). 💿

articulators. At the point of constriction, the integrity of the laminar airflow can no longer be maintained, causing part of it to separate. The vortices that are created as part of this turbulence radiate very high-frequency, aperiodic sounds. At two of the sites, if sufficient air pressure is supplied, the conditions may be right for the creation of a Bernoulli effect that can induce an oscillation of the velum (/x/), or uvula (/χ/).

Even though fricatives are aperiodic, the resonance of the vocal system still has a considerable effect on the radiated sounds. Each of these sounds has an area of the spectral envelope that will be magnified. Therefore, differences between them will be visible on the spectrogram. As was the case with vowels, the resonance of a fricative varies according to the positioning of the tongue mass.

Table 10-2. Fricatives in English.

Type	Turbulence Site Between	IPA Symbol Unvoiced	IPA Symbol Voiced
Interdental	Tip of tongue and upper/lower teeth	θ	ð
Labio-dental	Lower lip and upper teeth	f	v
Lingua-alveolar-palatal	Tongue and alveolar-palatal area	ç	–
Lingua-alveolar	Tongue (tip and blade) and alveolar ridge	s	z
Lingua-palatal	High, grooved tongue and the palate	ʃ	ʒ
Glottal	Narrowed glottis	h	–

In addition, there are several fricative sites along the alveolar-velar continuum where fricatives are produced for some of the principal non-English singing languages:

Table 10–3. Foreign fricatives.

Type	Turbulence Site Between	IPA Symbol Unvoiced	Language
Lingua-palatal	Tongue blade and palate	ɥ	French
Lingua-palatal	Mid-tongue and palate	ç	German
Lingua-velar	Posterior tongue and velum	x	German, Hebrew
Lingua-uvular	Posterior tongue and uvula	χ	German

Note: See the IPA table in Appendix A for examples of words that employ these sounds.

Resonance of the Unvoiced Fricative "CH" Class of Consonants

A series of fricatives share the commonality of the proximity of the tongue mass to the palate or velum (/ɥ/ /ɕ/ /ç/ /x/ /χ/). Differences between them are dependent on the position of the tongue on the longitudinal axis.

Utilizing the images in Figure 10–10 as benchmarks, spectrographic VRTF can be employed to help the student properly place these various phonemes in the oral cavity.

Possible Confusion Between Speech and Singing Terms

In speech, a number of fricatives (and their homogenic voiced twins) are referred to as *stridents* (/s/ and /z/, /ʃ/ and /ʒ/). This adjective is used to indicate that these phonemes involve far greater energy to create their characteristic turbulence. All other fricatives are called *nonstridents* (observe the differential in energy output in the spectrograms of /ʃ/ and /s/ shown in Figure 10–11).

However, the term strident is often used by voice teachers and coaches to describe a type of unwanted vocal production. Thus, use of the term in its speech meaning can lead to confusion in the singing studio. Strident should not be paired with the word fricative since it can be a potential source of misunderstanding.

To avoid this problem but still account for the increased energy in the production of the stridents, the author urges that voice practitioners adopt the use of the terms:

- **Sibilant** for the phonemes (/s/ and /ʃ/)
- **Fricative** for all other fricatives

The word sibilant is used by many voice practitioners to refer to high-energy fricatives. Also, the sound of the word has an activity to it that conveys the increased energy of the phoneme without the use of the speech term strident.

/x/, the Guttural "CH"

The /x/, the so-called guttural "ch," is a fricative that includes considerably more noise than simply the sound of turbulent air. It may be posited that the proper production of this phoneme might require the singer to induce a Bernoulli effect in

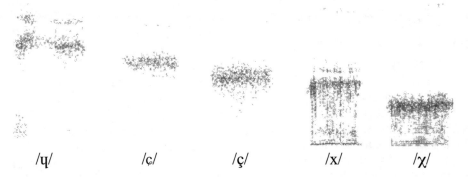

/ɥ/   /ɕ/   /ç/   /x/   /χ/

Figure 10–10. Spectrogram of the fricatives /ɥ/, /ɕ/, /ç/, /x/, and /χ/ (left to right) showing the resonantial shift as the tongue moves along its anterior-posterior axis. Note the vertical striations on /x/, and /χ/ indicating possible tongue-velum contact. 💿

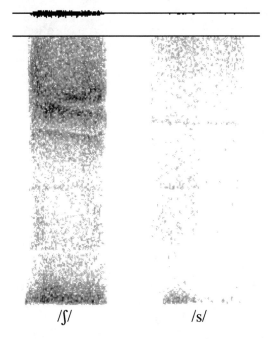

/ʃ/   /s/

Figure 10–11. Spectrogram showing the difference in production energy between the sibilant (strident) /ʃ/ and the fricative (nonstrident) /f/. 💿

the constricted area between the velum and the posterior area of the tongue. When the supraglottal pressure is sufficient for the Bernoulli to take place, the velum is drawn toward the posterior tongue. The velum's myoelasticity plus air pressure then return it toward its at-rest position. If the considerable pressure needed to create this phoneme is continued for some length of time, a velar oscillation is set up that gives this phoneme its signature sound.

Figure 10–12 features a spectrogram of the guttural "ch" (x) and shows its resonances and the noise-producing action of the oscillating velum (as indicated by the faint vertical striations in the spectrogram). Possible additional evidence of this periodic oscillation can be seen in the waveform shown at the top of the image. Many times, the bubbling of the saliva in the restricted area between the velum and the tongue also adds to the acoustical picture.

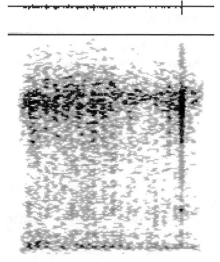

Figure 10–12. Spectrogram of the guttural "ch" (x) showing resonances and the noise-producing action of the oscillating velum as seen in the faint vertical striations in the spectrogram. 💿

A "Fricative Glide": The Special Case of the /ʍ/ as in "When"

This is a difficult sound to categorize. It could be placed in either Chapter 9 after the discussion of glides, or in this chapter with the unvoiced fricatives. Its placement in this chapter is due to the special fricative nature of its initial sound.

When this phoneme is pronounced as a true /ʍ/, one might be tempted to spell it as "hw," as the initial phoneme sounds something like an /h/ and then moves through a transitory /ᵘ/ on its way toward the primary vowel. Pronounced in this way, the word "when" could be written as ʰuɛn.

The use of /ʰ/ is not quite correct, however. The initial sound is actually an unvoiced fricative, written in IPA as /ʍ/, that sometimes seems to simultaneously combine elements of the bilabial /Φ/ and the frontal "ch" sound /ç/ that begins the word "hue." This sound is performed with some rounding of the lips, but that rounding is quickly relaxed, creating a glide, /ᵘ/, on the way toward the primary vowel of the word.

This wonderful packet of sounds has all but disappeared from American English (Americans simply employ the glide /ᵘ/). The /ʍ/ can be an additional phonetic delight when used by a singer, and this phoneme does not seem to sound stilted or out of fashion to most listeners.

travel the full gauntlet of the vocal tract, it is very difficult to perform with much amplitude.

Singers sometimes also narrow the pharynx and/or the oral cavity to create additional turbulence. Such a pharyngeal narrowing not only has a negative influence on the vowels that precede or follow, but may also be a contributor in the loss of mucosal moisture that seems to play a role in causing the dreaded "dry throat" about which so many singers complain.

AFFRICATES

Affricates are combination consonants. There are only two affricates in the English language.

Table 10-4. Affricates.

Written	IPA	Example
ch	tʃ	church
j	dʒ	judge

The IPA table in Appendix A makes a distinction between the two affricates because of technical problems in their execution that may arise in singing.

Aspirate /h/

The /h/, along with the glottal stop and stroke, are the only consonant made at the glottis in the English language. The narrow aperture that creates the fricative turbulence is created by the proximity of the vocal folds. To create this event, the arytenoids must move the vocal folds toward the centerline of the glottis so that they come to rest just outside the point where vocal-fold vibration would initiate. Because the sound of this phoneme must

/tʃ/

The /tʃ/ begins with the simple stop /t/. This part of the phoneme obeys all of the rules of a stop featuring a full closure of the oral cavity (as well as a closed velo-pharyngeal port), a buildup of pressure within that cavity, and finally a precipitous release. But, unlike the pure stop /t/, the tongue moves immediately into position so the released pressure sounds as the fricative /ʃ/.

The Prevoiced Affricate: /dʒ/

The /dʒ/ is classified differently because it begins with a prevoiced stop, /d/. Again, as with the /tʃ/, there is a full closure of the oral cavity (as well as a closed velopharyngeal port), a buildup of pressure within that cavity, and finally a precipitous release. Instantaneous with the moment of release, the tongue is moved into the /ʒ/ configuration. The difference between this phoneme and the /tʃ/ is that during the pressurization of the stop, the initial sound (a prevoicing) is phonation on pitch. That pitch then continues to sound during the release as the *voiced fricative /ʒ/*.

Because of the presence of the pitch event throughout the creation of this consonant, it must be considered with those where scooping is a possibility, and appropriate caution must be maintained.

OPTIMAL RESONANCE IN NONPITCH CONSONANTS

All of the principles of resonance optimization listed in the previous chapters apply to the phonemes discussed in this chapter as well. The reader is urged to review both the resonance creation checklist in Chapter 8 and the Target Jaw Elevation Table presented in Chapter 9. The principles of improving resonance are just as valid for nonpitch consonants as they are for vowels and pitch consonants.

Resonance Creation Checklist

☐ Low mandible (for more information on technique, see the Target Jaw Elevation Table that concludes Chapter 9)

☐ Proper tongue configuration

☐ Raised velum

☐ Pharynx open and relaxed

☐ Larynx relaxed low in the throat

SUMMARY

It should be obvious by now that the author believes that all phonemes used in singing can benefit from openness and resonance, not just the vowels.

The Diction Versus Tone Debate

A recurring debate in the world of fine singing centers on two opposing propositions:

• A singer can have great tone but must accept a lesser standard of diction to achieve it.
• Singers can have great diction, but only if they are willing to give up some tone.

Yet examples of singers whose artistry totally obliterates the need for this debate abound, embodied in the performances of both present-day stars and in the historic recordings of great singers from the past. *Tone and diction can coexist if enough care is taken in vocal training.* The addition of the concept of CR is the key.

While voice practitioners may marvel at the sheer magnificence of the genetic inheritance embodied in such voices, the *technique* by which they produce their art is available, both aurally and visually, to any voice practitioner who wishes to learn it.

CHAPTER

11

A SPECTROGRAPHIC MISCELLANY

The previous three chapters were built around the major classifications of phonemes found in the IPA table included with this book (Appendix A). But there are other nonphonemic vocal issues that can potentially benefit from the use of the spectrogram. This chapter includes a few of these to give the reader an introduction to the rich possibilities of spectrographic exploration in other areas.

PASSAGGIO

Usage of the Term

Most voice practitioners and voice scientists agree that there are multiple, tonally distinctive (if not mechanico-acoustical) areas of the singing voice.

The Strict Usage

Many singers and scientists use the word **passaggio** in the traditional way to denote the places *at which* a voice normally shifts to another register. These places have also been called lifts, or more pejoratively, breaks.

In this use of the terminology, a soprano may have her primo passaggio at E_4 (the shift point between chest and middle voice) and her secondo passaggio at F_5 (the shift point between the middle and upper voices). The bass or tenor has a primo passaggio and a secondo passaggio that encompass the interval of a fourth, during which the transition from the chest voice to the top voice must be accomplished.

Alternative Use of the Term Passaggio

One must be careful with the use of the term passagio because many singers have been taught (the author included) that the word refers to the *area* in which one modifies or blends the voice *between* registers. In this usage, the area between C_4 and F_4 in the female voice is called the primo passaggio and the area between C_5 and F_5 is the secondo. In traditional terminology, these blending areas would have been called the *zona di passaggio* or *zona intermedia*. Thus, in this broader usage, men would only have one passaggio (the primo) between chest and head voices, as opposed to women, who would have two (a primo and secondo).

This terminology can be used so loosely that the voice teacher would do well to determine a student's understanding of the terms, correcting them if desirable, before using the word passaggio or any of its Italian modifiers in the voice studio.

Defining Primo and Secondo Passaggi

The majority opinion holds that male singers have one principal area of register adjustment, the one between the chest and the top voice. By contrast, women singers possess two: the first is between the chest and middle voice, and the second is between the upper-middle voice and the top voice. In the male, the one zone of adjustment is between his primo and secondo passaggi; in the female, the adjustment zone between chest and middle voice is around her primo passaggio, and the adjustment between middle and top is around her secondo passaggio.

Figure 11–1 represents the ranges and registers of the common voice types for both sexes. Note that all ranges, beginnings and endings of registers, as well as

the placement of the adjustment zones (*zona di passaggi*) between registers are approximate. They are intended to serve as a general guide, not a rigid system.

Using VRTF To Deal with Passagio Problems

When discussing the use of computer feedback as an aid for working on passaggio problems, one must make a distinction between the passaggi of men and women. Based on work done to date, there are indications that the spectrograph can be useful when dealing with the woman's primo passaggio (chest to middle), but it may be of minimal use when dealing with the secondo passaggio or the man's zona di passaggio. For both men and women, the power spectrum appears to be the preferred tool when working with the passaggi (see Donald Miller's views on registration shift given in the following chapter).

Much more research is needed before definitive answers about the efficacy of using spectrographic VRTF to resolve problems of the passaggi can be determined. As of this writing, the Drew University Studio/Lab has used the spectrogram with good results when working on problems concerning the female primo passaggio.

The Woman's *Primo Passagio*: The Shift Between the Chest and Head Registers

A Three-Register Model for the Soprano Voice

Understanding the principles involved in shifts of register are complex and not particularly well defined in the literature. The graph shown in Figure 11–2 is based on spectrographic evidence and may help

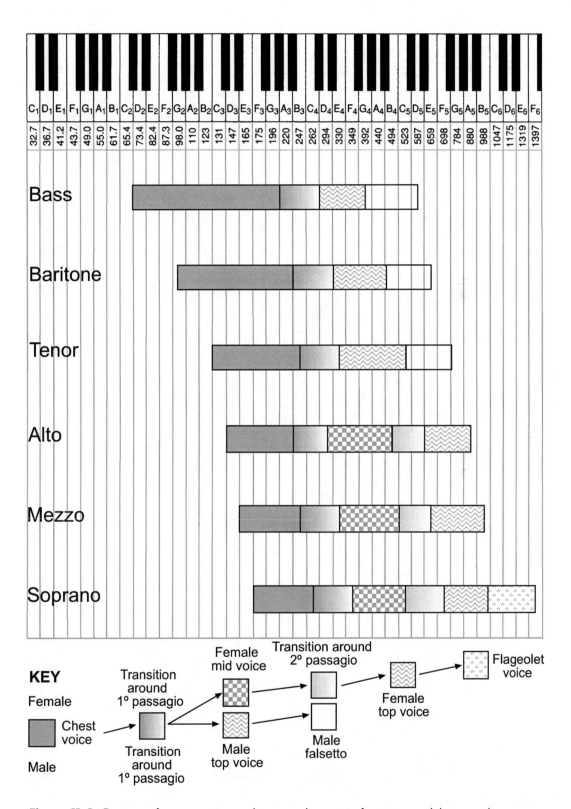

Figure 11-1. Diagram of approximate vocal ranges, placement of registers, and the *zona di passaggi*.

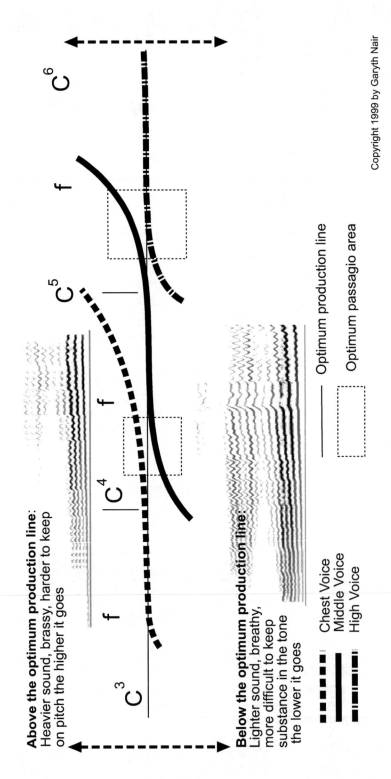

SOPRANO REGISTERS

Ramifications of taking a given register above or below its optimum production

C⁶

f

C⁵

Above the optimum production line:
Heavier sound, brassy, harder to keep on pitch the higher it goes

f

C⁴

f

C³

Below the optimum production line:
Lighter sound, breathy, more difficult to keep substance in the tone the lower it goes

―――― Optimum production line

⌐ ⌐
⌐ ⌐ Optimum passagio area

▬▬▬▬ Chest Voice
▬▬▬▬ Middle Voice
▬ ▬ ▬ High Voice

Figure 11-2. Schematic of a typical soprano three-register model showing the effect of carrying the voice too far above or below the optimal ranges of the registers. The two spectrograms shown in the *primo passaggio* area illustrate the head voice being carried down too far into the chest region (upper) and the chest being carried up too far until it finally breaks into the head voice (lower). The changes of pitch indicated by the spectrograms match the scale of the graphic's median line.

the reader understand the concept. The graph features the range of a hypothetical soprano, divided into chest, middle, and high voice. Each register is plotted against a median line that indicates the area of the best possible vocal production for a given register. Notice that the register lines remain in this ideal area for only a limited time. At either end of each register, the lines depart from the median, a departure that indicates a less desirable vocal production. Also notice that in this hypothetical representation, the register lines never meet or overlap on the median line. The two dotted boxes where the register lines are most approximate indicate the area in which the passaggio transitions should occur. Figure 11–2 contains two spectrographs of a female singer moving too far from her optimal chest and head ranges in the area surrounding the primo passaggio.

The Physioacoustical Problem

Before a woman learns to make a smooth transition between the chest and head voices, the shift between these registers is usually vividly apparent to the ear, an acute shift that also clearly shows up on the spectrogram (Figure 11–3).

When working with female singers on the primo passaggio, problems most often occur in one of two areas:

- The shift from chest to head voice is not performed as a deliberate action. When the shift does finally occur, it is actually a physioacoustical *abdication* that happens when the vocal apparatus can no longer sustain phonation in one register and must shift to the next adjoining one.
- The shift from chest to head may be consciously determined but occurs on the wrong note of the scale during the zona di passaggio.

Teaching the Location of the Shift Point

When singers are unable to shift between registers at will, they are participating in nothing less than a vocal lottery. Singers lacking this skill will stay in one register until the voice is forced to shift to the next register in order to continue making a viable vocal sound. Thus, the results of

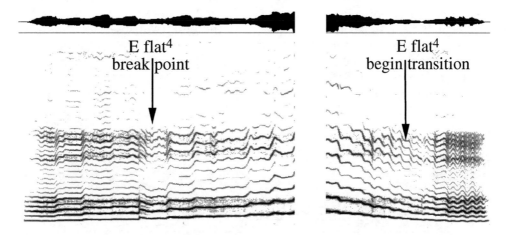

Figure 11–3. Spectrogram of a mezzo-soprano singing an ascending and descending scale through the first passaggio. On the ascending scale on the left, the singer allowed the voice to "break." On the descending scale on the right, she performed a smooth transition from head to chest. 🆑

each shift will be different as the shifting point is left to chance.

In the quest for a smooth primo passaggio transition the first technical skill that must be mastered is to make the singer's registration placement into consciously determined action. In the notes of the scale that immediately surround the primo passaggio (the zona), the singer should be able to sing, on command, each note in either chest or head voice at will.

Generally, the preferred switchover point by which the change between chest and head will be accomplished will lie approximately in the middle of the boxed area as shown in Figure 11–2. It is in this area that the two register lines experience their closest approach. For our hypothetical soprano, the best switchover point would probably occur on E^4 or E-flat^4.

Using the Register Extension and Toggle Exercises

Learning to sing any note in the zona di passaggio in either head or chest begins with the singer learning the feel of those notes when sung in either register. A classic technique to establish this is to purposely extend one register from an area where the other cannot be performed. If D^4 is desired in head voice, the singer should begin in head voice on D^5 and slide down to D^4 while remaining in head voice. Then the singer would be instructed to sing G^3 in chest voice and slide up to D^4 while maintaining that register.

When the singer is reliably aware of the difference in sound and feel, the toggle exercise can then be employed. The singer should switch between chest and head on a sustained note that falls within the boxed area in Figure 11–2 (in this case, E^4 for the soprano). In this way, the sensation of the two laryngeal configurations is experienced side-by-side and the student learns to place the note cleanly in one register or the other (see Figure 11–4).

Please note that this text does not advocate a rigid shift-over point for the passaggio. Differences in voice from singer to singer, as well as the musical and textual demands of the moment, may require that the switchover point be moved slightly in either direction. Still, the singer should be aware of her optimal area for the switchover and make decisions accordingly. Attempts to make the switch too high or low in the indicated box, where the register lines rapidly diverge, will most likely make the passaggio shift far more difficult to accomplish.

Blending the Transition

After a singer learns to switch between registers at will on any note in the *zona di passaggio*, work on blending the register transition can commence. When well executed, the gradual shift from one register to the other will resemble the transition between colors on a spectrum created by filtering light through a prism.

There is much variation in the approach to the problem of register shift in

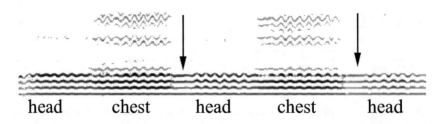

Figure 11–4. Spectrogram of a singer toggling between the head and chest voices on a single note (D^4). 🖭

the literature. One of the techniques that has had considerable success in the Drew University studio involves an attenuation of the brightness of the notes of the chest voice as the singer approaches the point for entry into the head voice (Figure 11–5). This attenuation is necessary because, as the chest voice is sung higher into and above the passaggio area, it becomes brighter and more forceful (some singers have described it as more raucous). Also, the head-voice notes neighboring the chest voice at that point fall near the bottom of middle-voice vocal effectiveness. Therefore, some of the brilliant timbre of the chest voice must be dampened in order for these notes to evolve smoothly into the head voice. This attenuation is achieved by slightly dropping the upper lip to remove some of the higher frequencies of the final chest voice tones before the switchover (see the discussion of *lip drop* in Chapter 8). When this transition is accomplished gradually, the ear of the listener perceives little or no tonal difference between chest and head.

Spectrographic VRTF is very useful in helping the singer learn the amount of

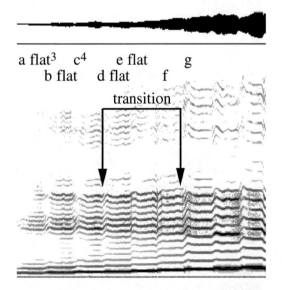

a flat^3 c^4 e flat   g
  b flat   d flat   f

transition

Figure 11–5. A smoothly executed transition from chest to head voice on an ascending scale. 🔘

attenuation necessary to make this transition happen in the smoothest possible manner.

VIBRATO

Vibrato is a quasi-periodic oscillation of pitch above and below the F_0-median line and occurs in voices that exhibit a free vocal production (free meaning that unnecessary musculature is not causing tension in the laryngeal-pharyngeal area).

Vibrato is one of the easiest facets of vocal production that can be recognized on the spectrogram display (Figure 11–6). Since the harmonics of the voice stay in lockstep with the F_0, the lines representing each harmonic will show the pitch oscillation of the vibrato. From this image, one can calculate both the **rate** (the number of vibrato cycles per second) and **extent** (degree of variation in pitch during each vibrato cycle). A third parameter of vibrato, **amplitude** variation, is not easily tracked with the spectrogram.

Barbara Doscher wrote,

To the ears of the average listener, a fluid vibrato is not heard as such, but is perceived as an integral part of the timbre. From an acoustical point of view, however, the "beats" of a vibrato define the musical texture of a tone. They add harmonic richness and give the impression that a tone is centered on pitch. Put another way, Benade says that a "fair amount of vibrato . . . adds a great deal of recognizability to the various sinusoidal components of the voice by providing them with a synchronized pulsation in frequency and amplitude (as they sweep across their various formants)." (Doscher 1994, pp. 199–200. The quote contained within this excerpt is from Benade [1990].)

Vibrato is not used by all cultures, and if it is used, it is not always employed the same way. Even in Western cultures, there are differences between vibrato use by jazz and pop singers and classically trained singers. While some might argue that vibrato is undesirable for certain styles of

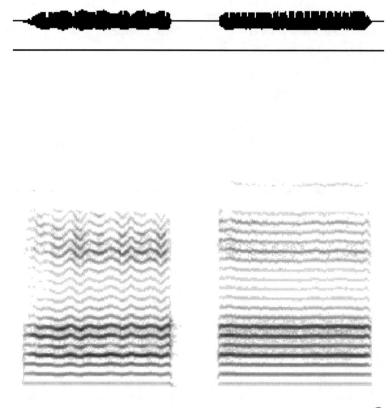

Figure 11–6. The vowel /a/ sung with (left), and without vibrato (right). 💿

music, it is the opinion of most mainstream voice practitioners that high-standard classical singing requires the presence of the vibrato.

Why Vibrato?

While one can measure vibrato and look for physiological factors that can alter it, no one knows with certainty why it occurs. Evidence is beginning to point toward a "stabilized physiologic tremor in the laryngeal muscles" (Ramig & Shipp, 1987; Titze, 1994). It has been observed that the average human vibrato rate is almost identical with that of muscle tremor speed such as shivering. This would seem to bolster the case that vibrato is caused by a neuromuscular oscillation (Hirano, 1995). Both Sundberg (1987) and Titze (1994) have excellent sum-

maries of current thinking on vibrato origin, and both point to this subtle neuromuscular cause and effect.

Muscle Tension and Vibrato

If the source of the vibrato is found in minor variations of muscle tension in the laryngeal musculature, then these muscle modulations would have to be very slight. By logical extension, if the musculature *surrounding* the larynx is overly tense, then it would seem feasible that such tension could disturb or cancel the minute vibrato-causing "tremors." Empirical evidence, gathered over years of observation in the voice studio, leads one to suspect such a correlation does exist.

There are other physiological factors that could cancel the vibrato event as well, but excessive tension in the anterior neck area would seem to garner most votes as the culprit in vibrato loss.

Using the Vibrato as a Muscle Tension Barometer

Even if the causes of compromised or missing vibrato turn out to be more complex than simple muscle tension in the laryngeal region, once can still use the vibrato as a barometer of the general state of tension in a singer's technique. By noting the areas where vibrato is missing in a sung line, it is possible to locate the root causes and correct them. When the spectrographic signature of the vibrato is suddenly compromised or missing in a line sung by a singer who is otherwise a good producer of vibrato, muscle tension in the instrument, especially in the tongue root-neck region, is usually the cause.

Vibrato Presence

Most singers, even at the most elementary level, can hear if the vibrato is absent from their production. This absence is easily seen on the spectrogram as straight harmonic lines (look again at the right image in Figure 11–5, which shows a vibratoless /a/ vowel).

The spectrograph can be intermittently used as an aid in guiding the student toward the desired goal of vocal relaxation (the expression used in the Drew studio/lab is, "the relaxed application of power"). As the singer gradually dissipates the unwanted tension from the vocal production, a tendency *toward* the vibrato state will appear as a slight, quasi-periodic wavering of an otherwise vibratoless, straight-line image. Spectrographic VRTF can be of enormous help to both student and teacher in the process of learning to recognize a vocal signal that indicates a *disposition* toward the onset of the vibrato. The area of muscle relaxation that per-

mitted the onset of the quasi-periodic vibrato must be identified and replicated repeatedly. As the singer learns to rid the instrument of unwanted muscular tension, such careful work will gradually lead to the production of a consistently periodic natural vibrato.

Vibrato Consistency

Most singers will probably be able to sing with the vibrato intact for most of their vocal production. They will be able to perform many phonemes in sequence with a natural vibrato but then it will suddenly disappear for one or more phonemes only to return again (see Figure 11–7).

The cause is often the improper production of a consonant immediately preceding a vowel. Once a student learns to recognize the visual marker of vibratoless production during VRTF, he or she can begin to correlate the physiological conditions causing its absence and correct them while singing in front of the display.

Quantifying the Vibrato

Gram is also useful in quantifying information about the vibrato. Vocal practitioners should calculate and maintain records of measurable parameters of singers' vibrati at regular intervals. Shifts in vibrato rate or extent may point to correctable problems in the technique that require intervention. The voices of older singers are especially prone to developing vibrato problems (see more on the aging vibrato later in this chapter).

The Singer's VRate

Each person has a natural vibrato rate that is determined by a highly complex relationship between anatomy and the laws of physics. The average vibrato rate (**VRate**) is between 4.5 and 6.5 Hz. However, Titze pointed out:

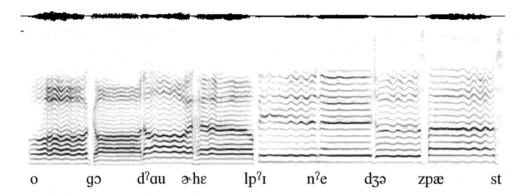

o   gɔ   dˀɑu   ɚ·hɛ   lpˀɪ   nˀe   dʒə   zpæ   st

Figure 11–7. Spectrogram of the sung line "O God our help in ages past" where the tense production of /g/ in the word "God" forces a following vibrato-less /ɔ/. The same problem occurs as the /ɛ/ in "help" progresses toward a tense /l/. The /e/ of "ages" suffers from the preceding misproduction of /n/ and the /zp/ combination spells trouble for the /æ/ in "past." The domino effect can be seen in the /ɪ/ of "in" following the tense /l/ (as well as potential problems with the /p/) of "help," and in the schwa /ə/ of "ages." 💿

But this answer needs many qualifications and explanations . . . vibrato frequency seems to increase somewhat with pitch and with the level of excitement for a given singer. On the one hand, nervousness, or excessive physical tension, is often manifested by a machine-gun vibrato, or *bleet*, in the 6- to 8-Hz range. On the other hand, lack of excitement, poor muscle tone, or fatigue may result in a *wobble* in the 2- to 4-Hz range. Regular exercises and good vocal conditioning seem to preserve the "acceptable" vibrato frequency range. (Titze, 1994, p. 298)

As various pedagogical techniques for the correction of VRate problems are explored, spectrographic VRTF can be used both as a diagnostic and a feedback tool to monitor efficacy and progress.

Calculating Rate of Vibrato

The task of calculating VRate is easy utilizing Gram. Save a sung passage sustaining a note in the middle voice (use Analyze Input on Gram's File menu). The file that results is called a .wav file. When the file is played back (by utilizing File/Analyze File), one can highlight a specific number of vibrato cycles. Begin by placing the cursor at the peak of the first

vibrato tracing and then depress and hold the left mouse button. While holding the button, move the mouse to the right, counting 20 cycle peaks. Do not release the button at the 20th peak. The resulting image will appear the same as the example in Figure 11–8. Before releasing the button, obtain the elapsed time of the 20-cycle highlighted box by reading the time in the information box at the lower left corner of the screen.

Once the elapsed time (in milliseconds) for the 20-cycle series is obtained, use the following formula:

(# of vibrato cycles/time in ms) × 1000 = VRate in Hz.

Example: (20/6089 ms) × 1000 = VRate of 3.284 Hz. Since most vibrati will present local variations of speed, the 20-cycle (or more) count is advisable in order to obtain a good average.

VExtent: The Dreaded "Wobble"

As long as the extent of the pitch traversal of the vibrato does not become too wide, the human brain happily focuses

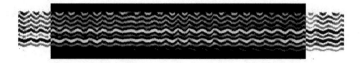

Figure 11–8. A vibrato pattern highlighted for 20 vibrato cycles for purposes of VRate calculation. (CD)

on the average of the extent and hears it as a single fundamental. Once the fundamental oscillates beyond a certain **VExtent**, the brain no longer performs the averaging and perceives the vibrato as an oscillation of pitch, known in singer's circles as **wobble**.

Wobble is normally defined as a VExtent extent greater than ±3% coupled with a VRate in the 2- to 4-Hz range. When confronted with parameters of this breadth, the brain of the listener can no longer average the extent and perceives the vibrato as an oscillation of two notes almost a semitone apart (±3% = ±.5 semitone). Figure 11–9 shows an abrupt shift from a normal vibrato to a wobble. When such a combination of Vrate and VExtent are encountered, the result is virtually unlistenable.

Measuring VExtent

VExtent is also easy to calculate on the spectrograph. Place the cursor at the top of a vibrato cycle and write down the frequency of the cursor position given in the lower left corner of the screen. Then move the cursor to the bottom of that cycle, note its frequency and calculate the difference between them. By measuring the VExtent for 10 or 20 cycles and calculating the average of the set, one can arrive at a reliable number.

Once a singer recognizes the difference between an acceptable extent and a wobble when viewed on the spectrogram, the teacher and singer can proceed to correct the problem.

The Aging Vibrato

As singers age, many changes may occur in the body that can have a detrimental effect on the singing product. These changes occur systemically throughout the body but the ones occurring in the larynx take on special significance for the singer. These changes include the loss of elastic and collaginous fibers that make the vocal folds stiffer and thinner (Sataloff, 1998, p. 128). Also, a potential loss of smoothness at the edge of the vocal fold mucosa can be experienced.

Sataloff, Spiegel, and Rosen wrote:

the notion that this decline occurs gradually and progressively (linear senescence) is open to challenge. It appears possible that many of these functions can be maintained at a better level than expected until very near the end of life, perhaps allowing a high-quality singing or acting career to extend into or beyond the seventh decade. (Sataloff, Spiegel, & Rosen in Sataloff, 1998, p. 128)

The reader is referred to the chapter in the Sataloff text for a more extended discussion and bibliography regarding this critical subject.

The challenges that may be presented to the singer during the aging process are not limited to those in the larynx. It is at the laryngeal level, however, that the voice practitioner may get the first hint of developing problems. It is recommended that voice practitioners track long-term trends in both VRate and VExtent over a singer's career. As a singer ages, these shifts in the vibrato parameters generally occur

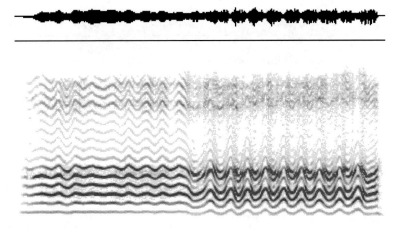

Figure 11–9. Spectrogram of a normal vibrato suddenly shifting to a wobble🔊

at glacial speed, and the only way to spot and correct them is long-term tracking performed at periodic intervals.

Teaching Trills

It may seem strange to move to a discussion of vocal trills just after a section on wobble, but they are related. A vocal trill can be described as a "vocal slight of mouth" created by a deliberate widening of the VExtent, purposely exceeding the point where the listener can average the normal vibrato's slight pitch variation into a single F_0. This intentional wobble, when well performed, can offer the illusion of separately sung alternating notes either a step or a half-step apart. In all but the fastest tempi, most singers take the time to actually sing the first two or three pitches that constitute the signature notes of a trill. This setup of the illusion causes listeners to imagine that they are hearing the separate pitches of the trill as the vibrato is widened.

It is ironic that a vocal "fault" in VExtent normally requiring intervention in the voice studio, can be exploited to produce vocal fireworks in the form of trill-based ornaments.

The illusion of the trill can be clearly seen on the spectrogram shown in Figure 11–10.

Since the rate and extent of the vibrato are so clearly revealed, most singers can quickly grasp the technique once they see a good example of the trill on the monitor (pay particular attention to the upper harmonic tracings that reveal fluctuations in the F_0).

A SUPPORT PROBLEM: "SUMMIT–ITIS"

Earlier chapters have already in dealt with issues regarding support, principally in discussions of vowel onset and exit in Chapter 7, and stop-consonant production in Chapter 9.

There is yet another subtle support problem that may appear in a singer's technique during the observation of spectrographic VRTF. The problem might be called "summit-itis" and is one of the most common problems encountered as singers make forays into their high voice. This problem is similar to that discussed in Chapter 7, the collapse of the vocal instrument during vowel exits. One may encounter two variants of the "summit-itis" phenomenon:

• acute loss of support at the end of a high note going into a rest, and
• after ascending to a high note, the singer may abdicate his or her support on the

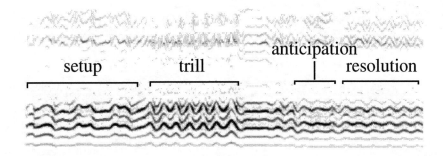

Figure 11–10. Spectrogram of a vocal trill. Note the three deliberate initial pitches used to set up the trill, then the widening of the vibrato extent to create the illusion of rapidly alternating pitches, and the final anticipation-resolution. 💿

way down, sometimes even before leaving the top note, thereby losing the quality of the production on the very notes that were performed beautifully on the way up.

Figure 11–11 shows such an event. The image at the top of the figure is a normally performed passage that is well supported both leading into and out of the highest note. The bottom image, however, clearly reveals the result of a premature lessening of support. It is almost as if the singer thinks, "We made it! Now relax." When this relaxation happens, the voice may "break" in the case of the single high note going into a rest, or tighten during the descending part of the passage, as shown in the illustration.

As more experience is gained with spectrographic VRTF in the future, other indicators of hypo- or hyper-support may be found.

INHALATION PROBLEMS

Proper breathing is always a primary concern in any voice studio. While proper inhalation involves the correct use of the musculature from the pelvic floor to the larynx and beyond, many problems that result in restrictive breath intake occur in the mouth and pharynx and glottis. Since

air stream turbulence, no matter where or how it is created, can appear on the spectrogram as noise, the computer can be used as feedback to help foster correct breathing habits.

Oral Constriction

A good breath for singing should begin with the oral and pharyngeal structures as much out of the way of the incoming airflow as possible. This goal gave rise to the admonition used in the Drew University studio/lab, "Breathe in the vowel you need." In other words, the singer should strive for quiet inhalations by opening the resonance structures as if a good vowel were already in progress. This vowel-like openness will reduce turbulence and result in a more efficient inhalation. To use the spectrograph in this way, the microphone must be placed extremely close to the lips at the centerline of the mouth.

The turbulence produced by insufficient openness occurs in three general areas:

- insufficiently opened mouth (turbulence being produced at the lips)
- constriction at the posterior portion of the oral cavity and the adjoining oropharynx
- reduced glottal aperture.

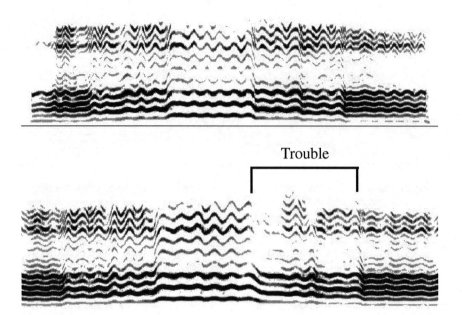

Figure 11–11. An arpeggio going up through the passaggio into the high voice and back. The spectrogram on the top shows the support applied equally during both the ascending and descending portions of the passage. The image on the bottom shows the result of the premature release of support. **CD**

The spectrographic images of these three types are shown in Figure 11–12. Each produces a noise that is centered in its own pitch area on the aural spectrum. By utilizing this feedback, the voice practitioner can offer more precise instructions to the singer in the pursuit open inhalation.

One must experiment with the lip-to-microphone distance to ensure that the passing air stream of a well-executed breath streaming directly by the microphone does not induce turbulence of its own and thus create a false result on the monitor.

It should be noted that when the spectrogram is used for this function, it cannot be used simultaneously for diagnosis and correction of other vocal faults. With the microphone placed so close to the mouth, the resulting analytical image will most likely be distorted.

Nose Breathing

Occasionally, one encounters a singer who has been taught to inhale exclusively through the nose instead of the mouth. The rationale usually given by such teachers, is that breathing through the mouth "dries the mouth and throat." Contrary to their opinion, a proper singing breath produced with optimally open oral, pharyngeal, and glottal spaces should actually produce *minimal* drying of the throat. A breath taken through the nose will almost certainly result in an insufficient volume of air for most sung phrases and should be avoided as normal singing technique.

If one encounters the habit of nose inhalation, Gram can help. By placing the microphone immediately in front of one of the subject's nostrils, the passing air stream will create turbulence around the microphone during the singer's desperate attempt to get enough air for the next phrase. This feedback technique actually creates turbulence by the interaction of the air stream passing between the microphone and the nasal port (not as in the case of improper inhalation through the

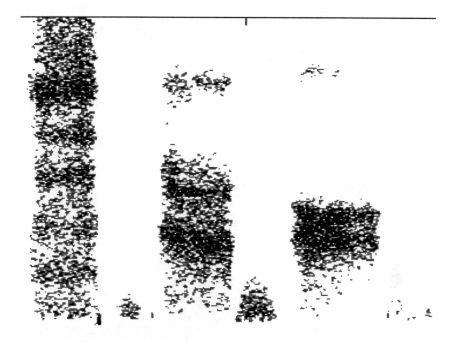

Figure 11–12. Spectrogram of orally created breath turbulence. The images (left to right) show the results of labial constriction, elevated tongue near the velum with tightness in the oropharynx, and an overly tight glottis. **CD**

mouth where the turbulence is created at some site in the vocal instrument). The resulting noise will appear as an aperiodic pattern on the spectrographic display. Its presence can be used as evidence that the inhalation is being made through the nose and not the mouth (Figure 11–13).

GLOTTAL STOP AND STROKE

A glottal onset features a full closure of the glottis as an articulative device at the initiation of a vowel. A perusal of the literature regarding glottal onset written by singers and teachers of singing reveals a significant divergence of opinion. The use of the terminology is not universal. There is no consensus on the question of whether such articulations should be used at all, and if they are to be employed, when and how.

To try to garner usable information amid the confusion, consider some facts that most

theoreticians would probably agree on regarding this type of onset.

- Glottal onsets are, as the name suggests, made at the glottis.
- Such onsets feature a full closure of the glottis before the first phonatory cycle.

One type of glottal onset is often called the **glottal stroke**. It involves a closure of the glottis at the beginning of phonation that involves a minor buildup of subglottal pressure. This type of onset is used to clarify diction in many languages. It is employed so subtly in English that native speakers use it hundreds of times a day without realizing it.

The other glottal onset type is much more active and is commonly called the **glottal stop**. This onset involves the buildup of substantial subglottal pressure which is then released to initiate phonation. Either of these definitions could place glottal onsets squarely within the definition of a stop consonant.

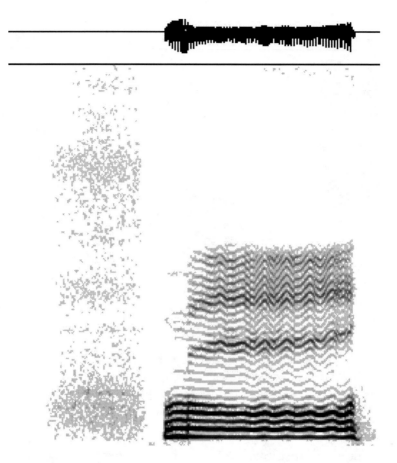

Figure 11–13. Spectrogram of a "nose" breath prior to phonation. ⓒⅅ

The glottal stop is actually a strong plosive and can be harmful to the voice. As such, it is justifiably prohibited in most pedagogical traditions. The prohibition against the glottal stop is so strict, however, that many voice practitioners have lost sight of the desirability of the glottal stroke as an acceptable and safe linguistic device.

Garcia's "Coup de la Glotte"

Manuel Garcia, the eminent 19th-century voice teacher, theoretician, and the inventor of the laryngoscope made a very clear distinction between these two types of onset.

Garcia (1984) defined *coup de la glotte* as "the neat articulation of the glottis that gives a precise and clean attack to the sound." Furthermore he wrote:

one must guard against confusing the stroke of the glottis with the stroke of the chest (*coup de poitrine*) which resembles a cough, or the effort of expelling something which is obstructing the throat. The stroke of the chest causes the loss of a large portion of the breath, and it makes the voice sound aspirated, stifled, and uncertain in intonation. The chest has no other function that to nourish the tones with air, and it should not push them or shock them. (Garcia, 1984, part one, p. 42)

As an example of the problems caused by the ambiguity of many commonly used vocal terms, this term ranks among the best. Problems with Garcia's clear distinction between *coup de glotte* and *coup de poitrine* began with later teachers, especially his star pupil, Mathilde Marchesi (1970). Marchesi seems to have permuted the meaning of *coup de la glotte* to mean a glottal stop. Even in our own time, Vennard (1967) cautions against the usage of the term glottal stroke, even though favorable references to this type of onset appear throughout his book. He seems to advocate the avoidance of the usage of any reference to a closure of the glottis as an onset articulation for fear of appearing to advocate the potentially harmful glottal stop.

Instead of avoiding all reference to glottal articulations, why not use the term glottal stroke as an acceptable description of a needed facet of vocal technique? Why not educate singers to recognize the difference between it and the potentially damaging glottal stop (or plosive).

Glottal Stop

The glottal stop onset is indicated by the IPA symbol /ʔ/ and can be approximated in English with the definite negative expression "uh-uh!" (written in IPA, ʔʌʔʌ). Figure 11–14 shows a glottal stop on the far left. Notice the amount of time it takes for phonation to settle (signified by the beginning of a regular vibrato pattern). It takes almost twice as long for phonation to settle than it does in the remaining two images of this figure.

As noted before, most teachers and clinicians wisely advise their subjects to avoid the glottal stop as it can be a major contributing factor in vocal injury (including the development of nodules). See CD Video 11–1 to view the action of a glottal stop.

Glottal Stroke

Vocal practitioners must remember that a glottal stroke is a far gentler, less disruptive momentary articulative closure of the vocal folds. Garcia calls for the "*delicate action of the lips,*" meaning a momentary light touch of the vocal folds and not the explosive release of high pressure air resulting from the full glottal stop.

The middle spectrogram in Figure 11–14 shows a little noise energy at the onset but the larynx quickly settles (taking 629 ms instead of the 801 ms needed for the glottal stop shown on the left). One can also easily see the difference in energy employed in these two articulations in the waveform at the top of the image.

The spectrogram on the right side of Figure 11–14 is an ASAI onset that shows even less time needed before stable phonation commences (405 ms). Video CD 11–2 shows the larynx performing an ASAI onset. (More information on ASAI can be found in Chapter 8.)

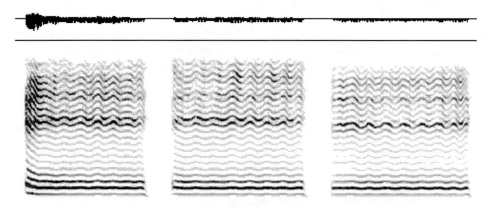

Figure 11–14. Three onsets: glottal stop (left), glottal stroke (middle), and ASAI (right). CD

Proposed IPA Symbols to Differentiate Between Glottal Stroke and Stop

To make the difference between the two degrees of articulation of this "consonant" when transliterating texts in IPA, the author proposes that the regular symbol for the glottal stop /ʔ/ be retained, and that the same symbol, printed in superscript / ʔ/, be reserved for the glottal stroke.

Glottal Stroke Usage

Many speakers of English use the glottal stroke as a means to differentiate a word-final vowel from a word-initial vowel. Consider the phrase "I answered." It is most often articulated as, /ai ʔænsɚd/. Without the glottal stroke between the two words, the listener might perceive the phrase as run-together, /ʔʌⁱænsɚd/.

The glottal stroke is also used in speech to differentiate the final stop consonant of one word from the initial vowel of the next, that is, "some ice" should be pronounced as /sʌmʔaⁱs/; without the glottal stroke it may be heard as "some mice" /sʌmaⁱs/ (Reid). Video 🄲🄳 11–3 clearly illustrates the difference in laryngeal action required for these two thoughts.

The glottal stroke should be used for clarity of diction in singing as well. In fact, the glottal stroke may take on greater importance in singing diction because of the singer's need to elongate and enrich the vowels. As long as both the teacher and the student are careful about the *degree* of articulation, no vocal harm should result from the use of the glottal stroke.

Voice practitioners should take care when reading the literature on this subject since the definitions for the two types of glottal onset are reversed in some writings about the voice. In those texts the glottal stroke becomes the more energetic and potentially dangerous act signified by the two terms. This makes no sense as the meaning of the word stroke would seem to carry less force than the word stop.

Dealing with glottal stops and strokes is an absolute requirement for both the teacher and the singer. Vocal practitioners must always keep the difference between the two onsets in mind; one can produce clarity of diction in a language for which such use is idiomatic while the other can cause vocal harm.

OTHER POSSIBLE USES FOR THE SPECTROGRAM

While the primary audience for this book will probably be voice practitioners, the type of intensive feedback utilizing the spectrogram being advocated here may be useful in some nonsinging fields as well.

Aiding in Accent Remediation

If one stops to think about it, the act of teaching singing is deeply involved with accent remediation whether it is the "correction" of the influence of a regional dialect or the effect of a native language on a foreign one. There are many phonetic idiosyncrasies that must be corrected on the journey to a fine singing technique.

It is not a great leap from the uses of the spectrograph that have been discussed thus far to the idea that the spectrograph could be used in the speech field to help alter regional dialects or accents. The same is true for its use in the learning of foreign languages. In the theater, the contrary is also true; the spectrogram could be used to help actors *create* a specific regional dialect or accent for a character role on the stage.

An unwanted accent, language-to-language, shares many of the same problems that occur dialect-to-dialect within a language. Needed remedial alterations may involve any or all of the following:

Vowels

- Shifts in vowel "color"
- Vowel substitution

- Vowel omissions
- Diphthong problems
- Missing secondary vowels
- Unnecessary secondary vowels

Consonants

- Shifts in consonant production (such as the use of an English stop /t/ in a language such as Italian where such a plosive spike is unidiomatic)
- Consonant substitution
- Consonant omission

This is, by no means, a complete list of the type of dialectal problems that can be seen and corrected by use of spectrographic RTF. The subject of accent modification is well covered in the speech literature and should be studied by every voice practitioner.

This view of the use of the spectrograph is not meant as a call to arms for teachers of singing to suddenly branch out into the accent-modification field. That field involves knowledge of speech phonetics, language, and technique that the field's practitioners acquire through years of intense study. These paragraphs are only meant to create an atmosphere of thought in which both singing and speech practitioners can share a dialog concerning concepts and methods.

Is the Spectrogram Under Utilized in the Speech Field?

The use of the spectrograph in speech is more problematic. Voice practitioners dealing with the singing voice have a distinct advantage because vowels in singing are, for the most part, performed for much longer periods of time than those in speech. It is, therefore, easier to locate and correct problems in a singer's production.

Having stated that, could speech therapists use more of the micro techniques presented in this text as part of their therapy arsenal? The reader is urged to read Robert Volin's chapter in this book for an overview of some of the possibilities.

SUMMARY

The discovery of nonphonemic uses of the spectrogram is just beginning. As the spectrogram is intensively used in day-to-day voice studio operations, one can expect that more uses will be found and shared in the future.

12

THE USE OF SPECTRUM ANALYSIS IN THE VOICE STUDIO

Donald Miller and Harm K. Schutte

In the interest of quickly getting to the practical application of feedback in singing instruction, the technical explanation of the signals will be kept to a minimum in this and the following chapter. It is assumed that those using the practical applications will, as curiosity prompts, expand their technical understanding of the signals by consulting other chapters in this book.

SIGNAL AND DISPLAY

The Power Spectrum

A typical power spectrum of a musical sound, such as that in Figure 12–1 (top), displays the complex components of the sound. These appear as a series of harmonics, each of which has a specific frequency. For the purposes of this text the display typically extends from a baseline of zero on the left edge to 5000 hertz (Hz; cycles per second) on the right. The first harmonic (H_1, or the fundamental frequency) is at 440 Hz; all higher harmonics are at multiples of that frequency, as is the case with all complex sounds that are harmonic (have a definite pitch). The relative intensity of each component is indicated in the vertical dimension, which in this case displays a range of 60 decibels (each vertical division equals 10 dB).

The configuration of the harmonics, each with its individual intensity, gives a visual equivalent of the sound quality. It is through the inspection and comparison of such visual displays that one may gain

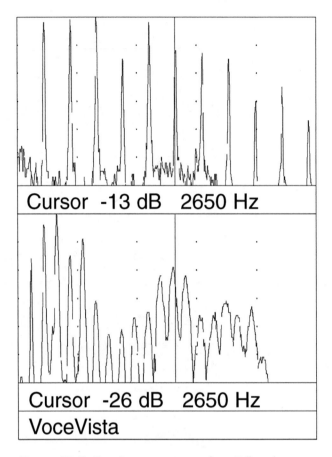

Figure 12–1. Top: Power spectrum of an E-flat alto saxophone sounding A^4 (440 Hz). Bottom: Power spectrum of a bass singing vowel /ɑ/ one octave lower at A^3 (220 Hz). The usual display is from 0 to 5000 Hz horizontally, with markers at each 1000 Hz. Vertical markers indicate differences of 10 decibels. The cursor is placed in the region of the singer's formant, here the 12th harmonic of the bass, corresponding to the 6th harmonic of the saxophone. Note the flatter declination in the spectrum of the saxophone toward the higher frequencies, as well as the wider-appearing harmonics of the bass, the consequence of frequency fluctuation in vibrato. **CD** 12-1a (top), 12-1b (bottom).

more insight into the sounds the ears hear. Important dimensions of sound not present in the power spectrum are time and the intensity of the complex sound as a whole. While intensity is partially reflected in quality (or timbre) of sound, the time dimension figures in the power spectrum only as the "slice" of time (the "time window") which is averaged for a given display. For analyzing sustained vowel sound (the sound that receives the most attention from singing teachers), the

time window is typically set for 200 milliseconds (0.2 sec). This averaged amount covers a single vibrato cycle, integrating all the changes in sound that occur within it. For more detailed segments of time, as well as for averaging longer stretches, the time window can be set to cover a shorter or longer segment.

An enormous amount of information is contained in a single power spectrum—far more than the singing teacher can utilize in a practical way. The practical value of the information only becomes apparent in comparing two spectra, because the differences between two spectra are far easier to identify and analyze than is the spectrum as a whole. This sort of analysis, easily provided by the VoceVista program, will be the basic modus operandi in the use of feedback for the voice studio.

Voice practitioners will find it useful to have the two spectra available for easy visual comparison, either by overlay of one onto the other, or by a split display with a single cursor extending vertically through both. Figure 12–1 is an example of the second type, comparing an /a/ vowel sung at 220 Hz by a bass (bottom) to the saxophone tone an octave higher (top). For examples of the overlay, see Figures 12–5 through 12–9.

Most of the figures in this chapter are made with the VoceVista program. The Gram program provides similar displays of individual spectra, both in real-time and "frozen" for close inspection, but it lacks the facility for easy comparison.

Harmonics and Formants

Sounds with pitch produce spectra consisting of a series of harmonics—labeled H_1, H_2, and so on—the frequencies of which are multiples of the fundamental. The intensity level of these harmonics, as they emerge from the vocal folds, diminishes regularly with increasing harmonic number. What causes the highly varying intensities of the harmonic components, the acoustic result of which is a particular quality of sound that reaches the ear?

The simplified answer to this is that the resonator of any musical instrument, including the voice, favors some harmonics while damping others. In the human voice, this source is in the vocal folds, which vibrate (open and close) at rates anywhere from about 60 to 1,200 times per second in singing. The resonator, which selects certain harmonics for amplification, is the vocal tract—the partially enclosed air space between the

vocal folds at one end and the openings at the lips and nostrils at the other. This complex resonator has a series of variable resonances, called formants, numbered from the lowest in frequency (formants are identified as Fx, x being the number of the formant). The first five of these are of practical consequence to sung sound. The first two, F_1 and F_2, are highly and precisely variable. In speech, the human brain recognizes specific vowels based on the relative frequencies of these formants. F_3, F_4, and F_5 are important in the production of a certain desirable high-frequency component that is characteristic of the quality singing voice.

Basic Information Concerning Resonances of the Vocal Tract

Traditional discussion of vowels and resonance in singing pedagogy is largely "unscientific," having developed without the benefit of advanced technology for the measurement of vocal sound. It is therefore useful to review some basic facts concerning the contribution of the vocal tract to the sung sound. The interpretation of spectra can be greatly advanced when the user is familiar with how the formants work together to produce and modify the various vowels, as well as to create the sounds that singers identify as "resonant."

Formants and Vowels

The relative frequencies of the first two formants, which account for most of the resonating power of the vocal tract, determine the vowel that listeners hear. Singers should understand the factors that influence formant frequencies as they cope with the twin tasks of producing clear vowels and modifying these to enhance resonance. One can place eight basic vowels in a schema that plots F_1 against F_2, and the result is a quadrilateral (Figure 12–2). These eight vowels can be divided into two series of four:

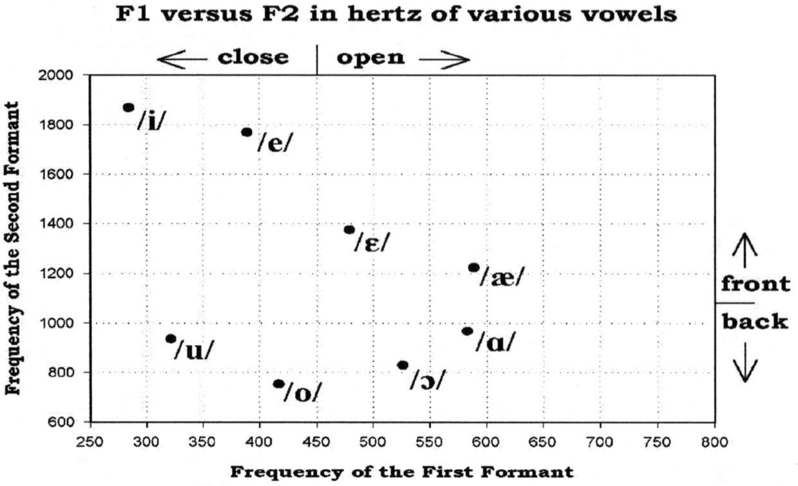

F1 versus F2 in hertz of various vowels

Figure 12–2. Schema of eight vowels, according to formant frequencies, in a plot of F_2 against F_1, measured at ca. 150 Hz in the author's (DM's) singing voice. The vowel dimensions "close" and "open" correspond to F_1 values, while "front" and "back" correspond to F_2 values. In the front series F_2 falls as F_1 rises. In the back series the variations in F_2 are much smaller. ⓒ 12-2a = Back vowels; 12-2b = Front vowels. Note that each vowel spectrum is followed by the same vowel performed using the Vocal Fry method (explained on pp. 193 and 194).

- front vowels, /i/e/ɛ/æ/, so called because the mass of the tongue is fronted,
- back vowels, /u/o/ɔ/ɑ/, in which the degree of lip-rounding plays a key role.

Both the front and back groups are characterized by a close-to-open dimension, reflecting the frequency of the first formant. Each group is given above in the order from close to open.

In moving through the front vowel series from close to open, one can feel the tongue constriction moving steadily backward, as it simultaneously becomes wider. Seen in terms of formant frequencies, the front series is characterized by a relatively high second formant and by the fact that in the front series an increase in one formant implies a decrease in the other.

Going from open to close through the back series, one is most aware of the increase in lip-rounding, accompanied by a less noticeable forward movement of the tongue constriction. With real-time spectrum analysis, it is possible to watch the effects on the formants as one goes

through the vowel series, moving first discretely and then continuously from one vowel to another. Likewise, one can experiment with lip-rounding or with changing the tongue constriction, jaw opening, and larynx height, while following the effects of these movements on the formant frequencies. Of course, all of these effects are at the same time modifications of the vowel sounds. (Other vowels can be analyzed as well, such as the front-rounded series /y/ø/œ/ found in French and German.)

The Higher Formants

The deliberate adjustment (whether conscious or not) of a formant to enhance a particular harmonic of the singing voice occurs almost exclusively with the first two formants. Nevertheless, the higher formants, F_3 through F_5, are also important. Spectrum analysis provides insight on higher formants as well.

The singer's formant, so called because it appears notably in the classically trained singing voice, is a strong high-frequency component, audible as a sort of "ringing." It appears in the spectrum as one or more high-level harmonics in the range 2.3 to 3.3 kHz, strongly enhanced by resonance(s) of the vocal tract. Spectrum analysis reveals that the strength of this resonance is the result of a particular approximation of two of the higher formants to one another. This produces a more powerful and broader composite resonance than a single formant could have in this frequency range. Better quality male voices, especially the basses and baritones, usually show an approximation of F_3 and F_4; an isolated F_3, separated by more than 500 Hz from the closest neighboring formant, is a typical characteristic of voices of lesser quality.

Identifying Formants in the Power Spectrum

Because the voice source and the resonator/vocal tract are largely independent of one another, they are often varied simultaneously. This makes the task of identifying and keeping track of harmonics and formants in spectrum analysis rather difficult for the beginner. (To acquire a feel for this double movement, it is recommended that the beginner experiment with first singing a constant vowel [resonator] and varying pitch [voice source], and then keeping pitch constant while varying the vowel, before going on to varying both together.)

The situation is further complicated by the fact that sound only appears in the spectrum at the frequencies of the harmonics. Relatively high intensity in a given harmonic (for example, H_3 in Figure 12–1, bottom) leads us to expect (correctly) a formant in the vicinity, but the center frequency of that formant cannot be precisely ascertained from the line (harmonic) spectrum. This problem is greatly aggravated in singing as pitch rises, and with it the distance between harmonics.

The sound that emerges from the singer's mouth is that of the voice source as processed by the resonances of the vocal tract. The proximity of a formant to one of the harmonics of the source can be crucial for both the size and beauty of a sung tone. There is a basic problem in using feedback from the power spectrum to achieve this desired proximity, however: As the pitch goes higher (and the stakes rise as the sound becomes more conspicuous to the public), the increased distance between harmonics raises the odds that a given formant will fall ineffectively into a gap between harmonics, where there is no sound to amplify. The sound literally loses resonance. At the same time, the increased distance between harmonics makes it more difficult to guess the location of the formants from the spectrum. The singer would like to know where his or her formants are located in order to align them better with the harmonics, that is, to use resonance more effectively.

Some computer programs with spectrum analysis offer an automatic computation of formant frequencies of voiced sounds based on linear predictive coding (LPC). Such programs function reasonably well at lower speech frequencies, in which approximate formant frequencies are also apparent in the harmonic spectrum. They become quite unreliable at about 350 Hz (first-line F in the treble staff), however. At much higher pitches, they are worse than useless because they falsely identify every harmonic as a formant.

Automatic programs are of little help in locating formants for the singing voice, but with practice, the user of this type of feedback can learn to determine formant frequencies with a practical precision.

Practical Technique for Determining Formants

Utilizing Vocal Fry

When the vocal folds are pressed lightly together and small quantities of air are allowed to "bubble" through the closed glottis, the resulting popping sound is called vocal fry. (It is also possible to produce a similar, but louder, sound by pulling the bubbles in the reverse direction through the glottis. The examples on the CD include both these methods for producing a continuous spectrum.)

Because vocal fry is nonperiodic—having unsteady or no fundamental frequency—it produces a continuous spectrum, with sound at all frequencies. From such a spectrum, it is possible to read with sufficient accuracy the frequencies of at least the first two formants, which generally carry the burden of the resonance. By directly comparing the spectra of the sung tone and its vocal-fry imitation, the singer can gain insight into how effectively the formants are used in that particular combination of vowel, pitch, and loudness (Figure 12–3, top and bottom).

Because the vocal fry spectrum shows the formants of a postural imitation of the sung tone, rather than of the tone itself, the user must be aware of the considerable possibility of error. Fortunately, direct comparison makes it possible to get a quick impression of the plausible correctness of a given imitation, aiding the learning process in the use of vocal fry.

Using Vocal Fry To Determine Formants

To see this technique in action, singers may try the following:

- Sing a sustained note on a specific vowel and pitch.
- Once the note is sounding, freeze the vocal articulators in that precise vowel position.
- Cease phonation while holding the articulator set used for singing the note.
- Initiate vocal fry while maintaining the set of the articulators for the vowel.

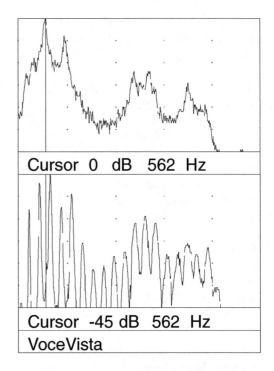

Figure 12–3. Top: Continuous spectrum of vocal fry (see text) with vocal tract maintained in the posture of the vowel and pitch of the bottom panel. Bottom: A bass singing /ɑ/, A^3 (same as Figure 12-1, bottom). The vertical cursor is placed at the peak indicating the first formant in the vocal-fry spectrum. This allows accurate reading of the location of the formant in the line (harmonic) spectrum. (The CD contains an additional example in which the singer alternates, without pausing, between a sung tone and vocal fry while maintaining a constant vocal tract.) 💿

On the screen the singer will see a continuous spectrum (without harmonic structure), having peaks at the frequencies where the formants are located.

It is suggested that the singer begin with relatively low pitches and nonextreme postures to acquire routine in the procedure before going on to the more difficult task of determining the formant frequencies of critical high notes.

RESONANCE STRATEGIES: EFFECTIVE ADJUSTMENT OF FORMANT FREQUENCIES

With the exception of voice literature that can be freely transposed, the composer prescribes the pitches the classical singer must sing. This means that all the other harmonics above the fundamental are predetermined as well. If the skillful singer is going to improve the alignment of formants and harmonics, the adjustment clearly must take place in the formants.

The composer constrains the formants as well by prescribing the vowel that must be sung on a given pitch. Still, a certain amount of "cheating" on the part of the singer is permitted, and even expected, in vowel (and thus formant) production. Particularly in the more difficult upper range, accomplished singers tend to adopt strategies both to avoid undesirable resonance effects and to enhance the production of notes where the "sound" of the voice is critically on display. The following paragraphs discuss some of the more common and useful of these strategies and the way in which spectrum analysis can help singers both to acquire them and to make them more effective.

Adjustment of the formants (and thus of the vowel) to achieve a desired resonance effect will be referred to as **formant tuning**. This can take several forms, the most common of which are:

- moving a single formant to coincide with, or approach, an individual harmonic and

- moving two adjacent formants close together to enhance any harmonic falling between them.

Cover in Male Passaggio

The management of the passaggio is one of the problems that arises early in the training of male voices and persists into professional practice as an item requiring careful attention and sometimes adjustment. This term refers to the approach, from the upper notes of what is usually called chest register, into the upper extension of the voice, often called the "full head" register. The passaggio is located in the note (or notes) where the voice "turns over," to use typical singers' jargon. In a textbook case, the tenor will have accomplished passaggio and arrived at the upper extension by the pitch G^4 (392 Hz), or at the latest, a semitone higher. Baritones and basses have correspondingly lower points of passaggio.[1]

The "Instinctive" Approach to the Top Voice: The Shout

The crucial point in a correct execution of passaggio is to avoid pushing the chest register beyond its natural limits by means of a forced, "shouty" production. This tendency, natural in most untrained voices, appears as a compulsion to tune the first formant to the second harmonic of the voice source in the attempt to extend the chest register upward. Singing

---

[1]Like many terms in singers' jargon, passaggio is not always consistently defined. It can be seen either as the note where the register change is accomplished (the "point of passaggio" here) or a series of notes in the transition between registers. In the latter case, the lower limit, where the singer enters the *zona di passaggio*, is called primo passaggio, and the upper limit is called secondo passaggio. This applies to the male voice. The female case is complicated by the fact that there are two major transitions, one where the middle register succeeds the chest register, and the other, described in detail in the text, approximately an octave higher than male passaggio.

teachers recognize this phenomenon in the undesirable raising of the larynx when approaching the upper range. As one discovers easily using feedback from spectrum analysis, raising the larynx (and thus shortening the vocal tract) increases the frequency of F_1. The larynx raising is thus a maneuver of last resort to get the first formant higher in order to add a semitone or two to the chest register. Voice practitioners describe the resulting vowel as too "open" (openness is the characteristic of high-F_1 vowels).

Spectrum analysis can confirm this description of the production of shouty high notes. The typical high note which is "forced" in this way has a second harmonic with a level 15 to 25 dB higher than the first harmonic. The vocal-fry imitation of the vocal tract when singing such a note (be sure the larynx stays in place!) shows a characteristic hyperextended F_1, tuned to H_2 (Figure 12–4).

The Trained Approach To the Top: "Cover"

The first essential in the solution to this problem of vocal technique is learning to resist the tendency to raise the larynx. A correct passaggio tone is shown in Figure 12–5. As can be seen from the vocal-fry imitation, F_1 has fallen below H_2, and this harmonic has consequently lost its dominant position in the spectrum. It has been suggested that the resultant production, with F_1 lower than H_2 and no longer dominant, be called, by definition, "covered" (Miller & Schutte, 1994). Note that the "darkening" of the sound need not involve an artificial lowering of F_1: The artificial lowering may take place, but it may also be sufficient that the singer refrain from raising F_1. This maneuver, incidentally, is an example of the avoidance of formant tuning.

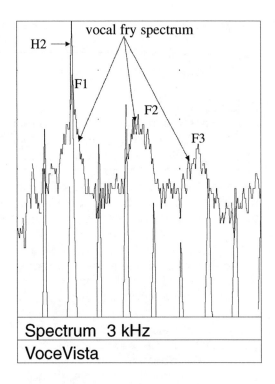

Figure 12–4. Bass singing "open" E^4 (330 Hz) on vowel /ɛ/, with overlay of vocal fry spectrum. F_1 is tuned to H_2, giving this harmonic a level of more than 20 dB above the others. F_2 and F_3, the smaller peaks in the continuous spectrum, fall between the harmonics. Note that the display has been reduced to 3000 Hz in order to show more clearly the relationships between formants and harmonics. 🔵

Finding a Different Resonance

One reason for the strong tendency to tune F_1 to H_2 on high notes in the chest register is that the resulting resonance is quite powerful. "Covering" necessarily implies a considerable loss of resonance from the first formant. A compensatory adjustment for this loss that most accomplished (opera) singers employ is the tuning of F_2 to a higher harmonic. At the point of passaggio this higher harmonic is H_3 in

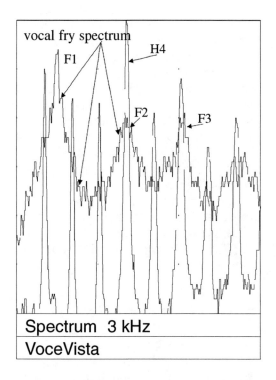

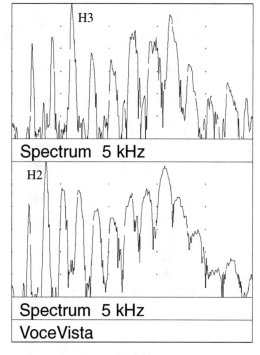

Figure 12-5. Bass singing "covered" E^4 (330 Hz) on vowel /ɛ/, with overlay of vocal-fry spectrum. F$_1$ falls between the first two harmonics, reducing the power of that resonance. F$_2$ is tuned to H$_4$, making this harmonic dominant. H$_6$, coinciding with F$_3$, is also enhanced. Note reduced frequency display. **CD**

Figure 12-6. Tenor passaggio. Top: Tenor singing vowel /ɑ/ on A^4-flat, with dominant F$_2$ resonance. Bottom: The same singer on the pitch F^4, where H$_2$, resonated by F$_1$, is dominant among the lower spectral elements, where the "vowel formants" (F$_1$ and F$_2$) are located. **CD** (Top window)

the case of a back vowel (/ɑ/ and /ɔ/) and H$_4$ in a front vowel (/ɛ/ and /e/). Figure 12-6, which illustrates the covered execution of passaggio, also shows this compensation for the loss of F$_1$ resonance. Although the tuning of F$_2$ in the upper extension of the range may occur naturally in some voices, it is more expedient to regard this, like cover itself, as an artificial adjustment of the vocal tract requiring practice.

Practical Hints

The ideal result in the teaching of cover includes not only the avoidance of the elevated larynx, but also learning the strategy of using F2 or the singer's formant. Such strategies not only keep the voice adequately bright and resonant, but also help to avoid an excessively lowered larynx. Finding F2 resonance will, in most cases, simultaneously overcome the compulsion to follow H2 with F1 (the shout). The approach through front

(continued)

vowels, with their higher second formants, often provides a breakthrough in finding the feel of F_2 tuning. For finer tuning of F_2, try varying the vowel in the direction of another vowel with a higher or lower second formant while watching the feedback in real-time. F_2 of the vowel /ɑ/ will rise for /æ/ and drop for /ɔ/, for example.

Female Passaggio and the "Back Strategy" in the Upper Voice

In the upper notes of the female "head" register (or falsetto—see Chapter 13 under Electroglottogram: Laryngeal Registers) there is a strong tendency for F_1 to follow H_1, or the fundamental frequency. Anyone seeking to make a full and resonant sound in falsetto will naturally gravitate toward this powerful resonance adjustment. It is small wonder that F_1–H_1 tuning in falsetto was the first type of formant tuning described in the scientific literature (Sundberg, 1977).

Classically trained female singers can carry this tuning all the way down to about D^4 (292 Hz) in the close vowels (/i/ and /u/). At the other end of what is usually called the middle register—from about F^5, where F_1 of the open vowels, when sufficiently "darkened," coincides with the fundamental (700 Hz)—the attraction of F_1 for H_1 is such that it occurs in all the vowels, whatever their normal first formants may be in speech. This generally recognized fact helps explain the lack of text intelligibility in the female high range.

The most salient difference between the male and the female voice is that of nearly an octave in frequency range, the result of the characteristic growth of the male larynx and vocal folds during puberty. Differences in formant frequencies, which reflect primarily the dimensions of the vocal tract, are much smaller. This basic similarity in resonance often makes it possible for the soprano and tenor to sing an octave apart, but with a resonance strategy involving a common formant. The similarity in resonance is not exact, however, and there are important parts of the range where male and female go their separate ways. One of these is the approach to the upper extension of the voice, occurring around F^4 (350 Hz) and F^5 (700 Hz) in the respective male and female cases.

A Typical Transition Strategy

Consider how a typical Italianate soprano manages her formants in singing through the fifth D^5–A^5. During this process an adjustment takes place which is analogous to the one discussed above, made an octave lower by the tenor. A series of figures below compares the harmonic spectrum of a sung /ɑ/ with its "imitation," produced with a vocal fry voice source. On the D^5 (Figure 12–7), our soprano is still in her middle register.[2] The first formant of this open vowel is higher than the fundamental frequency, and F_2 is close to H_2, contributing a strong resonance on that harmonic as well. By the time she reaches F^5 (Figure 12–8), however, H_1 has reached the frequency of F_1 (700 Hz) and now assumes the role of the carrier of the dominant resonance. The second harmonic, an octave higher, has moved beyond the reach of F_2. Thus, the balance between the first two harmonics undergoes a major shift in moving through the three semitones between D and F. On the G^5 (Figure 12–9) the first harmonic is even more

---

[2]As used in this chapter and the one following, the term middle register covers the range from the lowest pitches sung with a "falsetto" laryngeal adjustment up to the point where the fundamental frequency is equal to the first formant of an open vowel.

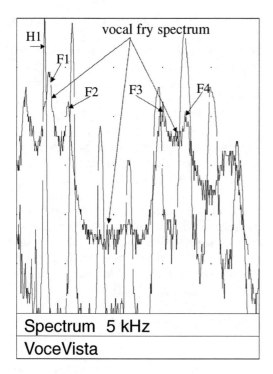

Spectrum 5 kHz
VoceVista

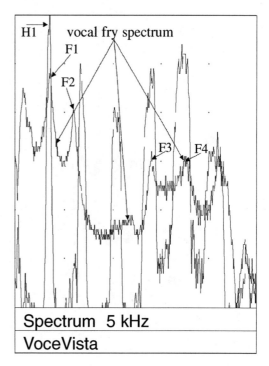

Spectrum 5 kHz
VoceVista

Figure 12–7. Soprano singing vowel /ɑ/ on D⁵, with overlay of vocal-fry spectrum. The fundamental frequency (H_1) is about 100 Hz below the first formant, and the first two harmonics are almost equally strong. F_3 and F_4 are positioned close to one another, creating the singer's formant. The first (low-frequency) peak in the continuous spectrum is not a vowel formant and has no effect on the harmonic spectrum. 🔴

Figure 12–8. Soprano singing vowel /ɑ/ on F⁵, with overlay of vocal-fry spectrum. F_1 and H_1 coincide, and F_2 draws away from H_2. The result is that H_1 is now 10 dB stronger than H_2. 🔴

registers is then run through stepwise from above (the easier direction) and only later in the opposite direction.

dominant, as F_1 follows H_1, and F_2 falls more into the position of supporting F_1.

Practical Hint

The resonant vocal tract of the upper voice, with F_2 closing on and supporting F_1, is usually easier to find by a light, direct onset with the vowel /ɔ/ on F⁵ or F⁵-sharp than by approaching stepwise from the middle register. The first formant of an open /ɔ/ typically tunes easily to these pitches, and the singer learns the feel of effortless resonance. Passaggio between the middle and upper

Larynx Elevation

Unlike the male strategy in passaggio, the female approach to the upper range accepts the raising of F_1 as it follows H_1 higher in pitch. The anatomy and physiology of the female vocal tract is such that it can accommodate a rising larynx without producing an unacceptable sound.

This is not to argue that it is incorrect to teach the "low larynx" in the case of sopranos. In the first place, the low larynx is possible throughout the middle range. In addition, the striving for a low larynx in the upper range may have a beneficial

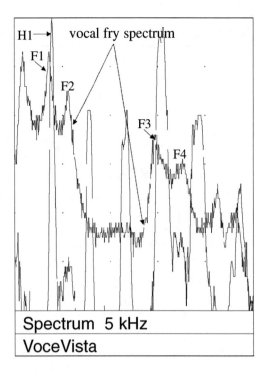

Spectrum 5 kHz

VoceVista

Figure 12–9. Soprano singing vowel /ɑ/ on G^5, with overlay of vocal fry spectrum. F$_1$ follows H$_1$ as this ascends, and F$_2$ draws still closer to F$_1$, contributing to the enhancement of H$_1$, which is now quite dominant in the region of the vowel formants. 🔘

effect, even if some elevation of the larynx is inevitable.

Rationale of the Back Strategy

The "back strategy" presented here has the following rationale: For an open back vowel (/ɑ/ or /ɔ/), from the pitch F^5 (top line, treble staff), where H$_1$ reaches the frequency of F$_1$, the second harmonic, at 1400 Hz, moves beyond the range of F$_2$. Further upward movement in pitch will raise the frequency of F$_1$, which necessarily keeps pace with H$_1$. F$_2$ rises less, and as a result draws closer to F$_1$. From this point on, the contribution of F$_2$ to the total sound is largely in strengthening the first formant by approximation. Thus amplified, F$_1$ has a particularly powerful effect

on H$_1$ of the high notes. This is especially noticeable in piano singing, where the strong resonator, concentrated on a single harmonic, yields a relatively high sound pressure level (and thus "carrying power") to a sound produced with little effort at the voice source. (Piano in this context means not so much a low sound intensity in decibels, as a perception of effortless production from delicately adjusted vocal folds.)

Both the approximation of F$_2$ to F$_1$ and the reliance on well-tuned resonance with a delicate voice source can be practiced by repeated low-pressure onsets with an sufficiently rounded /ɔ/ vowel on the notes F^5 to B^5-flat. The reason for the choice of vowel is that /ɔ/ (with varying degrees of openness) is the vowel in which the first two formants naturally occur closest together. With repetition, the singer acquires a feel for accurate tuning of this powerful resonance. As the soprano proceeds higher from G^5 (and the vowel increasingly opens), all back vowels will have much the same spectrum. A generalized front vowel, standing in for all four front vowels, may differ only marginally from this generalized back vowel.

This description of an approach to the female upper range, as well as the proceeding paragraphs covering the male upper extension, may sound quite complicated when read in the absence of the practical use of feedback. When each step can be seen directly in spectrum analysis, and particularly when the maneuvers are executed in one's own voice, the logic of the descriptions becomes quite clear. This practice also provides the advantage to teachers of gaining an objective insight into voices that differ essentially from their own. The soprano's back strategy and the tenor's F^2 tuning (a sort of "front strategy") are fundamentally different uses of resonance. This can be seen in Figure 12–10, where the two sing the same vowel an octave apart. If one of these singers attempts to teach his or her strategy to a pupil of the other sex, the results can be counterproductive.

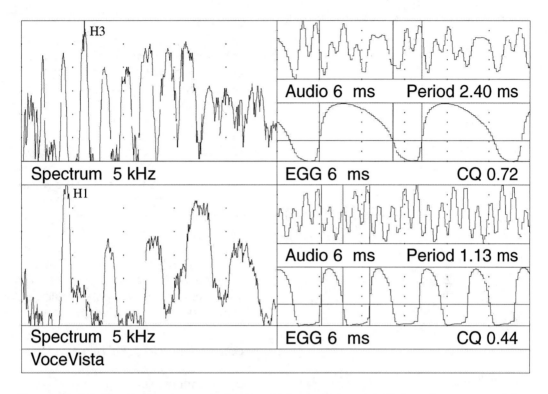

H3	Audio 6 ms	Period 2.40 ms
Spectrum 5 kHz	EGG 6 ms	CQ 0.72
H1	Audio 6 ms	Period 1.13 ms
Spectrum 5 kHz	EGG 6 ms	CQ 0.44
VoceVista		

Figure 12–10. Top: Tenor singing vowel /ɑ/ on A⁴-flat, with dominant H_3 from F_2 resonance. Below: Soprano singing vowel /ɑ/ on A⁵-flat, with dominant H_1 from F_1 resonance, supported by F_2. Both sounds have strong high-frequency components. For explanation of the time signals in the right panels, see Chapter 13. 🔘 12-10a = tenor; 12-10b = soprano.

The Flageolet ("Whistle") Register

The preceding two sections have addressed a basic problem of singing technique encountered by virtually all classical singers. This section, by contrast, illustrates how spectrum analysis can be used to gain insight into a type of voice production employed by an unusual voice type and occurring only occasionally in performance.

As noted, the soprano follows the fundamental frequency with her first formant as she sings into her upper range, allowing her larynx to rise in the process. Even that resource comes to an end, however. Usually by her high C (C⁶, or 1046 Hz), if not before, F_1 has reached the limit of its range. It would seem that the singer would have to sacrifice her greatest source of resonance in order to sing higher. At

this high pitch the harmonic spectrum, with its gaps of more than 1000 Hz between harmonics, reveals little direct information about where the resonances are located. A skillfully executed vocal-fry spectrum, however, shows us that the first harmonic remains resonant anywhere within the broader composite formant composed of the approximated first two formants (see Figure 12–11).

F⁶ (1400 Hz, and the highest pitch in the standard operatic repertory) would have to fall below the upper boundary formed by F_2, as it does in the figure. When F_1 approaches its limit at about 1000 Hz, the effort of the vocal tract to hold the shape of the formant increases. A portion of this effort may be eased a bit once H_1 has passed F_1. This can give the relatively relaxed sensation similar to that of playing a harmonic on a stringed instrument. This explains the choice of the name flageolet for the register (Miller

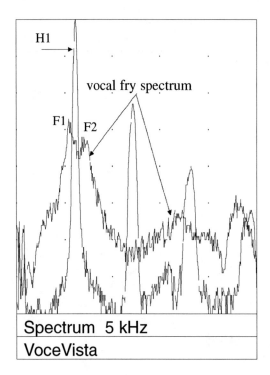

Figure 12–11. High soprano singing E^6-flat in flageolet register, with overlay of vocal-fry spectrum. F_1 and F_2 are closely approximated and straddle the very dominant first harmonic, whose frequency has moved about 100 Hz above that of F_1. 🔘

& Schutte, 1993). The term "whistle" is also appropriate, since the first two formants have merged effectively into one, removing any sense of vowel from the sound.

The Singer's Formant

In a treatise on the practical use of feedback from spectrum analysis, the singer's formant (SF) must receive special consideration. There are several reasons for this:

- Composite of formants: The singer's formant, insofar as that entity has been defined in the literature, is not one of the series of resonances of the vocal tract designated F_1, F_2, and so forth. It is a composite of at least two formants.

- SF is not adjusted: In singing, unlike F_1 and F_2, the SF is not adjusted with respect to fundamental frequency. It is left at a nearly constant frequency, being broad enough not to fall into the "gaps" between the harmonics, at least within the male singing range, when vibrato is taken into consideration.
- The importance of the singer's formant varies considerably from one voice type to another: In low male operatic voices, for example, the SF seems indispensable, while certain excellent sopranos show little evidence of it.
- Imaging the singer's formant presents different problems: The method used to make the SF visible in spectrum analysis can differ from the vocal-fry "imitation" used to locate the first two formants.

Locating the Singer's Formant

The continuous spectrum produced by vocal fry is usually less effective and accurate in revealing the configuration of the singer's formant than of the first two formants. An alternative method for investigating the SF is to sing a chromatic passage (a fifth, for example) setting the time window for a long enough period to capture and average the whole passage. While the lower formants, especially F_1, will often naturally adjust to accommodate pitch change, the upper formants tend to stay in place. A successful capture of a chromatic passage will result in a continuous spectrum that reveals the frequencies of the higher formants. One can measure the frequency "distances" between neighboring formants (Figure 12–12).

The fact that the singer's formant occurs relatively high in the spectrum makes it easier to locate with spectrum analysis. A consideration of vibrato explains why this is so. If a tone with a fundamental frequency of 200 Hz has an excursion of 10% (nearly a full tone) around the center pitch, the total sweep of the first harmonic is 20 Hz. The harmonic will appear in the spectrum to have a

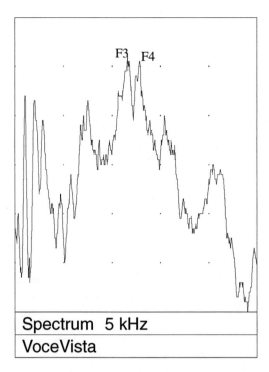

Spectrum 5 kHz

VoceVista

Figure 12–12. "Time exposure" (long time average spectra) of a bass singing a descending chromatic fifth, C^4-sharp to F^3-sharp on vowel /ɛ/. The dominant peaks around 2.5 kHz are F_3 and F_4, forming the singer's formant. These generally stay in place during the scale passage, while F_1 and F_2 adjust to changes in fundamental frequency, appearing as broader formants in the time exposure. The apparent strong dominance of the singer's formant is due to this difference in the behavior of formants with respect to changing F_0: The singer's formant keeps accumulating intensity in the same spot, while the vowel formants, F_1 and F_2, distribute their intensity over a broader frequency range as they shift their tuning with changing F_0. 💿

width of 20 Hz, provided that the time window covers the vibrato cycle (about 200 milliseconds). H_{10} (at 2000 Hz) of such a fundamental has a sweep 10 times as wide as that of H_1, or 200 Hz. The consequence of this is that at the frequency of H_{10} and higher, the sweeps will overlap one another and produce a continuous spectrum. (This can be demonstrated easily with feedback by varying the extent of the vibrato.)

Instead of counting on a wide vibrato to fill in the gaps, one can set the time window longer and sing a segment of a chromatic scale. (Producing a glide tone might seem an obvious method, but such production misses the characteristic muscular settings and the resultant sound of singing.) Even in the cases where singer's formant is not very strong, as in some female voices, it should be possible to determine the locations of formants 3 through 5 (Miller & Schutte, 1990). The female voice usually has a less sharply articulated singer's formant. Because of the shorter vocal tract, the distance between formants is generally greater than in the male voice, even when singing in the low range of fundamental frequencies. With the rising larynx accompanying the upper range, the increased spread of the formants tends to wipe out any synergistic effect between adjacent formants, although individual formants can still be effective.

Dimensions of the Singer's Formant

Because of the potential importance of the singer's formant in the professional singing voice, it is useful to keep certain quantifiable specifics of the SF in mind to characterize voices and follow their development in training. These are:

- Frequency: The most important factor determining frequency is whether the SF is formed by F_3–F_4 or F_4–F_5. Generally speaking, the approximation of F_3 and F_4 is found more often in quality voices. Some excellent tenors, however, have a strong singer's formant on F_4–F_5 at about 3.2 kHz. In female voices F_3–F_4 can produce a peak around this same frequency. A female SF of F_4–F_5 tends to exceed 4 kHz, and the resultant sound is less attractive.
- Compactness: The degree of approximation of the constituent formants is a key factor in determining the intensity

level of the resonance, which increases with diminishing distance between neighboring formants. When the distance between F_3 and F_4 is reduced below 300 Hz, the singer's formant often resembles a single peak.

- Level: This refers to relative sound pressure level of the harmonic(s) lifted by the SF resonance. It is usually given as the difference in decibels between the peak harmonics in the region of the vowel formants and those in the region of the SF. (Thus in Figure 12–3, bottom panel, the level of the SF is about 19 dB below that of F_1.) Sometimes a harmonic in the SF region even exceeds the peak harmonics among the vowel formants in level. There are tenors, including some who are well known, whose exposed top notes are regularly dominated by SF resonance (Figure 12–13, top panel). A well-tuned lower formant, however, can create such a dominant effect that the level of even a powerful singer's formant will appear unimpressive.

Resonance Strategies Determined From Commercial Recordings

Mention of the extraordinary singer's formants sometimes found in famous singers brings up the application of spectrum analysis to recorded material in general, and commercial recordings in particular. Is it possible to follow the resonance strate-

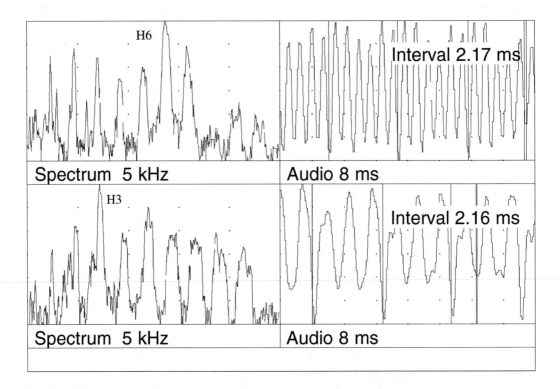

Figure 12–13. Spectra of the final note of "Celeste Aida" from Verdi's opera, taken from commercial recordings. The pitch is B4-flat, and the vowel is (nominally) /o/. (Vertical cursors mark the periodic closing points of the glottis in the audio signals in the right panels. For further explanation see Chapter 13.) Top: The tenor Placido Domingo, with a dominant singer's formant on H_6. Bottom: The tenor Luciano Pavarotti, with a dominant second formant on H_3. (The CD contains an additional example of this phrase, sung by tenor Enrico Caruso.) 🆑 12-13a = Domingo; 12-13b = Pavarotti; 12-13c = Caruso.

gies of exemplary singers in their recordings with any assurance that one is not being misled by the recording engineers?

Balances between singer and orchestra and among the various singers are adjusted at will by recording engineers, but this hardly constitutes deception. The question is whether the spectrum of the singer's sound is realistic, or is it deliberately manipulated during and after the recording process in order to make it more impressive? It is surely at least plausible that there might be some high-frequency emphasis in the singer's sound, which would affect the level (as described above) of the singer's formant. The sort of resonance strategies pointed out in these pages, however, resulting in the clear dominance of one or a few harmonics, would seem scarcely within the sound engineer's prerogative or knowledge. The crucial effects are so robust that they are equally apparent, regardless of the recording technique, even with early acoustic recordings with a high noise content (see the example of an acoustic recording on the accompanying CD). Simultaneous orchestral sound can hinder the reading of the singer's sound, and unaccompanied passages are preferred for analysis. But even when there is orchestral sound at the same frequencies as some of the singer's harmonics, however, the singer's "wider" harmonics (due to vibrato) can usually be distinguished. Moreover, much of what the singer enhances by resonance, and especially the singer's formant, is at frequencies where the orchestral sound is relatively weak.

While monitoring recordings, it is advisable to use a faster time window than the 200 ms recommended for direct experimentation with one's own voice because the user has to work with transient sounds of both singer and orchestra. Of course one cannot compare a harmonic spectrum with that of vocal fry, but extensive experience in locating the formants often makes it possible to interpret the results without a continuous spectrum for reference (see the following text). A good

example of this is the conclusion that the tuning of F_2 to H_3 is responsible for the salient resonance effect in Figure 12–13.

From an examination of Pavarotti's recordings one comes to the conclusion that he consistently employs a strategy of F_2 tuning from the passaggio point (usually G^4) all the way up to C^5. (This is the case, at least, for back vowels: for an /i/ he will sometimes use an approximation of F_2 and F_3, creating a broad formant with a center in the neighborhood of 2 kHz.) An alternative strategy employed by some tenors in approaching the highest notes is that of relying on a dominant singer's formant. This is a frequent strategy of Placido Domingo. These two tenors, who have dominated a generation of operatic heroes, are represented in Figure 12–13, (CD 12–13a and b) comparing their B^4-flats on the final note of Radames' aria from the opera *Aida*. Through the examination of recordings of other tenors, it becomes apparent that these two strategies are typical patterns of the most successful singers.

Whether the voice teacher or the singer can glean useful knowledge from such an analysis depends on a number of factors. Considering that voices such as these two tenors are not common, it would seem desirable to be able to ascertain whether a given voice utilizes one or the other of these exemplary strategies. If the answer is positive, the feedback can be used to develop consistency in the approach. If the answer is negative, one has the feedback to see if further experimentation might help a singer to develop such an approach. Of course, this may result in the unwelcome news that one's best sound will not bear comparison with the tenors preferred for such roles and that reassessment of voice type, or even career aims, is in order.

Similar comparisons can be made among other voice types taken from commercial recordings. Figure 12–14 compares two sopranos singing an A^5. Both have the indispensable strong fundamental, but one has a strong H_2 with a negligible singer's formant, while the other shows

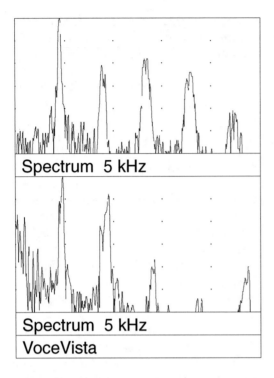

Spectrum 5 kHz

Spectrum 5 kHz
VoceVista

Figure 12–14. Spectra of sopranos singing A^5, taken from commercial recordings. Top: Maria Callas, from "Caro nome" in Verdi's *Rigoletto*. Bottom: Roberta Peters, from "Una voce poco fa," in Rossini's *Il Barbiere di Siviglia*. Both sopranos show the typical enhancement of H_1 by the first formant on high notes, but while Callas has strong third and fourth harmonics (here in the frequencies of the singer's formant), Peters' harmonics virtually disappear above H_2. (The CD contains an additional example of an A^5 by the soprano Renata Tebaldi.) 💿 12-14a = Callas; 12-14b = Peters; 12-14c = Tebaldi.

secondary resonance concentrated on H_4 at 3.2 kHz. Clearly there are fundamental differences with respect to voice type, technique, or both. The point is not to judge one or the other as wrong, but to reveal to the eyes, and perhaps to one's understanding of resonance strategies, what the ears are hearing. This is particularly important in the case of one's own voice, which is notoriously difficult to hear realistically. The contrast between these two famous sopranos provides another help-

ful lesson: As with the tenors, one can see there is more than one way to make a sound that thrills the public. This should give pause to those teachers who are convinced that they have discovered *the* way to produce the voice correctly.

Spectrum Analysis and Overtone Singing

One of the more obvious applications of feedback from spectrum analysis is in the monitoring of overtone singing. In the first place, it gives a clear picture of the acoustic basis for two sung tones issuing from a single voice organ. In its basic form, a single low fundamental is sustained, while the vocal tract—by producing exceptionally sharp and well-tuned resonances—enhances one after another of the higher harmonics, "playing" a tune on the pitches available in the harmonic series, much like a valveless trumpet. The upper harmonics usually employed, especially the octave H_6 to H_{12}, are carefully matched by the second formant. This is varied, as in whistling, by changing the volume of the front cavity of the vocal tract. The sound of the fundamental is damped behind the barrier presented by the tongue.

One of the chief elements of skill in such "singing" (which cannot control the vowel because F_2 is determined by the tune) is the accuracy and sharpness (narrowness of bandwidth) of the F_2 tuning (Schutte, Miller, & Svec, 1995). As with singing itself, this is usually monitored by ear. Spectrum analysis, however, allows one to see how well the desired harmonic is lifted above its neighbors, as well as its level relative to the suppressed first formant. In the example given in Figure 12–15, the virtuoso overtone singer Tran Quang Hai produces a remarkable 10th harmonic whose level is 10 dB higher than anything else in the spectrum. Try to match it!

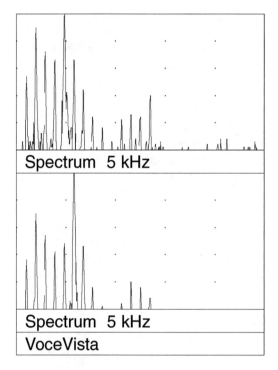

Figure 12-15. Spectra of overtone singing, showing the successive enhancement of the fifth and sixth harmonics, while the fundamental frequency remains constant. 🆑

ACQUIRING EXPERTISE WITH SPECTRUM ANALYSIS

This chapter has presented examples of the skillful use of vocal tract resonances, made visible and, it is hoped, intelligible by display in spectrum analysis. It may make interesting reading to those curious about the singing voice. A more practical knowledge of these phenomena will result, however, when one can make the connections among three elements:

- acoustic display
- perceived sound
- production of sound

Singing is a practical activity, and the highest use of singing theory is to improve the practice of singing. Real-time spec-

trum analysis provides a bridge between theory and practice, allowing both aspects to gain.

Language is quite limited in its ability to describe sound. This is even true of singers' jargon, which takes years to learn and means different things to different people. Considering this, it seems astonishing that not only singers, but voice teachers and even singing-voice researchers have made so little use of spectrum analysis in the decades since it became available. An explanation for this neglect may be found in the complexity and abundance of information offered by such a powerful tool: Those who could be profiting most from its use have not known what to look for in the glut of information. The practitioners who understand the difficulties of singing have not translated their knowledge into acoustical terms, while the acousticians have failed to grasp the practical use of sound in professional singing. This situation may change once acoustical understanding becomes commonplace among professional singing practitioners.

Instruction in the use of the singing voice usually takes place along these lines: The pupil sings; the teacher imitates, perhaps only mentally, using his or her own voice; the teacher analyzes and adjusts the sound; the adjusted sound is presented to the pupil either directly or by verbal suggestion; the pupil sings again, attempting to make the "same" adjustment as the teacher; the cycle is repeated. The expertise of the teacher who works in this way resides not only in knowing where he or she is heading with the pupil's sound (which at this stage may only faintly resemble the finished product as imagined by the teacher), but also in the ability to empathize with the voice of the pupil. The key point to notice is that the "model" of the voice used by the teacher for analysis and adjustment is always, to some extent, his or her own voice.

Visual feedback enters this process as a way of making the model more explicit.

Note that the pupil's spectrum need not resemble that of the teacher in all respects. On the contrary, there may be major differences with respect to gender, the type of voice, and so forth. Nevertheless, the teacher—and later the pupil—should know what details to look for in comparing the faulty with the corrected sound. The teacher learns what to look for just as he or she learned to sing: by paying careful attention to the results of adjustments. In the case of learning to use spectrum analysis, however, this learning process will be a matter of finding and understanding the visual patterns that correspond to the perceptions of the ear. The teacher must acquire a detailed knowledge of his or her own "model."

Formant Frequencies of the Vowels

As previously discussed, the tuning of resonances to enhance the sound is a form of vowel modification: adjusting the formant frequencies in accordance with the pitch sung. A most important element in the teacher's knowledge of vowel modification will be the "normal" formant frequencies, as well as their modified ranges, of all the vowels that the singer uses. There are of course references in the literature that give standard formant frequencies of vowels, and the learner does well to consult them. More important, however, is to make the connection (and notice the differences) between such standards and the formants of one's own voice.

Acquiring this knowledge is a fairly straightforward, if time-consuming, task. Visual feedback speeds the learning process, but anyone who has invested years in gaining expertise in the singing voice should realize that no machine is going to deliver such knowledge without considerable effort on the part of the learner. Once one has mastered the basic process of "imitating" a sung sound with vocal fry (see above), it is recommended that the learner carefully measure the frequencies of the first two formants of all the vowels, as sung in a comfortable, relatively low, part of the range. For each vowel, there will be a sung spectrum and a vocal-fry imitation from which the formant frequencies are extracted.

The selection of pitch for this exercise should be such that the sung spectrum offers relatively dense harmonics (thus lower F_0 is better). In this way, one can tell whether the vocal fry imitation is plausible. In addition, the pitch and vowel should be easy to produce in an effortless mezzo forte, presenting clear vowels in a singing, rather than a speech, articulation of the vocal tract (for the difference see Chapter 5 of this book).

The pitch D^3 (ca. 150 Hz) is suggested for male voices, although some tenors may be more comfortable a bit higher. For this exercise one should ideally avoid pitch levels where there is a strong tendency to tune the vocal tract, because the object is to locate "natural" and pitch-independent formant frequencies in a singing posture. For women's voices, it may not be possible to realize this ideal, because the distance between harmonics in the middle register is already large enough to make vowel modification natural for all pitches. Thus, it is suggested that women measure the formant frequencies in both chest and middle registers, for example, at B^3-flat and G^4, respectively. The differences between these two articulations can be quite instructive.

Effects of the Articulators

Once one has established a baseline of formant frequencies for the various vowels, the modifications effected by changes in articulation will make better quantitative sense. (For colleagues with an aversion to numbers and quantitative measurement it will still be useful to know which movements of which articulators raise and lower F_1 and F_2, respectively.)

Here the authors suggest exploring the effects of changing tongue constriction, jaw opening, lip rounding and spreading, larynx level, and the velum. One should also consider any other subtle adjustment of the vocal tract that is in the singer's personal arsenal. Although it is virtually impossible to change one of these articulators without affecting others, it is a useful exercise to manipulate them as independently of one another as possible. In this way, one learns to be more specific in modifying the vocal tract.

An example of the exploration one might conduct is to compare the effects of the factors' larynx level and jaw opening on the frequency of F_1 of the vowel /ɑ/. Record the formant frequencies for three larynx levels (normal-habitual, elevated, and depressed) times three degrees of jaw opening (normal-habitual, reduced, and extended). Such measurements do not constitute a scientific experiment, but voice practitioners might well be surprised by how such factors affect F_1. In any case, acquiring this practical knowledge offers one an advantage over the colleague who needs to consult textbooks or the scientific literature to determine how to raise and lower the first formant.

Passaggi of the Various Vowels

A rather advanced exercise, but one that yields information of great practical significance, is to plot the formant frequencies of several vowels through the passaggio (see above). These are relatively high pitches that are typically accompanied by marked muscular exertion in shaping the vocal tract. Thus, holding the vocal-tract posture for the vocal-fry imitation presents a challenge. One should carefully check for plausibility and error before accepting the results as realistic. In this exercise one seeks to discover at what pitches there are major adjustments in the use of resonance as the voice moves up the scale

into a higher register. The process of exploring these visually can also contribute to one's awareness of the "feel" of the changes.

It is important to know at what point the strong and natural coupling between F_1 and H_2 yields to a different adjustment and the voice "turns over." In exploring this, we can also experiment with moving the passaggio point higher or lower.

Of equal importance to locating the point of passaggio will be to discover what resonance strategy the voice finds to compensate for the F_1–H_2 coupling. Be sure to try both front and back vowels in this exercise. Frequently, voices will naturally take to one or the other in passaggio, as the traditional characterization of "ah tenors" and "ee tenors" indicates. This is also the place where one can see whether F_2 tuning takes place, as well as learn to tune F_2 to H_3 or H_4 for greater ease and fuller resonance. Be sure to experiment with moving F_2 by modifying the vowel (continuously between /ɑ/ and /æ/, for example) while watching the spectral display.

For the passaggio in the female voice, approximately an octave higher, the first thing will be to discover at what point H_1 reaches F_1 of an open vowel. In trained voices this typically occurs around F^5 (ca. 700 Hz), implying a certain degree of "darkening," because the female F_1 for /ɑ/ in speech is typically closer to 800 Hz. Another point to watch is the closing in of F_2 on F_1 as the voice ascends. This can have a beneficial effect not only in strengthening the first formant, but also in bringing F_3 and F_4 closer together, which will improve the singer's formant. A third point concerns the position of F_2 on the front vowels. It is difficult for those in the early stages of training to accept the degree to which front vowels must be modified in the upper voice. A young soprano, for example, will often want to sing a "real" /i/ at F^5. Acoustically, this is well within the realm of possibility, since F_2 can match H_3 at 2100 Hz without undue distortion of the vocal tract. In most cases, however, the ear of the experienced teacher will find the sound too shrill, and the singer's F_2 will have to be moved lower. This puts more of the burden on the first formant, where it seems to belong—at least in the classical tradition of training.

Estimating Formants From the Harmonic Spectrum

Up to this point the assumption has been that formant frequencies are ascertained by comparing the harmonic spectra with continuous spectra of vocal fry in the same vocal tract posture. The learner is strongly advised to acquire this skill, because it will form the basis of detailed knowledge of the use of resonance. Once one has become thoroughly acquainted with the behavior of formants in a given voice (especially one's own), it will not always be necessary to produce a vocal-fry spectrum to determine the resonance strategy behind a particular sound. This is especially the case when one or two harmonics are clearly dominant, that is, they emerge at least 10 dB above their neighbors. Experience will have taught that only the engagement of a particular formant with the dominant harmonic will produce a given pattern. By way of illustration, this is the basis for the interpretation of the resonance strategies implicit in the high B-flats of Paravotti and Domingo (see Figure 12–13)

The user of spectrum analysis must exercise due caution in making such interpretations, making sure that the method for locating formants is sufficiently mastered and that the knowledge of the behavior of formants is advanced enough to determine that there is no plausible alternative strategy to explain the result. The authors concede that this is a rather advanced degree of knowledge. On the other hand, it is far below the degree of knowledge represented by the expert ear of the practitioner, acquired over years of experience and experimentation with his or her own voice, as well as with the voices of others.

Detecting Nuances by Comparison

As already observed, the failure of practitioners to take advantage of spectrum analysis can be explained in part by the superabundance of information it provides in the absence of a simplifying scheme of interpretation. It is hoped that the few hints written here will encourage the voice practitioner to further explore the relatively unknown landscape of the vocal tract. Beyond some of the basic landmarks outlined above, there is infinite detail to examine in the nuances of sound that expert singers take seriously, sometimes to the bafflement of the layman.

To the extent that such nuances can be heard, and are not simply imagined by the listener, they will also appear in the acoustic signal and thus in the spectrum. The basic approach in identifying them, which will be the first step in explaining their production (the usual aim of singing teacher or theorist), is to examine two spectra for contrast. Here the 1% that shows consistent difference is more important than the 99% of two spectra that is in virtual agreement. Once contrasts have been identified, one can try to determine whether the difference is the result of the configuration of formants or is perhaps attributable to some other factor.

A word of warning to those who would explain what the singer does to produce a given sound: Singing teachers are notorious for giving explanations that are not, or cannot be, tested against facts. Objective feedback makes it possible to verify (or falsify) many would-be explanations, putting the discussion of the singing voice on a factual basis. For some, this will be cause to rejoice, but all voice practitioners will have to get used to the possibility of being proven wrong. The good news is that correcting a mistaken explanation or opinion is an opportunity for learning. The informed use of feedback can provide a chance to get voice practitioners closer to the truth about the singing voice.

CHAPTER

13

THE USE OF THE ELECTROGLOTTOGRAPH IN THE VOICE STUDIO

Donald Miller and Harm K. Schutte

SIGNALS IN (MICRO-) TIME

The **electroglottograph (EGG)**, also known as the laryngograph, is an electronic device for monitoring the contact area between the two vocal folds. The recorded or printed signal is called an **electroglottogram**. The principle on which it works is easily understood: A tiny, high-frequency electric current passes between electrodes fastened noninvasively to the neck at the level of the larynx. (This may sound sinister, but the user feels nothing.) The opening and closing of the glottis causes a variation in its electrical resistance, and the resulting signal displays this variation. This signal is typically shown together with the microphone, or audio, signal, which reflects the minute

pressure variations caused by, or constituting, the sound wave itself.

Unlike the signal for spectrum analysis, the EGG and audio waves show the time dimension, flowing from left to right. The vertical dimension in the two signals gives the amplitude of vocal-fold contact area and the relative air pressure respectively. Both signals are typically uncalibrated, allowing the gain to be adjusted to a level convenient for display. In contrast to the (real-time) spectrogram, which displays a segment of time more commensurate with what the listener experiences, the EGG and audio waves show the variation in microtime, typically only a few glottal cycles. (These cycles each last only about 1 or 10 milliseconds, respectively, in the cases of a soprano C^6 and a bass G^2.) Identifying the cycles in the EGG signal is a relatively simple matter, and computerized programs for tracking fundamental frequency often use this signal.

THE GLOTTAL CYCLE

The glottal cycle—the periodic opening and closing of the glottis, dividing the air stream into a series of puffs—is a relatively neglected aspect of the singing voice. The frequency of repetition of the cycle is fundamental in music, as it determines the pitch. There are other features of vocal fold vibration that singing teachers have paid little attention to, however, primarily because of their limited accessibility to inspection. Some of the grosser variations in vocal fold movement, such as the difference between chest and falsetto registers, have been visible since the invention of the laryngoscope nearly 150 years ago. Other factors have been more difficult to observe. The rapidity of movement of the vocal folds, together with the relative inaccessibility of the larynx, has presented a barrier to gathering factual information about its important details. In the past two decades the EGG has helped solve this problem—at least in the laboratory and clinic. Now it is available to furnish practical information in the singing studio as well.

Phases of the Glottal Cycle

The easiest phase to identify in the glottal cycle is that of the closing of the glottis. This is typically an abrupt occurrence, represented in the EGG signal by a sudden rise (or fall in the case of the inverted EGG), indicating an increase in vocal fold contact (Figure 13–1). From the slope of this rise, one can get a rough idea of the abruptness of the closing movement: Softer and breathier sounds will typically be reflected in a more gradual slope.

For the louder sounds of singing, it is important that the closing movement of the vocal folds be both complete and sufficiently abrupt. This is because the primary excitation of the resonator/vocal tract is caused by the wave of rarefaction ("thinning" the air) produced upon glottal closure, not, as was long supposed, by a compression wave emerging when the subglottal pressure bursts the glottis open. More abrupt closure not only produces a stronger excitation impulse, but also boosts the high-frequency spectral component necessary to produce the "ring" of the voice, the singer's formant.

Incomplete closure, on the other hand, softens the impulse delivered to the vocal tract and effectively eliminates any significant high-frequency component. While incomplete glottal closure may, without any pathology, habitually characterize certain patterns of speaking, particularly those of young women, one of the primary aims of training the classical singing voice will be to establish the habit of complete and abrupt closure, at least in mezzo forte and forte. The EGG can be an aid in monitoring exercises for establishing firm closure. It should be understood, however, that incomplete closure can be, and is, used to advantage in certain singing effects, particularly those of mezza voce.

The brief closing phase of the glottal cycle is followed by a longer closed phase of variable duration that is dependent on a number of factors, including loudness, register, and type of voice. Not only is the flow of air interrupted during this phase, but the quality of the vocal tract as resonator is improved with the glottis closed, particularly for the higher formants. The amplitude of the EGG signal remains high in this phase (vocal-fold contact is maximal), usually taking the form of a convex bulge between closing and opening.

The opening of the vocal folds is less abrupt than the closing and gives a far weaker acoustic impulse, if any, to the vocal tract. This makes it more difficult to locate precisely in the EGG signal. Nonetheless, it is important to pin down the opening moment so that one may identify the extent of the closed phase, as sound

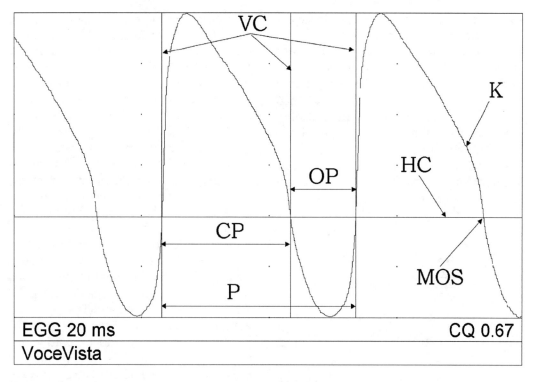

Figure 13–1. General explanation of the electroglottograph (EGG) signal as it reflects phases of the glottal cycle. The EGG signal is an indicator of vocal fold contact; thus an ascending line indicates closing, and descending indicates opening of the glottis. CP: closed phase, HC: horizontal cursor, K: convex "knee" in chest register, MOS: maximal opening slope, OP: open phase, P: period, and VC: vertical cursors. The horizontal cursor is adjusted manually to the estimated moment of glottal opening, which in this case is taken as the point where the slope of the descending curve is maximal. The closed quotient (CP/P) is calculated automatically and displayed (here CQ is 0.67), as is the length of the displayed time segment (here 20 milliseconds). The length of the glottal Period is taken from the interval between the outer vertical cursors, and this quantity is displayed under the audio signal (see Figure 13-2).

production differs considerably between the closed and open phases of the glottal cycle.

In the practical use of the EGG, the rule of thumb is to locate the opening moment at the point of the steepest falling slope. (Computerized programs for locating the closing and opening moments automatically identify them as the downward and upward spikes of the derivative of the EGG, corresponding to the maximal positive and negative slopes in this signal.) It is not always possible to determine this point unambiguously. Nonetheless, it can be helpful to scroll through the recorded EGG signal, looking for slight variations

in individual cycles that best reveal the opening moment. Since the most important practical use of the signal will be in comparing different phonations of the same individual voice, it is usually sufficient that the method used to pick the opening moment be consistent.

In the program used for the figures presented here (VoceVista), the horizontal cursor is manually adjusted to intersect with the point in the EGG signal selected as the opening moment. The vertical cursors then align with the points of intersection in both ascending and descending slopes. From this information, the closed quotient—the percentage of the glottal cycle in which the glottis is closed—is automatically calculated.

As the opening of the glottis occurs at a slower rate than the closing, it also spreads over more time. The EGG signal continues to fall after the point identified as the opening moment. In the following open phase, extending up to the following closing moment, the contact between the vocal folds is minimal. In this phase, it is difficult to extract useful information from variations in the amplitude of the EGG signal.

The Importance of the Closed Quotient

The closed quotient is defined as the percentage of the glottal cycle in which the vocal folds are pressed together, preventing any flow of air. There are two fundamental reasons for considering this measure one of the most important dimensions of a singing voice. One of these is that glottal resistance, and subsequently subglottal air pressure, are dependent to a large extent on this factor. The second, less obvious reason is that the vocal tract as a resonator has a superior quality with the glottis closed.

Sound waves, both at the fundamental frequency and the higher harmonics, are generated at the closing of the glottis. The resonation process consists primarily of the traveling and reflecting of these waves between the two ends of the vocal tract, the glottis and the opening at the lips. At the open end (the lips), the wave is only partially reflected, while part of the wave's energy, especially the higher-frequency components, passes the lips as radiated sound. At the glottal end, the returning wave is more fully reflected, provided the glottis is closed. If the glottis is open, however, the vocal tract acts as a pipe open at both ends. This can provide a good resonator in other instruments—although with different characteristics from those of the closed pipe—as in the case of a pipe organ. In the case of the vocal tract, the returning reflected sound that passes through the open glottis is completely damped in the bronchial space and therefore lost to the listener.

Thus, the strength of the acoustic signal (a fancy word for sound) is typically diminished in the open portion of the glottal cycle in the singing voice, as can be seen in Figure 13–2. At least for the chest register, it would be correct to say that the larger the closed quotient, the stronger the sound, all other factors being equal.

One should not conclude from this that the larger closed quotient is always better. First, it is possible to extend the magnitude of the closed quotient to the point where the voice is less efficient, a condition known as "pressed" voice. Second, the palette of the artistic singer contains any number of sounds that do not require the maximum of resonance. Finally, experience with the EGGs of various singers teaches that different closed quotients are characteristic of different types of voices, all equally good in their own way.

Information From the Audio Signal

As is the case with the EGG signal, the individual glottal cycles are relatively easy to identify in the signal from the microphone, especially when the two signals are displayed in parallel fashion in the same time scale. The audio signal is considerably more complex, however. The EGG gives information about the periodic variations in vocal-fold contact, but only at the basic repetition rate, that is, the fundamental frequency. The microphone signal also reflects the pressure variations of the harmonics, which, as seen in spectrum analysis, occur at multiples of that basic repetition rate. Before the days when fast computers became available to calculate the amplitude of the various harmonics, estimating the strength of the spectral compo-

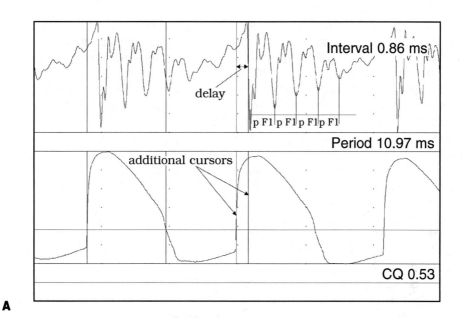

A

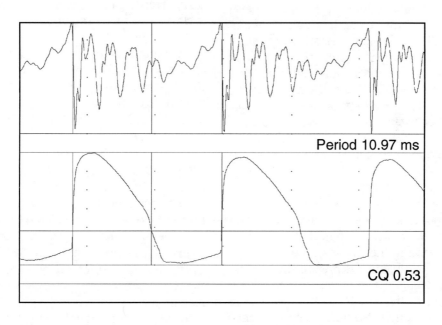

B

Figures 13–2. Microphone and EGG signals of bass, vowel /ɑ/, G²-flat, at speech intensity. Note how the amplitude of the acoustic wave diminishes (is damped) with each successive period of the first formant (pF$_1$) over the course of the closed phase. In the open phase this wave weakens greatly, and the acoustic energy carried over to the following cycle is negligible. The sharper rise just before the closing moment reflects the accelerating airflow just prior to glottal closure. **A**: Figure shows the two signals uncorrected for the delay in the audio. Additional vertical cursors have been placed at the moments of closure in the EGG and audio signals respectively (the first of these simply repeats the right-hand cursor programmed with the EGG signal—see Figure 13-1), to indicate the time delay of the audio. The time interval (here 0.86 ms) between the these two cursors is displayed in the upper right-hand corner of the panel. **B**: Figure shows the two signals adjusted to display the closing moments as simultaneous. (Subsequent figures in this chapter have all been corrected for this delay in audio.) 🆎

nents was a laborious and uncertain process, based on the appearance of this microphone signal. Today the form of the microphone signal is relatively neglected, but certain observations can nonetheless provide useful information about the voice that produces it, especially when it can be compared directly with the EGG signal.

Because sound must travel the distance from the glottis to the microphone through the air, the audio signal will arrive at the computer with a small delay after the EGG signal (see Figure 13–2). Thus, the first step in comparing the two signals is to adjust them to eliminate this discrepancy. Just as the closing moment is the most reliable point of orientation in the EGG signal, it is also usually the most readily detected landmark in the audio signal. If the polarity of the audio signal is correct, the phase of the cycle just before the moment of closure will usually show a relatively gradual, but accelerating, rise in the signal. Abrupt closure of the vocal folds ends this rise, causing a sudden drop in the audio signal. The largest peak-to-peak variations normally follow in the closed phase. With the vertical cursors aligned for the closing and opening moments, it is then possible to follow the development of the audio signal within the glottal cycle.

If the fundamental frequency is low and, correspondingly, the period is long, one can see the quick damping of the acoustic energy during the course of the cycle. It is usually possible to observe the effect of the weakening of the resonator caused by the opening of the glottis as well (see Figure 13–2). Finally, in another type of signal (see Figure 13–3), one can identify a dominant standing wave from the fact that the strong acoustic pattern continues through the open phase and is further propelled by the next closing of the glottis.

Singing and the Standing Wave

A standing wave is one in which the shape of the wave in a resonator remains virtu-ally constant, sustained by a force that is applied periodically, timed to reinforce the "standing" pattern. A common analogy for this is the pendular motion of a swing, maintained by periodic pushes at the recurring advantageous moment. If the push comes too soon, it cancels the motion; if it comes too late, the energy is wasted. The damping of acoustic waves in the vocal tract is quite rapid. At the relatively low frequencies and intensities of speech, the wave must effectively begin anew with each glottal impulse, the equivalent of starting from scratch with each push of the swing (see Figure 13–2). Singing generally occurs at higher frequencies than speech, however, shortening the period of the cycle. This makes it easier to set up a standing wave and to carry over the acoustic energy from one cycle to the next, much as one does in pushing the swing.

The condition for this vocal application of the law of conservation of energy is that the impulses be delivered to the vocal tract at exactly the right moment to sustain the standing wave within it. The adjustments that the singer makes cannot be in the frequency or its reciprocal, the period, because these are prescribed by the composer in the pitch. What the singer can adjust, however, is the frequency of the resonator, a process considered in Chapter 12 under the heading Formant Tuning. In terms of the swing analogy, this is the equivalent of shortening or lengthening the ropes of the swing in order to change its period.

In terms of the signals considered here, a strong standing wave is most apparent in the audio signal. In singing, the dominance of a standing wave can be such that it far overshadows any other component of the sound, although these other components remain an essential part of what one hears. The most common and obvious standing wave in singing is that of the soprano high note, where the first formant is aligned with the first harmonic (see Figure 12–10 in Chapter 12). Other

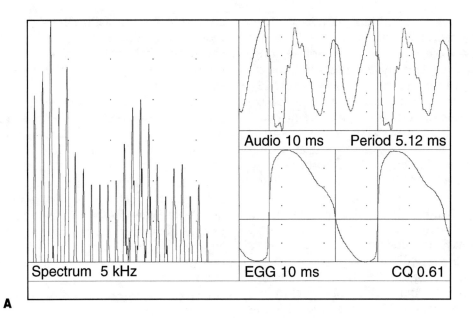

A

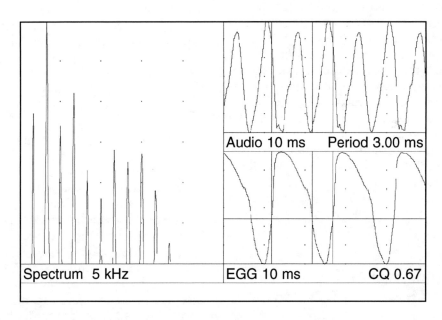

B

Figures 13–3. Signals showing how the audio signal reflects dominant standing waves in the vocal tract. In contrast to Figure 13-2A and B, the acoustic waves continue through the open phase of the glottal cycle with little visible loss of energy. The power spectra are included to show the dominant standing waves in another display mode. With the strongest harmonic ca. 15 dB above the rest, the sine wave at the frequency of that harmonic dominates the audio curve. In both cases it is evident how the acceleration and deceleration of the flow in the open phase reinforce the standing wave. **A:** Figure shows signals of a bass singing G^3 on the vowel /ɔ/. The first formant matches the third harmonic, thus completing three cycles within a single glottal cycle. **B:** Figure shows the same voice singing E^4 on the vowel /ɛ/. The first formant matches the second harmonic, completing two cycles per glottal cycle. This figure is made from the same "shouty" sound as Figure 12-4 in Chapter 12. (Other dominant standing waves, including one at fundamental frequency and one at $6 \times F_0$, can be seen in Figures 12-10 and 12-13 in Chapter 12.) 💿

examples of dominant standing waves are those of F_2 tuning, especially in the tenor voice (see the same figure), and, more exceptionally, the dominant singer's formant (see Figure 12–13 in Chapter 12). The reader has already observed above how this dominance can be seen in the power spectrum as well.

Such dominant standing waves have a marked effect on the overall sound-pressure level (SPL) of a given sound. If the audio signal is displayed with automatic gain control such that the maximum (displayed) amplitude remains constant, however, this effect of the standing wave on the SPL will not be apparent in the magnitude of the signal. One instead recognizes the dominance of the standing wave rather on the extent to which other details are diminished (see Figure 13–3).

While dominant standing waves greatly increase the efficiency of the vocal instrument as a sound generator, it is not implied that the skilled singer should always strive for this effect except, perhaps, in the soprano high voice, where F_1–H_1 tuning is generally expected. The very powerful standing wave of the raised-larynx shout in the male voice (see Figure 13–3B and Chapter 12) is explicitly avoided as a rule. As is generally the case in the cultivation of vocal sound, the final judge is the (expert) ear, not some physical measure of efficiency.

Laryngeal Registers: Chest and Falsetto

The recognition of "registers" in the singing voice can be traced back to the distinction between two fundamentally different types of mechanical action of the vocal folds. In the male voice, these vibrational patterns are generally known as chest and falsetto, with chest—the usual register for the speaking voice—being characterized by lower F_0s, larger closed quotients, and stronger high-frequency spectral components.[1]

This clear distinction between the two primary registers can be obscured in borderline situations and in certain types of voices, however. In female voices, for example, while this dual-register pattern has much in common with that of the male, the distinction between the two registers is usually less pronounced. Furthermore, the female frequency range is such that the "falsetto" vibrational pattern is appropriate for the larger portion of the classical singing range. By contrast, the male singer can usually dispense with falsetto altogether, extending the "chest" vibrational pattern upward (see Chapter 12, Male Passaggio). This major difference between the sexes has resulted in the reluctance of many singing teachers to apply the term falsetto to the female singing voice. In common parlance, the designations of the primary registers in women are chest and head.

With the information available from EGG technology the discussion of the primary registers can be put on a more factual basis, removing some of the heat from the controversy over terminology. In both sexes a characteristic feature of the "chest" vibrational pattern is a convex bulge or "knee" on the opening slope of the EGG signal (Figures 13–4 and 13–5). Increasing the loudness of the sound will typically sharpen the angle of the knee and raise the closed quotient. The "falsetto" vibrational pattern, in both male and female voices, typically lacks the knee, exhibiting a steep downward slope. On the one hand, the absence of the knee, which generally precedes the point of the steepest slope, makes it more difficult to specify the opening

---

[1]In this chapter, the use of quotation marks with the terms "chest" and "falsetto" will indicate that the authors refer specifically to the type of mechanical action of the vocal folds, not the sound in its entirety.

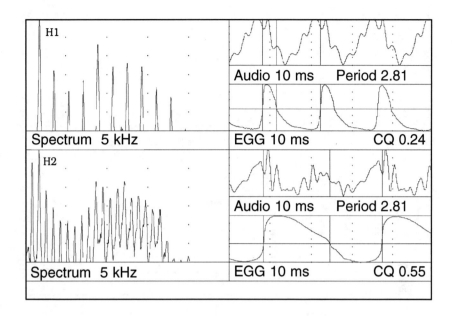

A

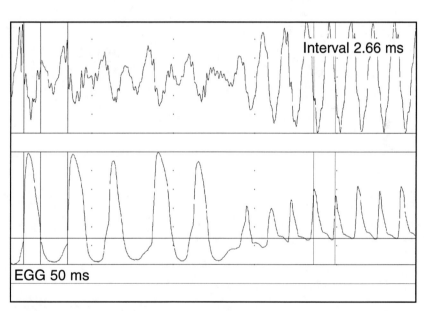

B

Figure 13–4. A: Signals showing a bass singing the vowel /i/ on F^3 in chest register (lower panels) and F^4 in falsetto (upper panels). Not only are the F_0s of the two tones an octave apart, but the closed quotients and shapes of the EGG waves are sharply differentiated, with the "knee" appearing clearly in the chest register. **B** shows the short time segment containing the rapid leap between the registers, located by scrolling back through the time signals. With both registers in a single display, the contrast in the amplitude of the EGG signals is evident. Note that the closed quotient is reduced just prior to the leap (compare Figure 13-4A). On the right side of the figure additional vertical cursors are placed to measure the period of vocal fold vibration in the falsetto portion. Visual inspection of the EGG signal shows that the repetition pattern of falsetto is established almost immediately, and the readout of the time interval (upper right) shows its period. (The period of the chest register portion is given automatically from the cursors on the left of the panel, and frequencies can be calculated as the reciprocal of the period.) 💿

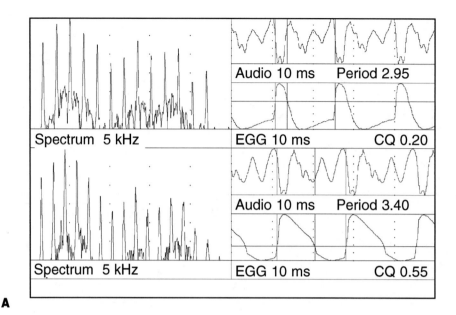

A

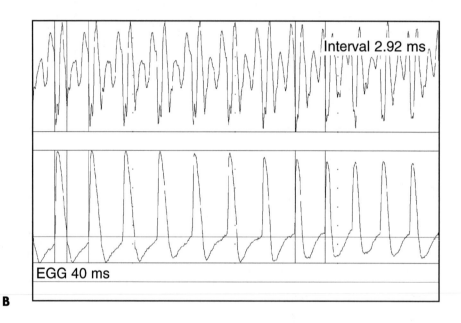

B

Figure 13-5. A: Signals showing a mezzo-soprano singing the vowel /a/ on D^4 in chest register (lower panels) and F^4 in "falsetto" (upper panels). Note the difference between the registers with respect to the closed quotient, as well as the "knee" in the EGG signal in the chest register. In the audio and power spectrum the differences between registers are less striking. (For a stronger "falsetto" sound at a high pitch, see Figure 12-10 in Chapter 12.) **B** shows the short time segment containing the rapid leap between the registers. This singer also reduces the closed quotient in preparation for the leap to falsetto, but here the contrast between the registers in the EGG signal is far more subtle that that seen in the bass voice. The difference in (vertical) amplitude of the EGG between the registers is small, visible after the sixth peak in the EGG. That the transition between F_0s is fully accomplished in this short time segment can be inferred from the respective measured time quantities ("period" and "interval"—see caption to Figure 13-4B). 💿

moment. On the other hand, the greater steepness of the slope narrows the time segment where the opening may occur. One can still make a useful estimate of the closed quotient, which varies in "falsetto" as it does in "chest," by arbitrarily setting the horizontal cursor at, say, 50% of the vertical dimension of the signal.

Before leaving the subject of the EGG signal and the laryngeal registers, mention should be made of another typical pattern one is likely to encounter. This has a sinusoid form, that is, one resembling a sinus curve, lacking the abrupt changes of slope. Such a signal typically indicates the absence of a closed phase of the glottal cycle (Figure 13–6). The motion of the vocal folds, while remaining periodic, is rather one of alternation between a more and a less open glottis. The modulation of vocal-

fold contact is thus quite small, and the EGG signal is correspondingly weak. Because of the automatic gain feature, however, the signal is amplified to fill the display space, a pattern that the beginner may mistakenly interpret as implying a closed quotient of around 50%. The relative "noisiness" of the signal that results from the amplification of a weak original signal is usually sufficient to distinguish this sinusoid from one indicating true closure.

The user of the electroglottograph should bear in mind that not all voices will produce EGG signals resembling the typical patterns examined here. For reasons not fully understood, the signals of a small minority of singers yield little useful information, even when the contact between electrodes and the neck is enhanced with electrolytic gel.

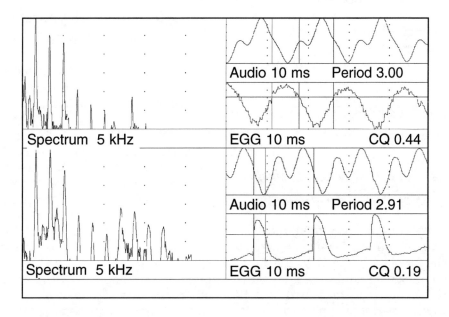

Figure 13–6. Signals taken at two points from a bass singing a sustained diminuendo E^4 on the vowel /a/ in falsetto. The EGG of the lower panels shows a brief closed phase, while the EGG of the upper panels is "noisy" and sinusoid, indicating a weak signal without closure of the glottis. Note that the readout of the closed quotient in the upper panel is misleading, a consequence of the fact that all signals are "normalized" to fill the vertical display space. 🆑

The Glottal Cycle and Subglottal Pressure

There is a considerable variety in the magnitudes of the air pressure that skilled singers use as a driving force for the vocal folds. Because concealment of effort is part of the art of the classical singer, the higher pressures sometimes used for loud high notes may not be apparent to the audience, or even to other singers not accustomed to using such pressures. A robust tenor voice, for example, may employ maximal pressures of up to three times the highest pressures of some lighter sopranos, yet both singers may be using a highly skilled and correct production. Subglottal pressure is thus an important variable in a given singing technique, and the informed teacher will want to be able to assess this factor on a factual basis.

Although it can be measured in the laboratory by means of a slightly invasive procedure, one cannot obtain an accurate estimate of subglottal pressure as easily as the formant frequencies or the closed quotient. Nonetheless, because subglottal pressure rises with glottal resistance, the closed quotient can still give important clues regarding the general level of subglottal pressures employed by a given singer.

The Closed Quotient and High-Pressure Singing

One of the ways in which the professional operatic singing voice differs markedly from the speaking voice is in the management of subglottal pressure. Pressures of 5–10 cm water (as measured in a U-tube manometer) are typical for quiet conversation, and in loud speech these rise to around 15 cm. By contrast, maximal pressures used in sustaining forte high notes vary, according to the singer, from about 35 cm to well over 100 cm of water. The higher pressures are partly due to the higher fundamental frequencies (F_0s) of singing: Subglottal pressure rises systematically with F_0. These higher pressures can also be reached momentarily by nonsingers in shouting, but there the sound is not sustained.

To create the pressures at the upper end of this range, it is necessary for the larynx to present a high resistance to the subglottal air. One way of achieving this is to increase adduction of the vocal folds and raise the closed quotient up to two-thirds or even three-quarters of the glottal cycle. Although such values look like hyperfunction, or "pressed voice" to those accustomed to investigating the speaking voice, they are quite common among male opera professionals (see, for example, Figure 12–10 in Chapter 12, where the closed quotient is above 70%). Some singers habitually employ high closed quotients, even for mezzo piano sounds, making a virtue of the resulting low airflow.

Acoustic Backpressure in "Falsetto"

Male opera singers can raise their closed quotients up to extraordinary levels to produce the high subglottal pressures of singing. What can women do, who employ a "falsetto" vibrational pattern of the vocal folds in which the upper limit of the closed quotient is not often much above 40%? A second way to create and manage relatively high subglottal pressures is by utilizing the natural acoustic resistance presented by the glottis when the first formant is tuned to the fundamental frequency in the "falsetto" vibrational pattern (see Chapter 12). Under the conditions of this sort of formant tuning, which happens quasi-automatically in the female high voice, the phases of supraglottal pressure variation are timed in such a way that the phase of the open glottis coincides with high positive supraglottal pressure, greatly reducing the escape of air. (The reader who wishes to comprehend this phenomenon more fully is referred to Schutte, H. K., and Miller, D. G., The effect of F_0/F_1 coincidence in soprano high notes on pressure at the glottis, *Journal of Phonetics*, 1986, *14*, 385–392.)

High subglottal pressures in the "falsetto" mode are thus created with less vocal-fold adduction than those in "chest" mode. The soprano also enjoys the great acoustic advantage of the standing wave when F_1 is tuned to H_1. This means that the soprano can usually produce an elevated sound pressure level with considerably less effort than her tenor colleague when both are sustaining the "same" high note, an octave apart. Such a fact can have important consequences in the studio where one type of voice is teaching the other.

Variation of the Closed Quotient and Voice Type

One of the important ways in which emotion is communicated vocally is through the listener's empathy with the speaker's or singer's vocal organs. In this respect, variation of both closed quotient and subglottal pressure is an important carrier of the emotional message—even more so than changes in the decibel level that accompany such variations. Ideally speaking, the classical singer should be able to adjust the closed quotient continuously from zero to maximum at all pitches. In practice, this is of course not possible. Not only do high and low F_0s present obvious limits to the full range of closed quotients, but the smoothness of transitions between soft and loud is sometimes interrupted by stepwise adjustments in vocal-fold contact. The perfect *messa di voce* (swelltone) throughout the entire frequency range is an elusive goal, particularly in male voice, where the pattern of vocal-fold vibration at the soft extreme has much in common with "falsetto."

The EGG provides an excellent means of monitoring the changes—not only in the closed quotient, but also in the pattern of contact between the vocal folds and especially in identifying minute abrupt transitions between one pattern and another. The point is not so much to aid in the achievement of the perfect swelltone as to identify and come to terms with the natural limits of the instrument. Some voices can easily achieve a high closed quotient, while others have difficulty establishing even an instant of complete closure of the glottis. Those with a tendency to the large closed quotient often have difficulty in smoothly reducing vocal-fold contact on a *diminuendo*, while other voices with natural closed quotients of limited magnitude are particularly adept in handling glottal adjustments appropriate to the gentler areas of expression. Not all well-trained voices can achieve everything desirable in singing. It is helpful to be able to explore the factual basis for the variety of gifts and limitations. As the use of EGG becomes more widespread and more voices of high quality are examined, understanding of the variety of voice types will increase.

Closed Quotient and Resonance Strategy

As already observed, the primary acoustic impulse to the vocal tract is furnished by the closing of the glottis, with only a minor impulse, if any, proceeding from the opening. The timing of the glottal opening can play an important role in determining the strength of the impulse, however. Consider again the discussion of standing waves and the metaphor of the child on a swing. It is apparent that the push of the air escaping on the opening of the glottis will contribute positively to the size of the puff of air escaping if this push is timed to occur within the phase of rising supraglottal pressure. If it occurred in the opposite phase, when the supraglottal pressure has begun to fall, it would reduce the abruptness of the fall in pressure and thus weaken the impulse to the vocal tract.

The typical closed quotient of 50–60% in the "chest" vibrational pattern presents the opening moment at a point in the glottal cycle where it is most favorable for a standing wave at twice the fundamental frequency, that is, with a dominant second harmonic (Figure 13–3B). In this pattern the first cycle of the standing wave proceeds entirely on acoustic energy, occurring within the closed phase, after the impulse has been delivered to the vocal tract, while the second cycle has both a well-timed push from the glottal opening and a "pull" from the closing. Similarly, the smaller closed quotient of the "falsetto" pattern implies that the most favorable standing wave is the one in which the first formant is equal to the fundamental frequency. Here the push occurs early enough in the cycle to contribute to the rising phase of the standing wave. If, on the other hand, the first formant is tuned to the fundamental in the "chest" pattern, the open phase of the glottal cycle is too short to deliver the most effective push-pull. For this reason the tuning of F_1 to H_1 is acoustically considerably more efficient in "falsetto" than in "chest." This also helps explain the difference between the tenor and soprano resonance strategies in Figure 12–10 in Chapter 12.

This same reasoning can be applied to the situation in which the tenor tunes the second formant to H_3. This resonance strategy is most effective only if the closed quotient extends over two-thirds of the glottal cycle, leaving an open quotient of one-third to drive the standing wave. From this example, it is apparent that the F_2–H_3 strategy for the B-flat in "Celeste Aida" (see Figure 12–13 in Chapter 12) works best for a robust voice with a high closed quotient.

Monitoring Registration Events

Some singing teachers attach particular importance to the achievement of a smooth transition between "falsetto" and "chest," or vice versa, practicing such transitions in special exercises. Whether the transition is truly continuous, or, alternatively, a small "click" between registers that is skillfully concealed, it can be revealing to monitor such events with the EGG in real time. Still more instructive is to store the short passage in which the event occurs and then to scroll back through the recorded signal, searching for stepwise or continuous adjustments in the pattern of vocal-fold contact.

The storing and scrolling capability can also be used to obtain a realistic sense of the amplitude of the EGG signal. For practical reasons, this signal is set to use 100% of the display space. Using such automatic gain control has the disadvantage of obscuring differences in the relative magnitudes of the EGG signal in different vibrational modes, however. In most male voices, for example, the signal in "chest" has a markedly higher amplitude than in "falsetto." While this difference is not immediately apparent when only one register or the other is displayed, a moment of abrupt transition in a time segment long enough to include both registers will clearly show the relationship of EGG magnitude. It will also display the speed of the transition between the two registers (see Figures 13–4B and 13–5B).

Monitoring Larynx Height

Many teaching methods give an important place to the vertical position of the larynx, and a "comfortably low" position is often recommended. From a scientific viewpoint, this is not surprising because the low larynx results in a longer vocal tract and thus in the relatively low formant frequencies characteristic of the "classical" singing technique. Furthermore, there are probably sound physiological grounds for connecting the low larynx with a less stressful production of high-intensity sound.

In many male singers, it is possible to monitor larynx level visually. This method is somewhat haphazard, however, considering that the singer's attention must be on other things at the same time. In addition, laryngeal movement of another sort is simultaneously present, such as the small modulations of larynx height that often occur in vibrato. The larynx is visually more elusive in female singers. Its movements can be followed to some extent kinesthetically, but one suspects that the lack of visual prominence can explain why larynx height traditionally seems to get less attention in female singing technique than it does in the male case. Nevertheless, the effects of adjustments in larynx level on the formants of the vocal tract are similar in both sexes.

The electroglottograph with dual electrodes offers a simple means of tracking larynx height. Because the electrode near-er the larynx gets a stronger signal, the modulations in the relative signal strength between the two electrodes can reveal laryngeal movement. The resulting signal can be used to follow vibrato, which has the same frequency as the laryngeal movement (although it may differ in phase). More significantly for instruction in singing, it is possible to detect both laryngeal rigidity and larger movements, such as raising the larynx in executing an upward leap.

The monitoring of laryngeal height shares the great advantage of all well-designed objective feedback: It helps to remove adjustments in voice production, as well as pedagogical admonitions, from the realm of vague words and wishful thinking, giving a factual basis to the discussion of "what the singer does."

CHAPTER

14

SOME CONSIDERATIONS ON THE SCIENCE OF SPECIAL CHALLENGES IN VOICE TRAINING

Katherine Verdolini and David E. Krebs

Any voice teacher faces challenges in training. In this text, Professor Nair has emphasized two particular challenges. One is the possibility that speech patterns may interfere with singing. A second is the certainty that the singer perceives his or her voice differently than others perceive it. The purposes of this chapter are to provide background in the science behind these two challenges and to describe how the spectral analyzer may be used to overcome them.

Before proceeding, we would like to make a few special introductory comments about "performance," "science," and how we use science in this chapter. Both

of us (KV and DEK) come to science with performing backgrounds, one of us in singing (KV) and one of us in athletics (DEK). As such, we are acquainted with the ephemeral nature of performance and the mystery inherent in the pursuit of excellence. At a philosophical level, it is reasonable to ask: "What is the role of science in such an endeavor?" Does science serve to concretely explain and reduce mystery and magic in performance? Does science seek to be concrete and "know," where performance tends to defy clear answers? We think the answer to those questions is emphatically "no." In fact, the situation may be reversed in some ways. In our view, performance, and especially performance pedagogy, critically require a sense of *knowing*, or confidence. We need to be certain about our next note; we need to exude confidence that what we are teaching is right. In contrast, modern science is philosophically set up to *doubt*, to raise questions. Contrary to popular impression, science is not configured to "prove" anything; instead, it is configured to disprove. Stated differently, where performance must be deeply trusting, science must be deeply speculative.

These observations explain our approach to science in this chapter. In our comments, we are cautious and, at times, tentative. Some of our suggestions are particularly speculative, based on scientific literature but as yet untested in the voice and speech domain. We will emphasize potential uses of the spectral analyzer in voice training, but also caveats to those uses. An important principle to emphasize is that performance and science are not opposing but complementary. Performance's confidence is balanced by science's caution; science's hesitancy is balanced by performance's trust. We invite you into this chapter with an appreciation of this balance.

CHALLENGE 1: HYPOTHESES ABOUT SPEECH INTERFERENCE WITH SINGING

In voice pedagogy, there are two polar opinions about the relation between speech and singing. Most classical singers are familiar with the Italian adage, *Si canta come si parla* (One speaks as one sings; as described, for example, by Miller, 1977, with reference to buccopharyngeal adjustments in vowels). An alternative opinion, expressed in this book, is that speech patterns are not only different from singing, they can actually interfere with singing. In the next paragraphs, we

will examine the two separate hypotheses inherent in this view: First, that speech and singing do differ; second, that the difference may produce an interference relation. Later, we will come back to these topics and discuss how spectrographic analyses may help to address difficulties arising in voice training as a result of speech interference.

Similarity and Differences Between Speech and Singing

There is little doubt that speech and singing are similar in some fundamental ways. At the most superficial level, singing essentially can be seen as "sung speech." Motivationally, speech and singing both arise from the same global impetus, which is verbal expression and communication. Anatomically, speech and singing activate identical peripheral structures, including respiratory, phonatory, and resonatory structures. Technically, the degree of similarity between speech and singing depends on the type of speech and the type of singing. Similar vocal-fold vibration patterns are used in female chest voice in speech and belting, for example, while vibration patterns are different for female chest voice in speech versus falsetto singing (e.g., Estill, 1995). Despite such surface similarities, there are differences between speech and singing that extend across all or almost all styles of speech and singing. Discussion of some of the most salient differences follows.

Duration of Pitch and Loudness

Perhaps the most obvious difference between speech and singing regards the duration of pitch and loudness variations. In speech, specific pitches are rarely sustained at all, but fluctuate continuously within and across words. In contrast, a critical feature of virtually all singing—except perhaps "Bob Dylan"-style singing—is that target pitches are sustained without fluctuation, even if briefly, for a period of time that may range from a few hundred milliseconds for rapid, staccato, or melismatic singing, to 10 seconds or longer for heroic "money notes."

Relative Timing

A second, more critical difference between most speech and singing regards the relative timing of consonants and vowels. In speech, a typical ratio is approximately 1:5 (for example, 50–60 milliseconds [ms] for many consonants in comparison to about 150–300 ms for a vowel). In singing, consonant duration probably changes very little compared to speech. However, as every singer knows, vowel duration is usually markedly lengthened in singing. The result is a large change in the relationship of consonant-vowel durations, which may become as small as 1:200 or less in singing (50 ms for a consonant versus 10 seconds for a sustained vowel).

On paper, this relational difference may not seem impressive. In the human brain attempting to produce skilled behavior in singing, the result may be pure havoc. The experimental literature is clear that relative timing is a fundamental parameter, if not *the* fundamental parameter, of skilled behavior in general. Stated differently, when people acquire a skilled behavior, as much as learning which specific muscles to activate, they learn a relative timing of muscle activation. Relative timing is so essential to skill that it frequently transfers to new absolute timings, or speeds (e.g., adagio versus andante in singing), and to entirely new muscle sets (e.g., left versus right arm in some sports), with little if any practice (Carter & Shapiro, 1984; Raibert, 1977; Shaffer, 1980, 1984; Terzuolo & Viviani, 1979). Conversely, similar-appearing skills with different relative timings may transfer more poorly. The point is that relative timings of consonant-vowel durations in speech are wrong for almost all types of singing.

Coarticulation

A third important difference between speech and singing, called coarticulation, is related to timing issues. Coarticulation refers to the physical and acoustic influence of a given sound on neighboring sounds. In physical terms, coarticulation refers to anticipatory gestures made by the articulators in preparation for upcoming sounds, or conversely, lethargy in the articulators after a sound has been produced. Coarticulation is at least partly the result of mass and inertia properties of the articulators.

A concrete example is the following. In isolation, the vowel "o" is made with the velum relatively raised, preventing air from entering the nose (Figure 14–1). In running speech, the vowel "o" during a stressed syllable might last about 250 milliseconds. Now consider the case of the word "on." As already established, the velum should be relatively raised for the production of "o." For the "n" that follows it, however, the velum must be lowered, otherwise it will be perceived as a "d." From a raised position it takes the velum about 125 ms to lower for the production

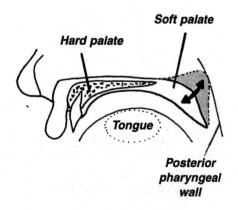

Figure 14–1. View of the action of opening and closing the velo-pharyngeal port. (From *The Speech Sciences*, by R. Kent, 1997, San Diego, CA: Singular Publishing Group. Adapted with permission.)

of "n" (Keefe & Dalton, 1989; Kuehn, 1976). Clearly, if the velum is to be lowered by the beginning of "n," velar lowering has to initiate at least by the midportion of "o," if not earlier. The result is that the "o" will be relatively nasalized in normal running speech. Indeed, nasalization may occur over two or three vowels prior to a nasal consonant (Zemlin, 1998). Equally important, the lowered velar position will likely persist in sounds that follow the "n" ("on a . . .") because velar raising similarly requires about 125 ms (Keefe & Dalton, 1989; Kuehn, 1976) and will not be completed by the time the "post-n" sound begins.

In singing, the situation is quite different. Take the sung phrase "on a . . ." (clear day?). The duration of "o" is likely to be much longer than for speech, on the order of 500 ms or longer. Therefore, coarticulatory movements required for "n" will not have to initiate midvowel or earlier, as for speech. Rather, velar lowering can initiate at the tail end of the "o" vowel. Similarly, once "n" has been produced, only the very initial portion of the next sound ("o") must be produced with the persistent lowered velar position from "n." The remainder of the vowel can be free of the necessary coarticulatory influence. Thus, both vowels that precede and follow "n" can be relatively denasalized. A corollary is that denasalization may be a technical goal to maximize the voice's carrying power; all other factors being equal, non-nasal sounds are more intense than nasalized sounds. In sum, coarticulation, which is essentially pervasive in speech, may have very different relative timing qualities in singing. In idealized singing, many coarticulatory effects may disappear altogether. The result for the performer may be a substantially different "feel" (and sound) to singing, as compared with speech.

Voice Quality

A fourth difference between speech and singing relates to voice quality, reflected by the sound spectrum, described in Chapter 12. In speech, the most important acoustic information lies in the lower range of harmonics, in which different energy clusters (formants) distinguish one vowel from another. In Western classical singing, vowels are of course important. However, equally important is the special, ephemeral "ring" in the classical singing voice. This ring defines most classical singing aesthetically, and indeed is probably required to project into a big house or over an orchestra. The singer's ring corresponds to the presence of unusually intense harmonic energy in the range of approximately 3000 Hz. Most evidence indicates that the "ring" is produced by manipulating the shape of the resonating cavity right above the vocal folds (narrow) in relation to the size of the pharynx right above it (large) (Sundberg, 1972a, 1978; Yanagisawa, Estill, Kmucha, & Leder, 1989). Further, many good singers routinely shift vowel "formants" (intensified clusters of acoustic energy in the sound spectrum, which define vowels) to coincide with the voice's fundamental frequency or pitch to boost the overall sound amplitude or intensity (see for example, Titze, 1994). Such manipulations do not occur in regular speech.

Neural Substrates

A final difference between speech and singing is worth mentioning. Although both vocal forms arise from similar macroscopic motivations, such as expression and communication, they may fundamentally depend on different cognitive and neural substrates. Recent evidence suggests that two distinct brain systems may regulate speech versus nonspeech vocalization. Experimentally, speech-type vocalization is obtained with stimulation of a specific area in the brain's surface, Broca's area in the left cerebral cortex—the top, outside portion of the brain (Figure 14–2, top). An important nonspeech vocalization center is located in a deeper, phylogenetically "older" area of the brain,[1] called the periacqueductal gray (Figure 14–2, bottom). At least in animals, stimulation here does not produce speech vocalizations as occurs for stimulation of Broca's area; rather, stimulation in the periacqueductal gray produces emotional, nonspeech vocalization. It is reasonable to think that some singing may at least partly arise from this older, more primal system. Other evidence derived from brain-damaged individuals suggests that whereas speech is usually governed by Broca's area in the left frontal cortex (Figure 14–2), singing heavily utilizes right hemisphere brain functions, at least in nontrained voice users (Curry, 1967; Kimura, 1964). The upshot is that although at the broadest level speech and singing appear grounded in similar motivations, the specific cognitive and neural substrates may be different. If a singer comes to the singing task with a speech "mentality," the entirely wrong neural system may be set into motion.

THE INTERFERENCE HYPOTHESIS

The fact that two activities—such as speech and singing—are different from each other does not mean that one necessarily interferes with the other. Tennis and swimming are different; yet there is no reason to think they interfere. It turns out that the degree of interference between any two behaviors is probably partly related to the behaviors' similarity and to the automaticity of one or both behaviors. Take, for example, the case of a racquet swing. Consider a tennis player on a racquetball court for the first time who initiates a swing in response to an approach-ing ball. For the sake of argument, let's say that the ideal initial portion of the swing is the same for both tennis and racquetball. So far, so good. The tennis player should fare well. However, the final portion of the swing may need to be different for racquetball than that for tennis. Because the tennis player's swing is a highly automatized, unitized behavior, it is likely that the final portion of the swing will continue according to tennis standards and may fail with respect to ideal racquetball form.

A similar situation may exist with respect to speech and singing. The singer sets about the task of verbally communicating and emoting. It is entirely reasonable to think that the highly automatized, unitized speech response may be spontaneously activated, with unintentional imposition of speech's relative timing, coarticulatory, spectral, and other characteristics.

Before proceeding further with this discussion, some background may be useful. What are automatic behaviors? Why might they interfere with the development or performance of other, nonautomatized behaviors?

In the scientific literature, automatic behaviors are described as "habits" that arise from massive repetition. They are initiated rapidly, without conscious awareness, in response to a given stimulus, as the result of practice or exposure. They are thought to be governed by a mental machine with enormous capacity, which processes vast amounts of information in parallel, that is, all at once (Posner & Snyder, 1975). Automatic, habitual behaviors are fluent (effortless) and stereotypic (uniform). As such, they are well suited for survival, as they allow for rapid, complex responses to common, environmentally challenging situations. Because

---

[1]"Phylogeny"refers to the evolutionof the species. Thus, "monkeys" are phylogenetically older than humans. Phylogenetically old structures are those that appeared relatively early in evolution. In the case of the brain, and particularly in terms of the specific structures discussed here, the phylogenetically older structures are still present in the newer species (humans) and are supplemented by newer structures such as the cerebral cortex, which apparently allow for consciousness.

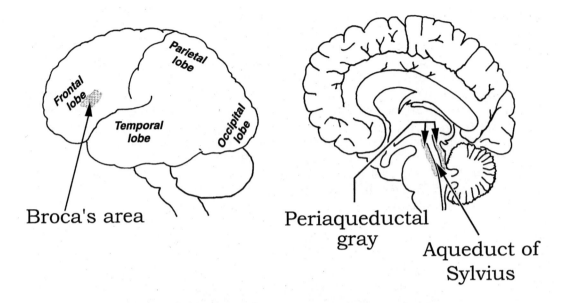

Broca's area

Periaqueductal gray

Aqueduct of Sylvius

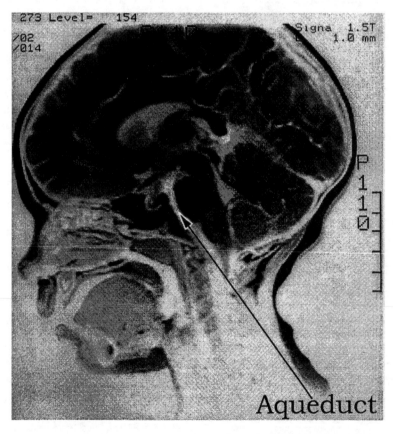

Aqueduct

Figure 14–2. Top: Inverted view of a CAT scan of Bottom: midsagittal view of human brain, a child's head showing the aqueduct. Broca's area is just anterior to the front part of the shadowed area. The basal ganglia are deep inside the brain and are lateral to as the shadowed area. Darkened areas adjacent to the aqueduct (arrow) indicate the periaqueductal gray.

they do not use conscious resources, such resources are available for other needs such as ad-libbing during an orchestra bridge because one's partner has missed an entrance (see Epstein, 1994, for an excellent review). Automatized habits may depend on various neural systems depending on the task. Brain structures called the basal ganglia (see Figure 14–2), however, often appear to play a central role (Salmon & Butters, 1995).

A key issue in all this regards the mechanisms by which automatic responses are called up, and speed with which automatic behaviors are activated. Confronted with an habituated stimulus, execution is initiated within a few hundred milliseconds or less (e.g., Neely, 1977). It takes considerably longer to initiate newer, as yet unhabituated responses. The experimental literature suggests that the response time here is on the order of *seconds*, not *milliseconds* (e.g., Neely, 1977). Let us return to the example of the singer who approaches the task of verbally communicating via song. Given the stimuli "communicate!" and "emote!," there can be little doubt that the quickest, most available response for many singers is the highly practiced speech response. A series of concatenated speech mechanisms are rapidly set into motion and carried out. Without a slowed, conscious mental effort to interrupt this process, the singer can hardly help it. The wrong cognitive, neural, physiological, and acoustic mechanisms are activated. What is the theoretical solution? This is the topic for the next section.

What Is a General Solution for Speech Interference?

Luckily, our brains are not entirely governed by the system controlling automatized, stereotypic habits, called the "implicit" or "procedural" learning and memory system (for review, see Verdolini, 1997). An alternative system also exists, called "explicit" or "declarative" learning and memory. In contrast to the procedural system, the declarative system depends on midline brain structures called the hippocampus and amygdala, and also the thalamus (see Figure 14–2) (e.g., Damasio, 1989; Milner, 1962; Scoville & Milner, 1957; Squire & Moore, 1979; Victor, Adams, & Collins, 1971; Zola-Morgan, Squire, & Mishkin, 1982). Of note, the declarative system is a phenomenally slow, effortful mental machine. It can only process about seven items—plus or minus two—within any given brief time frame. Further, information is not processed in parallel in this system, but is rather processed "serially," one item at a time (Posner & Snyder, 1977). Slow, effortful processing of this type lays the groundwork for what one usually thinks of as "thought," or "awareness." Stated more simply, the slow, laborious declarative learning and memory machine allows for the unfolding of human consciousness. The point for this chapter is that although the declarative system is phenomenally slow, it is flexible. It is well suited to inhibit automatized responses (e.g., Neely, 1977) and to institute new behaviors.

Relative to vocal pedagogy, the ultimate point is that slow, effortful, conscious processing may be not only well suited, but also necessary in singing training to interrupt speech habits and to institute new singing gestures. In a later section of this chapter, we will consider how the use of electronic devices in voice training may favor the evocation of slow conscious processes and thus stop short speech patterns in singing training.

CHALLENGE 2: FALSE PERCEPTION OF SOUND

Most of the sounds that one hears are "airborne." That is, sound sources such as vocal folds or violin strings generate patterns of disturbance in the conduction medium (air, for example), similar to water molecule disturbances in the ocean.

These disturbance patterns impinge on membranes and bones in the ear, which in turn stimulate the auditory nerve. Nerve impulses are then transmitted to the brain, where they are perceived as sound.

A critical issue regards the medium for sound transduction. When other people produce sounds, the disturbance patterns travel through air to impinge on one's auditory apparatus. However, people perceive their own sounds primarily through bone conduction. Bone conduction favors low frequencies in the spectrum. Also, the part of one's own sound that one perceives via air conduction favors low frequencies; low frequencies have a broad angle of radiation from the mouth and essentially "bend" around the head to the ears and therefore one hears them. In contrast, high frequencies have a narrow angle of radiation and jettison forward away from the individual. In sum, the net result of bone conduction and radiation properties is that people perceive the sounds that they make with boosted low frequencies and attenuated high frequencies, compared to how others perceive the same sounds. A corollary is that the high frequencies are responsible for the brilliance or "ring" in the voice. Thus, singers fail to normally perceive the brilliance in their own voices, which is the very target of much formal voice training.

In short, we perceive the sounds that we make differently from the way that others perceive the same sounds. The transformation of self-sound is not a small problem in voice pedagogy. One would be hard pressed to identify another type of training that encounters the same problem; in voice the learner is attempting to train a phenomenon that he or she cannot directly perceive the same way that others do. Compare this situation to pole vaulting, for example. In pole vaulting, the goal is to clear a bar stabilized at some distance from the ground. Performance relative to this goal is patently obvious and identically perceived by any ob-server, including trainer, performer, and sports enthusiast. The pole is either cleared and remains aloft, or it is not cleared and cascades. Singing is a very different situation. The singer-"athlete" perceives goal performance—"good singing" (however defined)—differently than others. When our own ears tell us that we are singing "well," the sound may be distinctly "not well" to others. Conversely, when our ears tell us that the sound is not good according to our standards, listeners may indeed perceive the sound as good, as we would if we heard it by way of normal air conduction.

Sound transformations are not a small issue in voice training. They essentially foul up a critical and important parameter of training: feedback. In the tradition-al skill-acquisition literature, feedback refers to sensory information—auditory, visual, kinesthetic, and so forth—that learners process relative to their own performance. In classic terminology, feedback is distinguished from another type of information about learning: knowledge of results. Knowledge of results (KR) refers to information provided to the learner by an external source, such as a teacher, about performance results relative to some goal. Both process feedback and KR are required for learning. Without them, learning does not occur (e.g., Bilodeau, Bilodeau, & Schumsky, 1959). It follows that to be useful for learning, feedback and KR must be valid and stable across trials. Altered auditory feedback, that is, altered perception of one's own sound in singing, seriously undermines the feedback principle in singing training. Therefore, the importance of and dependence on KR in singing is greater than in other types of training. Essentially, the student needs to substantively rely on KR from the environment for accurate information about performance relative to the goal of "beautiful singing." Some singers acknowledge that, in a voice teacher, they are essentially hiring a good set of "ears."

If the teacher could be a reliable, steady source of KR, then the problem could be solved relatively simply. Singers rely on the teacher to supply accurate information about their performance relative to goal, or KR, and training proceeds. Unfortunately, there is evidence to indicate that even the best teachers may necessarily fall short of this goal. Several solid studies indicate that listeners, including trained listeners, fail to perceive sounds consistently from one trial to the next. One reason may be attentional fluctuations. Another, equally important reason for perceptual instabilities is that listeners' criteria for "good" or "bad" sounds shift from trial to trial, depending on which sounds they have just heard (see, for example, Kreiman, Gerratt, Kempster, Erman, & Berke, 1993).

For this reason, the problem of deformed auditory feedback in singing cannot be wholly solved by a reliance of KR from the teacher in voice training. In the next section of the chapter, we will consider ways that the spectral analyzer may help to augment KR and thus learning in the voice studio.

USE OF THE SPECTRAL ANALYZER AS A POSSIBLE SOLUTION

The spectral analyzer offers a partial solution for the special challenges in voice pedagogy addressed in this book. In this next section of the chapter, we will discuss this claim relative to the two special challenges addressed in this text: the speech interference challenge and the challenge of altered auditory feedback.

The Speech Interference Challenge

As discussed in a previous section, a general solution to the speech-habit interfer-

ence problem may be to interject slow, conscious, effortful processes in voice training. Many tools could be used for such interjection and indeed are routinely used in some approaches to voice pedagogy.[2] The spectral analyzer is one tool. Essentially, by displaying acoustic information on-line and making it available to the student for inspection, analysis, and discussion, cognitive processes during singing become slowed and effortful. The groundwork is laid for the development of conscious inhibition, which may be needed to interrupt automatic speech habits. As discussed in detail elsewhere in this text, the spectrogram is useful for time-based information about voice and speech (e.g., relative timing, coarticulation) and can be useful for examining voice quality as well. Both the spectrogram and the sound spectrum, which displays information about the harmonic intensities at one moment in time, are well suited to address harmonic information and thus the "singer's ring."

The Challenge of Altered Auditory Feedback

A second challenge in voice training regards the deformation of auditory feedback in singing—that is, the deformation of one's own sound, as one perceives it under usual circumstances. As already established, one cannot fully rely on the teacher's ear (i.e., auditory perception) in training. Assuming that the ultimate goal of voice training is acoustic, the spectral analyzer is especially well suited to address feedback and KR problems. The spectral analyzer is neither subject to feedback deformation nor attention or bias shifts across trials. Thus, the information arising from the spectrum should be entirely reliable, repeatable from trial to trial, if

---

[2]An example is the Alexander Technique, which incorporates the notion of inhibiting old responses before proceeding with attempts to produce new ones (see, for example, Alexander, 1974).

data are collected in a consistent fashion. The potential is great for voice training. KR is a critical component of skill acquisition of any type. It stands to reason that KR's effectiveness increases with its stability. In this regard, the spectrum wins hands down over auditory feedback (singer listening to himself) or auditory-perceptual KR (teacher giving student information about performance based on auditory perception). Furthermore, the spectrum provides information about performance extremely rapidly, which voice teachers cannot do.

Having said as much, there are some theoretical caveats that should be discussed if the spectral analyzer is to be used responsibly in the voice studio.

Caveats

Reliability

Reliability is defined as the extent to which a measure consistently yields the same information for identical performances. For the spectral analyzer to yield consistent, reliable KR—which is indeed one of its major advantages—stable data collection procedures must be followed. Microphone-to-mouth distance must be constant, for example. The microphone angle also may be important.

Validity

Validity refers to the extent to which a measure accurately reflects the phenomenon it is supposed to reflect. Assuming adequate equipment and constant data collection procedures, the spectrogram should reveal valid time-based information about vocal performance. Thus, the spectrogram should provide valid information about the relative timing of consonants and vowels and about coarticulation. Where voice quality is an issue, the situation is somewhat more complex. Although formal perceptual studies have

not been conducted, anyone scrutinizing a spectral display can easily see that the display reflects important aspects of voice quality, in particular the "singer's ring" (see Chapter 4). It is also true that voice quality is a complex phenomenon. No single spectral observation can capture its totality. Thus, spectral information cannot be seen as a wholly "valid" or complete indicator of voice quality. Spectral information should be used together with the teacher's (and student's) judgment to complete the picture.

Considering the picture even more globally, voice output can be seen as the product of several converging production factors, including the relative timing of each component's movement during a task, or coordination. How each structure coordinates its mass and momentum is the subject of much study. If one could identify the voice's spectral "signature" of the tongue or vocal folds' movement, then one could study their coordination directly using techniques called cross-correlation or coherence techniques. Currently, however, we cannot identify individual structure's contributions from the voice spectral record alone, so one must measure the movements of each individual structure—something most people would find quite invasive. Perhaps video techniques will exist one day that permit such coordination analyses applied to vocal structures, as are used routinely on the arms, legs, and trunk by the second author (DK). Until then, the listener and expert teacher's information retains hegemony.

Lag Time

Successful feedback depends on speedy responses. Whether the feedback loop is from the thermostat controlling a furnace and room temperature or from a spectral analysis of singing, to be effective the information must be accurate, salient (relevant), and timely. We describe the accuracy and saliency of the spectral analyzer in other sections of this chapter. As to timeliness of spectral feedback, one must consider both instrument and human sensor lags. The device takes between 40 and 120 milliseconds (just over one-tenth of a second) to acquire, process, and display the voice signal. The human sensor (vision, in this case) acquires this information from the spectral analysis device and requires at least 200 milliseconds more to respond to its information. Thus, from the time one speaks or sings, the minimum time before one could possibly "correct" voice production is a quarter second. Most often, however, the lag time will be greater, perhaps as long as a half second. For a rapidly delivered musical piece, the notes will be shorter than a quarter or half second. In such cases, the singer cannot correct the note during actual singing. In such cases, the spectral feedback is not considered to be "biofeedback," which assumes on-line corrections, but rather "knowledge of results." In other words, a student can learn about what to do or not to do next time from the spectral feedback. In the case of slow singing, on-line corrections are possible.

The quarter- to half-second lag described in the prior paragraph corresponds only to neural delay times. One must also consider the mechanical factors impeding rapid responses. These considerations mainly concern mass, inertial, and coordination factors. Changing the movement of the comparatively massive tongue or lips must be slower than changing the vocal folds' vibration rate. How much slower the response time to feedback must be will depend on the type of changes desired and inertial factors. Inertia refers to the speed and direction of the mass' movement. As Newton tells us, a body in motion tends to stay in motion (in the same direction, i.e., momentum); thus, if the tongue must move one millimeter more in the direction it was already headed, the change can be easily and rapidly effected. But if tongue direction is to be reversed, a pause is required along with a complete reversal of momentum, and thus

much more lag will be required for such a correction.

Such considerations do not compromise the use of spectral analyzer in voice training. They simply alert the user to qualifications so that the device can be used most effectively.

Transfer

An important concern inherent in the use of the spectral analyzer—or any electronic equipment in voice training—regards the transfer of gains made in training to "no-instrument" performance conditions. In this chapter, we have talked about the role of the declarative, conscious, explicit memory system in altering intrusive habits such as speech. As a matter of fact, the alternative procedural, *nonconscious*, implicit memory system is not only deeply involved in the regulation of habits the conscious system can interrupt, it is also involved in the acquisition of new perceptual-motor skills that are instituted once the habitual events have been suppressed (Squire, 1986). A corollary is that the procedural or implicit memory system involved in both habit management and skill acquisition appears strongly dependent on modality and context consistency from training to test trials. This means that a transfer from one modality to another—say visual to auditory modality—or a transfer from one environment to another—say voice studio to stage—may be poor.

We will focus on the modality problem. The spectral analyzer provides visual information about sound. Often people assume that visual information is somehow more meaningful or precise than auditory information. With the visual display afforded by the spectral analyzer, vocal practioners "see" sound. Therefore, we feel that it is more "objective" (and "good") than information that we "hear." The inherent assumption is that visual information is somehow "better" than auditory information. There is some precedent for this assumption, both anecdotally and experimentally. Anecdotally, one can consider the example of wave length perception. Most humans readily identify visible energy wave lengths, that is, color, in a reliable way across observers. Observing a Red Delicious apple, almost all humans will describe it as "red" rather than some other color. In contrast, only a few, special observers correctly identify audible wave lengths as specific pitches (perfect pitch; Bb_3 confidently and reliably perceived as Bb_3). In this regard, visual information does seem more certain and more replicable than auditory information.

Based on such observations, visual displays of voice production should indeed be more concrete and precise than auditory information alone. The principle of modality specificity in training tempers conclusions about the unqualified superiority of visual information in voice training however. As noted, the learning and memory system that governs both habit production and skill acquisition appears fundamentally linked to modality specificity (Jacoby & Dallas, 1981; Verdolini, 1997). This means that behaviors trained in one modality (visual, for example) do not necessarily transfer completely to a different modality (auditory-kinesthetic, for example). The upshot is that skills acquired with the use of the visual information provided by the spectral analyzer do not necessarily transfer to situations in which the visual information is not relevant, such as skilled performance on a stage far away from any equipment. The principle of modality specificity is a serious one to consider in any voice training utilizing spectral information. We do recognize, however, that motor skills are often successfully taught in physical rehabilitation using visual and auditory biofeedback (Krebs & Behr, 1994).

Indeed, Nair has emphasized elsewhere in this text a means to address the transfer problem. Wherever the spectral analyzer is used in voice training, systematic "withdrawal trials" should be incorporated. That is, after exposure to visual information afforded by the spectral analyzer and conscious awareness of the issues displayed by it, the student should attempt repeatedly to replicate the same behaviors without visual support. That is, the teacher should record the data for the student's later inspection and verification of goal attainment without machine support. Visual and nonvisual (auditory, kinesthetic) trials should be systematically alternated in training. The alternative, that is, a full reliance on visually supported information in training may enhance immediate performance, but may inhibit learning for the final acoustic goal. The same principle applies to any techniques used in voice training, electronic or otherwise, that do not closely recapitulate the final performance situation.

SUMMARY

- Speech and singing are similar in some ways, particularly in their dependence on a similar global motivation and their dependence on the same peripheral anatomical structures.
- Speech and singing also differ in some ways, including the stability of prosodic variations, relative timing of consonants and vowels, coarticulation, and the acoustic output spectrum. Speech and singing also may partly depend on different brain structures in some cases.
- Virtually all singers come to the project of voice training with deeply engrained speech habits, which have formed over a decade or longer of constant daily use. It is reasonable to think that the impetus to "communicate!" verbally may inadvertently trigger the strong speech response, which is then partially played out in place of the intended singing response.
- Slowed mental processes and conscious inhibition may be useful if not needed to block the automatized speech

response, and institute the developing singing response, at least in early stages of training.

- The spectral analyzer may be useful to introduce slowed mental processes and consciousness important for inhibition of an unwanted speech response in singing.
- All persons perceive their own voice differently from others. Low frequencies are boosted and high frequencies are attenuated in the perception of one's own voice as compared to others' perception.
- Particularly given the deformation of auditory feedback in singing training, external sources of information become especially important. The most important source is knowledge of results (KR) provided by the voice teacher. At the same time, it must be acknowledged that the teacher's own perception of the student's sound is subject to a series of degrading influences, including attentional and bias shifts.
- Feedback and KR are essential to perceptual-motor learning. Without them, learning does not occur. The deformed auditory feedback in singing and the necessary fluctuations in KR consistency inherent in any teacher's responses pose a notable challenge in voice pedagogy.

- The spectral analyzer can be used to increase the consistency (reliability) of KR provided to the student about his or her vocal productions. An assumption is that data collection procedures remain invariant across trials.
- Spectral information captures some aspects of sound in the visual modality, but sound's totality is perceptually captured by the ear. The teacher's ear remains the final and supreme judge of any sound event in training.
- In rapid singing, information from the spectral analyzer can be used to learn how to improve the next performance, but not the current one. On-line corrections of current productions are possible with slow singing.
- If spectral information is to be used in voice training, the transfer problem should be addressed by introducing systematic "withdrawal trials" during training, whereby visual and auditory-kinesthetic trials are alternated until the student has been reliably "weaned" from the electronic display. Other stabilizing techniques are discussed in Chapter 6.
- The routine successful use of biofeedback tools in physical therapy provides precedent for the use of similar tools such as the spectral analyzer in voice pedagogy.

CHAPTER

15

APPLYING GRAM TO COMMON SPEECH PATHOLOGY AND VOICE THERAPY TECHNIQUES

Robert A. Volin

Speech-language pathologists, as they work to help their clients replace aberrant speech patterns, confront the same challenges as those encountered by teachers of voice. The first of these is that habituated speech patterns interfere with the acquisition of new patterns. The second is that speakers do not perceive their own speech as others do.

SPEECH HABIT INTERFERENCE

Habituated speech motor patterns interfere with the acquisition of new patterns because normal speech production is usually controlled without conscious attention (Borden, Harris, & Raphael, 1994), and conscious control of speech production is difficult to maintain. The influence of habituated control patterns is strong even when the speech mechanism is disrupted, as in dysarthria, and motivation for change is high. Recently, a patient whose intelligibility was severely compromised by Parkinson's dysarthria spoke for many others when he protested, "But in my head it [my speech] feels normal!" Indeed, one can argue that speech-language pathologists are needed precisely because so many individuals with phonological, voice or motor speech disorders seem to be unable to modify engrained speech patterns, even when highly motivated to do so.

SELF–PERCEPTION OF SPEECH

Another problem encountered by speech-language pathologists is that many clients seem unable to perceive their speech productions as others perceive them. This problem may be due in part to the "deformation of auditory feedback" in singing that is discussed by Professors Verdolini and Krebs (see Chapter 14), but there is a language-based component as well. Speakers of various languages use different acoustic criteria to recognize phonemic boundaries. Japanese speakers, for example, do not recognize the English-language distinction between /r/ and /l/ (Strange & Jenkins, 1978). Similarly, speech-language pathology clients who have developed nonstandard phonology fail to perceive distinctions between their aberrant phonemes and standard productions. When an 18-year-old student, who had been frustrated by previous therapy, produced /ɝ/ correctly with the help of real time spectrographic feedback, he complained that his correct production didn't sound right to him (Shuster, Ruscello, & Smith, 1992).

Visual feedback provided by the spectral analyzer can be used during training to neutralize and replace habituated motor speech patterns and to supersede inefficient or obstructive perceptual cues. Let us briefly review some principles of motor learning to see where visual feedback fits into the process and how it might be used most effectively.

PRINCIPLES OF MOTOR LEARNING: A BRIEF OVERVIEW

Schmidt (1988) defined motor learning as "a set of processes associated with prac-tice or experience leading to relatively permanent changes in skilled behavior." Motor learning progresses through three generally recognized phases, called *cognitive*, *associative*, and *autonomous* (Fitts & Posner, 1967). These phases are not separate and distinct; they gradually merge into one another.

Cognitive Phase

At the cognitive phase, a learner's primary task is to determine what is to be done, how performance is to be assessed, and how best to attempt the first few trials. Early comprehension of the task is aided by explanations, demonstrations, other teaching materials, and initial trials. Emphasis is placed on perceptual mechanisms, with extensive use of visual, auditory, and kinesthetic cues. These cues may come from internal (sensory) feedback or from *extrinsic* feedback, which generally consists of visual or auditory displays. Performance during this phase is highly variable, and progress is most dramatic. Most improvements at this phase can be defined in terms of learning what to do rather than consolidation of the motor patterns themselves. Eventually, the learner manages to integrate the separate components of the activity and begins to form a plan for initiating each of the component parts in proper sequence.

The cognitive phase, although crucial, encompasses a relatively short period in the overall learning process (Fitts & Posner, 1967; Oxendine, 1984; Schmidt, 1988). As the process continues, the learner must develop *internal representations* of performance goals if permanent learning is to take place (Schmidt, 1988, Schmidt, Lange, & Young, 1990; Wulf, Schmidt, & Deubel, 1993). At this transitional phase, the cognitive and associative phases overlap.

Associative Phase

In the associative phase, learners begin to refine their skills. Although they receive less extrinsic feedback, they gradually eliminate errors and make fine adjustments. Movements become consistent, and errors decrease in frequency and magnitude. In this phase, learners develop internal error-detection and correction mechanisms that supplant external feedback in guiding their actions (Schmidt et al., 1990). At this phase, the speech-language pathologist's client produces a target phoneme consistently in words, phrases, and even sentences in the structured atmosphere of the clinic. The student of voice begins to achieve an optimal resonance on a single vowel, at a single pitch, and then attempts to generalize the performance to other sounds, other pitches, and eventually to song. Many hours of practice under favorable conditions are required during the associative phase, which takes significantly longer to complete than does the cognitive phase (Oxendine, 1984).

In advancing from the cognitive to the associative phase, the structure of practice is critical. Extrinsic feedback is important for establishing and improving performance, but long-term learning will not be effective if subjects are allowed to become dependent on extrinsic feedback. As Verdolini and Krebs (see Chapter 14) have emphasized, retention of recently acquired skills is demonstrably improved by reducing or fading the delivery schedule of guiding information (Schmidt et al., 1990; Young & Schmidt, 1992; Wulf et al., 1993). Effective long-term learning is enhanced when reduced guidance induces the development of subjective error detection capabilities and internal information processing to replace external guidance from feedback.

Autonomous Phase

In the autonomous phase, which is gradually reached after extended periods of practice (Schmidt, 1988), the skill has become largely automatic. Schmidt (1987) described a model of automaticity in which the motor system, through practice, shifts its mode of operation from a closed-loop, data-driven style to an open-loop system in which motor programs are developed that control movement and reduce the need for sensory information to guide error correction. Conscious attention is not required and in fact may interfere with effective performance of well-learned actions (Oxendine, 1984). For a speaker or singer at this level, conscious attention may be devoted to higher order elements such as voice quality or projection, or to fine points of meaning rather than to elements of speech production per se.

USING GRAM AS AN EXTRINSIC FEEDBACK INSTRUMENT IN THERAPY

A Tool for the Cognitive Phase

From the foregoing it is clear that extrinsic feedback is principally an instrument of the cognitive phase. The extrinsic visual feedback provided by Gram can be viewed as a substitute for internal sensory cues that provide knowledge of performance. It provides specific action-event information that is outside the normal sensory channels, making normally unattended behavior observable. Once behavior becomes observable and a focus of attention, it can be brought under voluntary control (Basmajian, 1982).

Withdrawal of Feedback

We have seen that extrinsic feedback can help clients acquire the desired skills, but we have also seen that long-term learning will not take place unless feedback is carefully withdrawn as soon as there is consistency of performance under continuous feedback conditions. How does one do this? An initial approach would be to use the Gram program alternatively as a direct real-time feedback (RTF) device and as a modality for knowledge of results (KR). Withdrawal from RTF can be readily accomplished by shielding or turning the screen while clients perform the task. Upon completion of 1, 5, 10, or 20 consecutive correct productions without RTF, clients can again view saved samples on the screen for post-trial KR. In this way, correct performance, supported by the client's internal representation rather than by external feedback, may be reinforced and maintained.

When using extrinsic feedback, the clinician should remember that there will be those who catch on to the activity quickly, and those who have considerable difficulty. The majority will fall somewhere in between. Clinicians can use RTF with all their clients as long as they bear in mind that criteria for withdrawal of RTF must be based on individual performance.

SOME GENERAL NOTES ON USING GRAM FOR SPEECH AND VOICE REAL-TIME FEEDBACK

Delay

There is a nominal 75 millisecond delay between any utterance and its visual representation on the screen by Gram. That nominal delay is extended, however, when the user places additional signal processing demands on the system. Thus, the most immediate display will be one in which the FFT size is set to 512, and the Frequency scale is set to Linear. As FFT size is raised, particularly to values of 4096 and above, the delay is increased and the value of the program as a provider of RTF diminishes.

Display Modes

The most recent version of Gram (version 4.2.10 at this writing) offers three display modes, Scroll, BScope, and LScope. Each display offers advantages. The scope displays can be configured as either BScope, a histogram bar display where amplitude is represented at each frequency by a vertical bar, or LScope, a continuous line plot of amplitude at each frequency. The scope displays are particularly useful for helping individuals to acquire continuous vocalic sounds, such as the ever-elusive /ɝ/. The scope modes are similarly effective in helping individuals who wish to modify their accents to acquire the vowels of a phonological set that differs from their own. The clinician may find LScope more useful in that it permits the placement of frequency markers for formant targeting, while the BScope display does not. Either display is, of course, an acontextual snapshot of a vowel shape. Once the isolated target has been achieved consistently, it would be advantageous to transfer the display to the Scroll mode and, from this display, continue to work on the vowel target in varying phonemic contexts.

Signal Acquisition

Verdolini and Krebs (see Chapter 14) point out that data acquisition procedures must be consistent if the system is to yield consistent, reliable KR. From a clinical standpoint, it is important to appreciate that standardization must be established *for each client*, and *for each separate task* that the client may perform.

Microphone placement is often critical. The microphone should usually be relatively close to the speaker and (usually) oriented toward the speaker's face. At times, the clinician may want to place the microphone within millimeters of the client's lips, while at other times it may be advantageous to position it 12 or more inches away. The clinician might consider using a headset-mounted microphone as a way to ensure within- and across-session consistency of signal strength.

Simple Arithmetic

For some of the applications described here, it will be helpful to have a calculator available. The Windows calculator accessory is very handy for this purpose. To access this utility, click on Start, then Programs, then Accessories, and finally Calculator. Once accessed, drag the calculator to the lower left-hand corner of the screen (Figure 15–1). The calculator is usually in the background, unseen, until it is needed. To access it, simply click on its icon in the Taskbar. When finished with it, click anywhere on the Gram display to make the calculator disappear.

Parameters

Gram users can alter the settings in the Scan Input or Analyze Input dialog boxes to adjust the program's signal acquisition and performance.

Frequency range is primarily determined by selecting the Sample Rate (Hz).

The faster the sampling rate, the broader the frequency range. Generally, 5 kHz or 11 kHz are fine for voice and the vocalic formants, while rates of 22 kHz or 44 kHz tend to display the fricatives best. When FFT is set anywhere above 512, the user will usually be able to make an additional selection of pitch ranges, using the Band (Hz) scrollbar.

Adjustment of frequency range to accommodate the F_0 ranges of men, women and children is accomplished most readily by increasing or decreasing Sample Rate. You can also consider changing FFT values as well. One can also adjust the frequency range (Band [Hz]) directly when FFT size is set to 1024 or higher.

Adjustments in the FFT Size affect frequency range, display latency (delay), and duration of the Scroll mode display. Latency and duration vary directly with FFT size.

Adjustment of Spectrum Average is particularly helpful in smoothing the Scope displays, which tend to be too unstable for feedback display at values lower than 15 or 20.

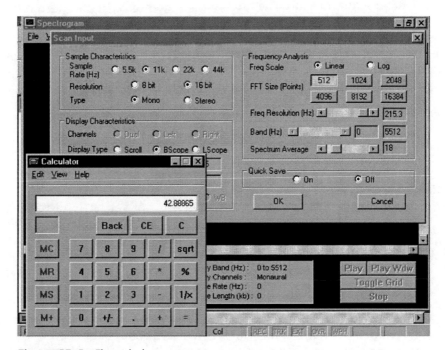

Figure 15–1. The calculator.

Additional adjustments will be discussed in context of particular applications, below. A table of useful settings has been compiled (Table 15–1) to simplify these adjustments for the reader.

SELECTED SPEECH AND VOICE THERAPY TASKS ADAPTED TO GRAM

The remainder of this chapter will be a how-to manual, representing methods for using Gram to supply RTF and KR for a range of commonly employed speech and voice therapy tasks. The tasks will be organized in terms of (unavoidably overlapping) speech production parameters as follows: articulatory accuracy, duration, intensity, pitch, prosody, rate, breath support, and voice quality. This section of the text is best followed at the computer with the Gram program active.

Articulatory Accuracy

Spectrographic displays are most helpful with continuant sounds, such as vowels, fricatives, and glides. Because these sounds extend over a considerable duration, they are readily represented on a screen and are accessible for on-line monitoring and adjustment based on RTF. Plosives are difficult to display in real-time because of their brief duration and relative paucity of acoustic energy.

Targeting Vowels and Vocalic Continuants

To target specific vowels and vocalic continuants, begin with the Scope display. Set the parameters to the Vowels (LScope) setting in Table 15–1. Select Scan Input (F4), then set the frequency marks to the average F_1 and F_2 (or F_2 and F_3) values of the target. Average formant values for men, women, and children are readily

obtained from several sources, for example, Chapter 9 in Baken (1992). Frequency Markers are set by clicking on Pointers at the top of the screen, then clicking Freq Mark. The frequency markers will be displayed as vertical lines on either Scope display (Figure 15–2). As the client attempts the target sound, peak frequencies will appear. The client is then instructed to adjust the articulators to move the peaks onto the target markers. Contrastive drill is often helpful at this stage. Once consistency is reached in this display, then the RTF should be gradually withdrawn, as suggested above. When consistency is reached without RTF, then the task should be moved from production of the isolated sound to production of the sound in various phonemic contexts. Start by presenting CV and CVC targets using the Scope display, then move to the Scroll display (Figure 15–3).

In Scroll, reset the parameters to the Vowels settings, if need be (see Table 15–1). There is no need to reset the frequency markers, which will now be displayed as horizontal lines. As the display begins, look for formant strength and for the presence of higher harmonics at onset. Practice alternating between the target vowel/continuant and other continuant sounds. Choose alternate targets for their value in contrastive drill (in sound or articulatory positioning). Later, practice a prolonged production of the target in CVC contexts. Withdraw RTF as the client progresses in consistency.

Plosives

Gram is not very helpful in discriminating the various plosives, but attending to the presence of the F_0 frequencies (voice bar) works well in distinguishing voiced from unvoiced consonants. This is readily seen in the Basic Scroll configuration (see Table 15–1).

The clinician might prefer to use the waveform bar at the top of the screen to display the voicing distinction. Voiceless

Table 15-1. Gram Parameters.

Task	File Type	Sample Rate	Display Type	Attenuation	Linear/ Log	FFT Size	Frequency Resolution (Hz)	Band (Hz)	Spectrum Average	Frequency Mark
Basic Scroll -a	Analyze/Scan Input	5.5k	Scroll	0	Lin	512	10	0-2756	4	
Basic Scroll -b	Analyze/Scan Input	11k	Scroll	0	Lin	1024	10	0-2756	4	
Vowels	Analyze/Scan Input	11k	LScope	0	Lin	1024	107	200-2956	25	F_1/F_2
Pitch Range -a	Analyze Input	5.5k	Scroll	0	Lin	2048	2.7	60-749	4	
Pitch Range -b	Analyze Input	11k	Scroll	0	Lin	4096	2.7	60-749	4	
Habitual Pitch	Analyze/Scan Input	11k	Scroll	0	Lin	4096	2.7	60-749	4	
Prosody	Analyze/Scan Input	11k	Scroll	0	Log	1024	11	100-5512	4	
Fricative Scroll	Analyze/Scan Input	44k	Scroll	0	Lin	1024	43	1980-13005	4	3.5kHz-9kHz
s/ʃ Scope	Scan Input	22k	Scope	0	Lin	512	200	0-11025	30	

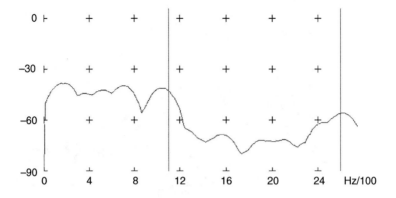

Figure 15-2. Frequency markers set for vowel targeting.

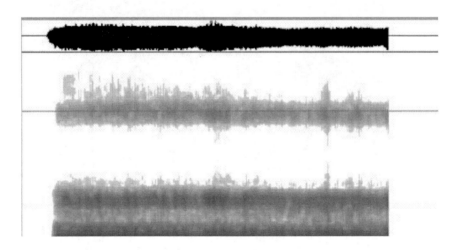

Figure 15-3. Frequency markers in the Scroll display.

plosives should produce a momentary absence of waveform energy, while there should be some energy present during all or most of the closed phase of voiced plosives. The user will find that microphone placement is a very sensitive aspect of data acquisition during this activity. By placing the microphone obliquely against the neck at the level of the thyroid cartilage, one can acquire a clear distinction between voiced and unvoiced conso-

nants. In Figure 15-4, the microphone was about one inch from the speaker's lips.

Fricatives

f/θ Contrast

Because their places of production are so close, these fricative sounds are difficult

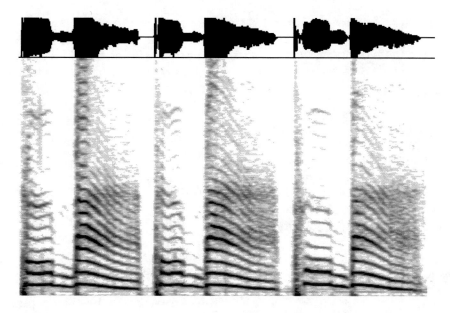

Figure 15–4. Voiced/voiceless distinction [pu/ba]. (CD)

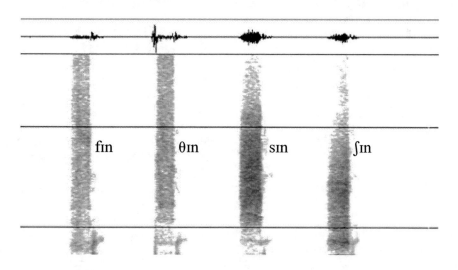

Figure 15–5. fricative distinctions: "thin/fin", "sin/shin." (CD)

to distinguish (Figure 15–5). /f/ presents as a very diffuse noise source with no truly prominent bands of energy. On the other hand, /θ/ presents as diffuse noise with a distinct band of increased amplitude in the range 5 kHz to 9 kHz. To display this contrast, select Scan or Analyze Input, then set the parameters as shown in the Fricative Scroll row of Table 15–1. Frequency markers can be set (or reset) any time the main display is active.

s/∫ Contrast

This contrast can use the same parameters as f/θ. Set Frequency pointers at roughly 3.5 kHz and 9 kHz to frame the energy in /s/, and to 2.2 kHz and 6 kHz to frame the major energy in /∫/. To frame only the major energy of /s/, try setting the frequency marks to 4900 and 8000 Hz.

Voice and Respiration

Duration

Maximum Phonation Time

Before beginning this task, access the Windows calculator program to help determine and record maximum phonation time. Now, select Analyze Input (F2) and set the parameters as in the Basic Scroll configuration (see Table 15–1). You may wish to change FFT to 1024, which will narrow the frequency range and enhance your view of the vocal harmonics. Have the client take a comfortable deep breath, then click on OK (or press Enter) and cue the client to begin. Click STOP (or press Esc) when the client stops. This brings up the Analyze File parameter window. Notice that the duration of the file (Beginning and End in milliseconds) is displayed on the left side of the screen. At this point, you will use the calculator to help you place the entire sample on a single screen so that it can be measured accurately. Click on the calculator from the Windows Taskbar. Enter the "End" number, and divide by 590. Round this product up to a whole number, and use it to set the Time Scale. This will place the entire sample on one screen. Click on OK, then measure the voiced area with the

mouse. Using the calculator again, subtract the end time from the beginning time to determine MPT in milliseconds.

This application serves multiple purposes. It provides an accurate measure of MPT, it records the sample for later comparison, and it provides a voice sample for visual analysis of harmonic strength and noise (see Vocal Clarity on p. 254).

S/Z Ratio

For both sounds, follow the MPT sequence using the Fricative Scroll parameters. While it is certainly easy and sufficiently accurate to record s/z durations with a stopwatch, the clinician may prefer to have a record of the client's production. This is particularly true if there is suspicion of difficulty in sustaining consistent levels of phonatory or respiratory effort.

Phrase Length Targeting

This activity is commonly employed in the management of various types of dysarthria, vocal fold paralysis, alaryngeal speech, diminished respiratory control, and other speech and voice disorders. In the Basic Scroll configuration, a full Scroll screen represents about seven seconds of time. Using the Analyze or Scan Input modes, you can use the cursor to represent a time interval from one to seven seconds from the *right* margin of the screen (Figure 15–6). Select Scan Input (F4), check parameters, and click OK to begin. Use the mouse to position the cursor and simply "left-click." Now, let the scrolling display reach the right side of the screen and cue the client to begin a phrase. The onset of the phrase will appear at the right of the screen, scrolling leftward toward your cursor target. The client's task is to maintain production until the onset display reaches the cursor. To extend the duration of the screen display beyond seven seconds, change the FFT value. An FFT of 2048 yields about 13 seconds, and an FFT of 4096 provides about

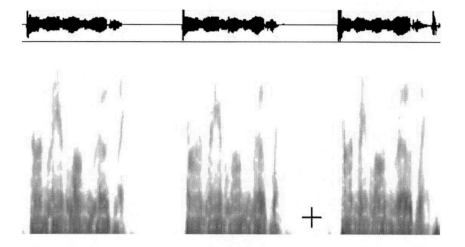

Figure 15–6. Setting a marker for phrase length targeting.

20 seconds per screen. While this application of cursor placement cannot be precise in Gram, a rough approximation is generally adequate for therapeutic phrase length targeting.

Intensity

Intensity assessment and targeting can be problematic on many current generation computers because the software drivers that control audio operations may have built-in automatic gain control features that cannot be turned off. To determine if a computer has this problem, go to Scan Input (F4) and select the Scope display mode. If the display automatically rises to a consistent level every time this screen is opened in a quiet room, then the system has built-in automatic gain control (Figure 15–7). In this situation, the user cannot trust the display to reflect absolute changes in intensity, but it can still be used to display relative changes.

Intensity Targeting

Select Scan or Analyze Input, with Scope display. At the left margin, relative dB levels are displayed. Amplitude changes in F_0 (at the left of the display) can be measured and used for RTF. It may be useful to adjust the relative sensitivity of the display using the vertical scroll bar at the right side of the display.

Pitch

Pitch Range (Assessment or Expansion)

Use Analyze Input (F2) with the Pitch Range settings. Have the client start from a comfortable pitch, then produce ascending tones until the limit is reached. Repeat the process, moving from the highest to the lowest sustainable pitch (Figure 15–8). After **STOP**ping the signal acquisition, use the cursor to mark highest and lowest fundamental frequencies. Remember to distinguish modal from loft registers!

Habitual Pitch

It is possible to obtain a rough approximation of a client's habitual pitch with Gram. Open Analyze Input (F2) with settings for Habitual Pitch (see Table 15–1). The client may read sentences, count from one to ten, or perhaps recite the first sentence or two from the Declaration of

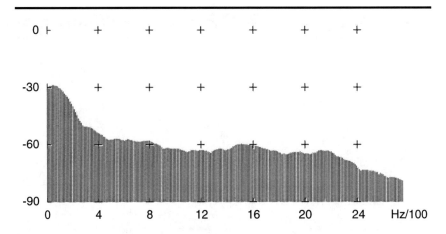

Figure 15–7. The effect of automatic gain control (BScope).

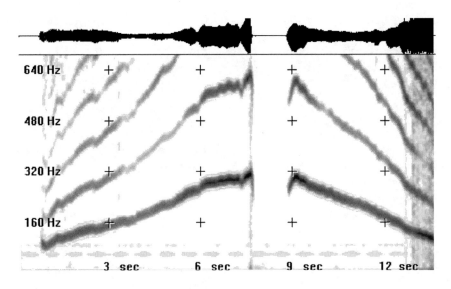

Figure 15–8. The pitch range task. 🆔

Independence (Figure 15–9). When the client has finished, STOP signal acquisition, then use the cursor to mark the apparent median F_0. Some users find it more accurate to measure the frequency of the second harmonic and then divide by 2 to obtain the estimated habitual F_0.

Pitch Targeting

Use Scan or Analyze Input (F2 or F4), with the settings for Pitch Range. Before the client begins, set a frequency mark (Poin-

ters/Freq. Mark) to the desired frequency (Figure 15–10). The client's task is to match the lowest harmonic to the designated pitch range. Alternatively, use a Scope display after setting the frequency marker.

Prosody and Rate Control

Use the Prosody parameters in the Analyze or Scan Input modes. With a sample rate of 5.5kHz and an FFT of 512, there is

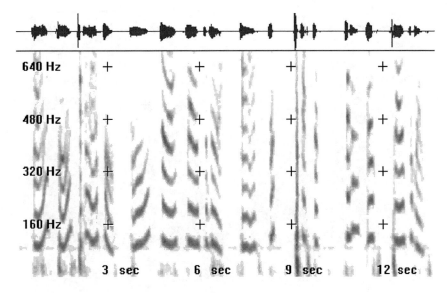

Figure 15-9. Habitual pitch estimation. 💿

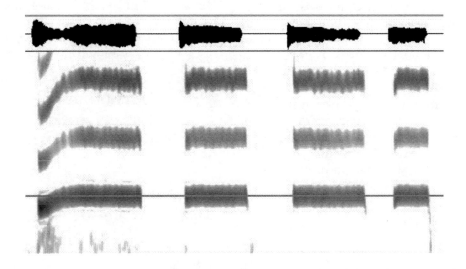

Figure 15-10. Frequency marker set for pitch targeting.

minimal delay. Use the Log scale to accentuate the F_0 and lower harmonics (Figure 15–11). When the Log scale is used, the display is a bit blocky, but it gives a rapid and readable representation of inflectional change. This configuration can also be used to provide feedback for rate control. Use the Linear scale to eliminate the blocky display.

Vocal Coordination and Control

Continuous Phonation

This technique is commonly used in the management of hyperfunctional voice disorders and disfluency. Use Scan Input

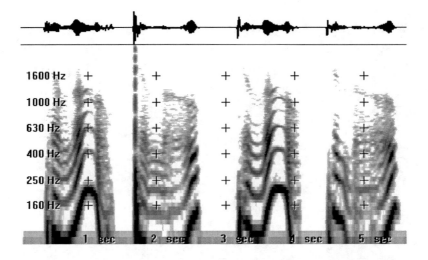

Figure 15–11. Log scale display for prosody and rate control. CD

(F4) with the Basic Scroll display parameters (Figure 15–12). In the initial phase of this work, the client repeats stimulus phrases and sentences that contain only voiced sounds and plenty of vowel-initial words. The client's task is to produce phrases in legato fashion, with no voiceless breaks. The client may attend to the waveform at the top of the screen, which should reflect continuous energy, even (if not especially) at word boundaries. Alternatively, the client's attention may be directed to the spectrogram display, particularly toward the lower formants, which should be uninterrupted in this task.

Vocal Clarity

Use the Basic Scroll display parameters in Scan Input mode to generate a narrow band spectrogram. This display allows the client and clinician to examine the harmonics for consistency of intensity and relative freedom from noise (Figure 15–13). Set for 1024 FFT size for men and 512 FFT size for women and children.

Effort Closure Exercises

Use the Basic Scroll screen. Good performance will be manifested as a strong verti-

cal display of harmonic energy, whereas poor effort closure will probably result in "blooming," in which the lower harmonics, related to F_0, appear early in a syllable, while the higher harmonics appear after a significant lag (Figure 15–14).

Reduction of Vocal Hyperfunction, Hard Glottal Attack

Alternate Voiced and Unvoiced Continuant Cognate Pairs

This task serves to induce a sense of voice-induced vibration for the client while viewing the difference between voiced and unvoiced continuant pairs (s/z, f/v, etc.). Use the Fricative Scroll setup with a 22 kHz sampling speed to show higher formant frequencies. Call the client's attention to the prominent voice bar during voiced phonemes (Figure 15–15).

Prephonation Airflow

This technique is used to soften glottal attack at the moment of voice onset. In one

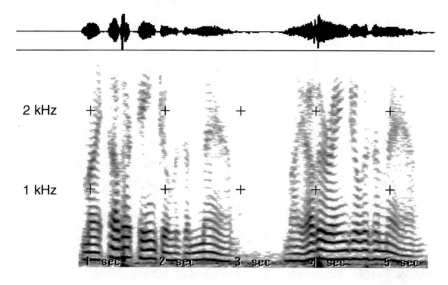

Figure 15–12. Discontinuous and continuous phonation. 📀

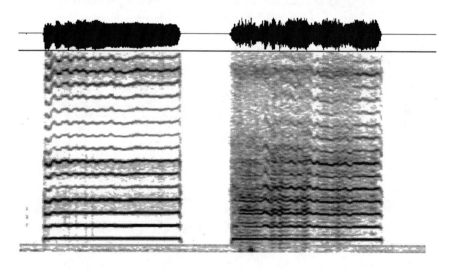

Figure 15–13. Clear and hoarse voice qualities. 📀

variation, the client begins the utterance with a gentle /h/, followed by a vowel. In this variation, the client will see a broad (1k) band of noise from about 500Hz to 1.5 kHz reflecting the /h/ prior to the onset of the phonated vowel (Figure 15–16). Gradual onset of the vowel will be clearly differentiated from the frication by the appearance of the harmonics. Attention should also be drawn to the gradual increase of intensity, reflected in the waveform display.

Whispered Onset

In a second variation (Figure 15–17), the client whispers the target vowel, producing turbulent noise in the region of the prominent F_1 for that vowel, until gentle

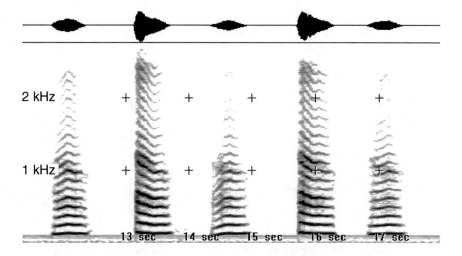

Figure 15–14. Sharp vowel onset contrasted with "blooming." 🔘

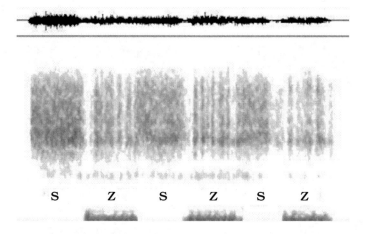

Figure 15–15. Contrastive voicing drill with sibilants. 🔘

phonation produces a voice bar and gradual sharpening of the waveform display.

Yawn-Sigh Technique

If this common strategy for laryngeal relaxation is successful, the spectrograph display will show reduction of energy in the range above the F_0 area (conservatively, above 500 Hz). In contrast, a hard glottal attack will show substantial energy in the F_1 and F_2 regions, originating in a sharp vertical line.

Gram Can Grow with You

These past few pages offer some preliminary suggestions for the use of the Gram program to provide extrinsic feedback in the practice of speech and voice training in a speech-language pathology practice. Gram can be configured to display most of the parameters of speech and voice that can be captured acoustically. As the clinician becomes familiar with the program by using it in therapy, other methods and other applications will undoubt-

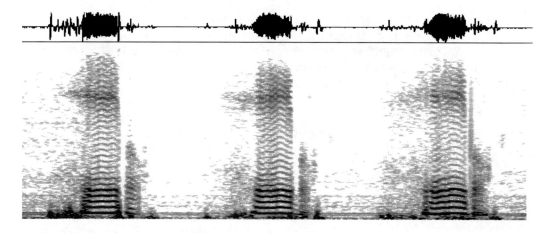

Figure 15–16. Prephonation airflow for soft glottal onset. 🆑

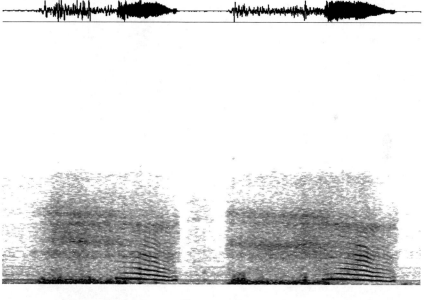

Figure 15–17. Whispered onset. 🆑

edly spring from the natural creativity that is part of the therapeutic process.

OTHER COMPUTERIZED FEEDBACK SYSTEMS

There are several commercial computerized feedback systems on the market as of this writing. Should the reader desire sys-

tems with more sophisticated and dedicated functions than Gram can offer, a full listing of these systems can be found in Appendix D.

SUMMARY

- Speech-language pathologists confront the same challenges in training that are encountered by teachers of voice. The first of these is that habituated speech patterns interfere with the acquisition of new patterns. The second is that speakers do not perceive their own speech as others do.

- Visual feedback provided by the spectral analyzer can be used to neutralize and replace habituated motor speech patterns and to supersede inefficient or obstructive perceptual cues.

- A review of principles of motor learning indicates that extrinsic feedback, such as that provided by Gram, is most effective in the cognitive, or early skill acquisition phase. Furthermore, long-term learning will be effective only if the extrinsic feedback is systematically withdrawn as the new skill develops.

- The Gram program can readily be configured to provide speech and voice biofeedback for a substantial variety of common therapeutic tasks. To do so, the user must become familiar with the program and its control features.

- The tasks for which Gram can supply essentially real-time extrinsic feedback extend to practically every domain of speech and voice production. The boundaries of its utility may be determined as much by the imagination and creativity of the clinician/teacher as by the limitations of the program itself.

- While there are other excellent computer-based systems that provide real-time feedback for speech and voice parameters, Gram stands alone in its cost-free availability to anyone with a computer and Internet access.

CHAPTER

16

CREATING A STATE-OF-THE-ART VOICE STUDIO

When considering the setup of a voice studio practitioners must pay close attention to three areas:

- studio atmosphere
- equipment required for the task
- environmental concerns.

FIRST IMPRESSIONS COUNT

To understand the critical nature of these three areas of concern, imagine trying to decide if one should retain the services of a certain doctor or lawyer. While people may not be consciously aware of it, when walking into a professional workplace for the first time, the choice of furniture, decoration, and functional placement all work together to help build first impressions. Seemingly insignificant details observed consciously or unconsciously, contribute to an initial feeling of trust—or lack thereof.

If one sees old, poorly maintained equipment, or doesn't find equipment that is standard in such a facility, one may decide to look elsewhere. Other concerns, such as the temperature, humidity, and cleanliness of the air in the facility can factor into the overall impression as well.

The trust level that is required for a successful professional relationship between singer and teacher is just as critical as that necessary between a doctor and patient. The amount of thought and care that a voice practitioner invests in setting up a new studio (or refurbishing an established one) becomes a critical concern.

Even after the time for first impressions are over and a trust bond has begun to develop, the atmosphere of the office should continue to reinforce, during every working session, the atmosphere of professionalism and trust.

WORKING ATMOSPHERE

Many well-designed professional offices balance an almost home-like comfort with other indicators that simultaneously declare the space as a serious business site. If the ratio between these two seemingly conflicting extremes is skewed too much to the home side, the client may feel insecure. On the other hand, if the space is too businesslike, the client may sense an off-putting, unwelcoming sterility. One needs to strike a ratio that does not stray too far from the center but yet reflects the philosophy of the voice practitioner's approach to the profession.

Comfort and Professionalism

Furnishings

It will be up to the teacher to decide how many amenities he or she needs for the individual studio. Matters such as furnishings, carpet, wall hangings, window treatment, color of the walls, and so forth are all matters of individual taste and style. With very little work (and expense) the comfort level of a voice studio, and the sense of well-being it conveys, can increase significantly.

Plants

Plants, as long as the teacher has the time and interest to care for them, can add much to the atmosphere of a studio. Foliage such as ivy and philodendron are perhaps the least expensive and are the most forgiving if care is not lavished on them on a regular basis. If plants are not a burden to the voice practitioner, then by all means bring them into the studio. Try to avoid flowering plants as they may provoke allergic reactions in your students.

Professional Decoration

Designated areas in a professional office often prominently feature the professional's diplomas, certificates, photographs capturing career highlights, awards, and so forth. These additions go a long way toward the establishment of the professional nature of the office (see Figure 16–1).

Studio (Business) Name

Practitioners should have a name for the studio, and if possible, a logo. The author's studio is called *VoiceQuest*, a name that seems to inspire more trust than if it were called, Garyth's Voice Studio. Consider the reaction one may have when looking for a good auto mechanic. AutoCraft may convey a better image than Bob's Garage. It is no different when considering the reaction of a potential client to the name of your vocal training business.

Nameplate on the Door

A brass or wooden nameplate on the door to the studio greets the student with the message, "This is a professional space and the work that goes on in here is serious and trustworthy."

Stationary, Business Cards, and Receipts

Once practitioners select an appropriate name for their business, they should print stationary, business cards, and receipt books with:

- studio name
- address
- phone number
- fax number
- email address

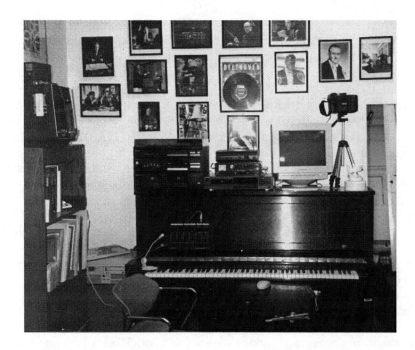

Figure 16–1. Picture of the author's voice studio at Drew University, Madison, New Jersey.

- owner's name
- logo

Product engineers call this "look-and-feel" bonding. Voice practitioners *are* offering a product: their knowledge, skill and experience. Attention to all aspects, no matter how insignificant they may seem, will pay off in the kind of clients practitioners attract thereby impacting on the success of the studio.

STUDIO EQUIPMENT

Piano

A piano is an indispensable piece of equipment for the voice studio. The choice of the type of piano has a lot of influence on the layout of the studio furnishings. Of course, the piano must be of high quality and be *always* well tuned. One can choose among an upright, studio piano, or a grand piano.

Sight Lines and Choice of Piano

Most musicians, when confronted with a decision of what type of piano to choose for their work, quite naturally consider the sound of the instrument as their principal concern. But the choice of piano for a voice studio must also take sight lines into consideration.

Upright Pianos

Many teachers who use an upright piano are confronted with two choices: placing the student either behind the piano, facing the teacher, or to the side of the piano, facing the keyboard.

The decision between these options depends on how much of the student's body the teacher wishes to observe. Those teachers who pay as much attention to the abdominal wall musculature as they do to the face, will want to see the entire person, from the feet to the top of the head.

Grand Pianos

There is no doubt that a grand piano, because of its greater string length, sounds better than upright pianos. The grand piano also conveys an impression of greater professionalism because it is the instrument that is used in concert life.

The grand piano solves the sight-line problem, but only if the singer can be persuaded to stand somewhat back from the crook. Whether they are facing the teacher at the keyboard or facing an audience, singers love to nestle into the crook; it is a very comfortable place. There is an undeniable emotional security in that space, but a singer standing there is invisible to the teacher from the waist down.

One additional consideration: If practitioners do use a grand piano in their studio, they should make sure to protect its top. Piano tops quickly become temporary desks and even tables for food and drink. Despite the most strongly voiced prohibitions by the teacher, some student will eventually manage to damage the surface of the lid.

The best protection is a thin sheet of plastic that can be purchased at a hardware store and then cut to the size and shape of the piano lid. If the finish of the piano is in flawless condition, it is advisable to put a beautiful soft cloth between the piano lid and the plastic. Make sure that the cloth itself is soft enough to avoid marring the surface if it is shifted.

Floor Loads

It is not uncommon for a professional to establish a voice studio only to find out, some months later, that the weight of their piano cannot be carried by the floor of the studio. Floor loads (the term used by structural engineers) can be determined precisely. The concern with the weight of a piano is not so much its total weight, but the *point load* weight because the weight of the piano is concentrated on its wheels. Voice practitioners must be sure that the flooring structure of a proposed studio can bear the weight of the piano, themselves, their students, and all ancillary equipment. If they do not own the studio space, they should get a written OK for the placement of the piano before renting, buying, or borrowing studio space. They should also make sure that the space will be safe and that they will not be liable for any damage to the floor if the estimated load-carrying capacity is incorrect.

Audio Equipment

A good audio system is a necessity for three reasons:

- recording lessons
- closed-loop feedback
- playback of historical recordings as reference

Recording Lessons

Benefits

Many students consider it helpful to leave the teaching/coaching session with a recording of the entire lesson for use until the next session. Few singers ever have time to take notes during a lesson and the availability of the tape can help them reconstruct solutions for problems that occurred during the session. Also, listening to recordings of one's voice can accelerate the process of learning to accept the actual sound of the voice, that which would reach the audience versus the student's internal hearing. One of the greatest challenges faced by voice practitioners is to wean singers away from believing that what they hear internally is acoustical truth.

Instant Playback During the Lesson

The practitioner can stop the tape during the session and play back short passages to illustrate pedagogical points. Thus, the student gets to hear the voice as it actually sounds, good or bad, from an external vantage point.

Closed-Loop Feedback

Closed loop feedback was mentioned in Chapter 5. It is an audio setup where the singer's voice is picked up with a good microphone, amplified, and sent back to the student through earphones. Hearing themselves sing, *while they are singing*, helps them correlate how the instrument *feels* with how it actually sounds to the audience.

This real-time feedback is invaluable, but, care must be taken so that it does not become a crutch; see Chapter 5 for details.

Playback of Historical Recordings

Today's singing students and their teachers have access to examples of the greatest singing that has occurred since the advent of recording in the early years of the twentieth century. One can listen to technical facets such as:

- tonal production
- performing styles
- Klang of foreign languages
- acting through diction
- ornaments and alternate passages (especially in opera)
- how an aria fits into the whole fabric of a larger work

Often the habit of learning by listening to others starts in the studio under the teacher's guidance. (Also remember the wise admonition that one can learn as much from a poor performance as a good one.)

Equipment List for the Studio's Audio Equipment

The equipment needed to utilize the electronic audio potential is listed as follows:

- a high-quality amplifier

- a cassette recorder (preferably a dubbing deck to permit fast duplication of examples) that includes the following:

Microphone inputs: Note of caution: the designers of recording equipment apparently have decided that nobody needs microphone inputs anymore, so most of the cassette recorders on the market cannot be used to record the voice in the studio. When one does find a machine with microphone inputs, the machine is generally very expensive. As a result, this piece of equipment may constitute a voice studio's largest single expense (other than the piano). Given the constant demands that will be made on the mechanics and circuits of this machine, buying a top-of-the-line recorder may be a good idea.

Input volume controls and metering: Voice practitioners should make sure that the machine has recording input controls and a way of metering the sound being recorded. Many inexpensive tape machines are meant for automatic speech recording and have circuitry that raises the level of soft sounds and reduces the level of loud ones so everything is homogenized into a sort of mezzo forte.

Dolby noise reduction: The machine should also have Dolby noise reduction (it now comes in several types).

- Name-brand tape should be required for use in the studio. Be sure to specify the brand and type of tape that the student should bring to the session. Cheap cassette tape is inferior, especially in terms of the abrasiveness of the magnetic coating. Running cheap tape across the head of a high-priced tape recorder is the equivalent of running a continuous strip of fine sandpaper across those delicate surfaces.
- good microphone (a single unit, stereo microphone, if possible).
- CD player (if one uses historical recordings in his or her practice).

- turntable (if the teacher has an extensive collection of vinyl recordings).
- reel-to-reel tape recorder (if the studio possesses a tape library made on such machines during the period preceding the advent of good cassette decks). If a practitioner intends to do research, a reel-to-reel recorder is also valuable as it offers a way to slow signals down for closer observation (recording at 7.5 ips and playing back at 3.75 ips for analysis).
- connecting cables and power cords for all of the above.
- power strips to plug in equipment— power strips also make it easy to turn whole systems on and off with one switch instead of many.
- surge protectors at the wall outlets to protect expensive equipment from damaging line surges.
- velcro cable ties to bundle the systems' cables so the studio space doesn't wind up looking like Medusa's head.

One need not spend a mountain of money for good equipment. Modest expenditures, because of advances in miniaturization and mass production, can yield equipment of a quality unthinkable at that price just 20 years ago.

A Procurement Schedule May Be Right for You

Voice practitioners who are just starting out or are replacing obsolete equipment don't have to buy everything at once. Set a priority list and stick to it.

VIDEO EQUIPMENT

The reasons for owning video recording and playback equipment are the same as those given above for audio equipment. The ability to videotape a student during the session and then play the passage back is a great aid, especially when dealing with technical matters such as breathing, stance, use of facial expression, body language in acting, and so forth. While one may have a mirror in the studio in which students can observe their performance while singing, one must remember that the students' attention is divided between what they are doing (singing) and what they are supposed to be observing. Seeing a replay of the event is often a better pedagogical technique.

COMPUTER

If one wishes to employ computer analysis as VRTF in the voice studio, a computer system, including the following, is a necessity.

Equipment List

- CPU (IBM-compatible)

  A 486 is a minimum; a Pentium processor is preferred, the faster the better. The computer has to make unbelievable numbers of mathematical calculations per second in order to present the VRTF image on the monitor. The faster the CPU, the faster and cleaner the image.

- mouse (comes as standard equipment with most computer systems).
- operating system: The CPU must be running Windows 95 or Windows 98 to take advantage of much of the analysis software on the market today.
- memory (as much RAM as possible): The minimum is 16 megs; the Drew University Studio runs its computers with 64 megs of RAM.
- monitor: For use in the voice studio, the larger the better as both teacher and student will be looking at the display from a distance. A 17" color monitor should be the minimum size for VRTF use. If the monitor is located on top of

the piano be sure to protect the top of the piano with a felt or rubber pad.
- sound card: A 16-bit sound card is minimum.
- microphone

The microphone need not be expensive. Fidelity is needed only up to c. 15,000 Hz. But, before purchasing a microphone, read the section that follows on microphone placement.

The microphone should have a wind screen (a foam bonnet) that cuts down unwanted "pops" and transients from the subject's breath as it leaves the mouth.

- hard drive

Buy as large a hard drive as is affordable. Sound and graphics files, should one wish to save them for future reference, are *very* large (a *.wav file can easily go over 1 meg in just a few seconds of recording). Consider a hard drive that is 5 gigs or larger.

- software: A fully functional spectrogram program can be found on the CD that accompanies this book. Other programs are on the market that can perform more complex technical operations which reveal facets such as:

jitter

shimmer

LPC

EGG

The spectrogram that accompanies this book should be adequate to enable the reader to get his or her working knowledge and studio up and running. The vast majority of analyses that one will need to perform can be done with this program. Also, because the program is straightforward and user friendly, it is easy to learn to use.

Setup of the Computer

CPU

The CPU should be out of the way, perhaps on the floor but still easily accessible to the teacher during the session. One may have to buy extension cables in order to accomplish this.

Mouse

Be sure you will have a horizontal surface upon which you can operate the mouse.

Monitor

Place the monitor on top of the piano in a position where it is possible for both the teacher and the subject to see it clearly.

Computer Microphone

The microphone need not be a top-of-the-line model since one will not be concerned with extremely high frequencies (as you would in an audio recording for archival purposes). This microphone should be *in addition* to the one used to make the recording of the session.

Microphone Placement

From session to session, the microphone must be at the same relative distance and position in front of the subject's mouth. Microphones are maddeningly susceptible to mal-positioning.

The intensity of sound that the microphone senses decreases in proportion to the square of the distance from the source, so an improperly placed microphone may result in an ill-defined spectrogram that is not as useful as it could be.

The microphone should not be too close to the mouth, or the spectrogram will be distorted. It should not be too far away, as the weaker harmonics will not be read.

Experiment with the microphone to find the optimal distance.

There are three possible solutions:

- Place the microphone on a floor stand (preferably a boom stand so the microphone can be stabilized in the proper position in front of the singer).

  This solution will work, but it is the most difficult of the three to accomplish. Singers like to—and should—move, so the ideal microphone positioning will be lost very quickly. If the singer is told to stand still in front of the microphone, bad habits of stance and vocal production may result.

  A better solution is one that lets the microphone move with the subject (Figure 16–2)

- Use a headset (a combination of a microphone on a boomlet attached to a head band). *Important:* If one uses a headset, it should **not** have an earphone. An earphone covers the students ear(s) and will result in a skewed sense of the sound being produced.

Several manufacturers sell quality headsets at reasonable prices. Look for a headset designed for speech recognition (computer dictation programs). This type of microphone is fully adjustable, has a windscreen, and has sophisticated noise cancellation capabilities that make sure the singer is the prime source of the sound being analyzed.

Make sure the cord that connects the headset to the sound card is long enough to permit the performer free range during the lesson. Also, make sure that the cord, after it leaves the sound card, is secured to a heavy object. That way, if the subject forgets and moves too far, no damage to the inputs on the computer's sound card will occur.

- Place the microphone in a harmonica holder. This simple but elegant idea comes from Robert T. Sataloff's medical practice in Philadelphia. Sataloff uses an inexpensive harmonica holder (of the type that Bob Dylan uses) that can

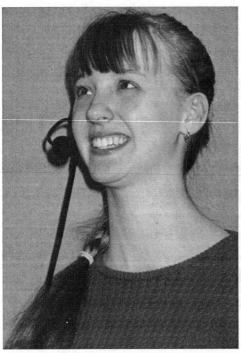
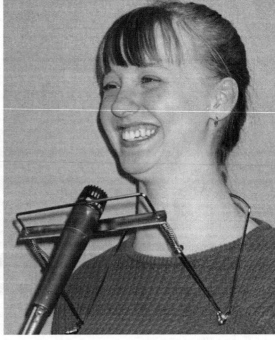

Figure 16–2. Student wearing a headset (left) and a microphone in a harmonica holder (right).

be purchased from most music stores. Again, as in the case of the headset, once it is set up, the student will not have to worry about proper positioning and can get on with the session (Figure 16–2).

As was the case with the headset, make sure the cord that connects the headset to the sound card is long enough and properly secured.

Ancillary Equipment

Clock

A large clock should be placed where the student *cannot* see it. Also, for studio use, quartz-action clocks that do not produce an audible tick are the best.

Phone Machine

Students need a way to leave messages for their instructor. A phone machine, especially if one can change the outgoing message remotely, is invaluable in case of lesson-canceling bad weather or the teacher's illness.

Teacher's Chair

Especially if one teaches a long schedule, his or her chair should be as comfortable and ergonomic as possible. Purchase a chair at a business furniture store. The chair should have:

• a swivel base
• arms that will allow support but not get in the way of piano playing
• ergonomically designed back and seat
• adjustable height and back controls

One should not stint on this expense. If the price of the right chair seems too high, practitioners should estimate how many hours they will spend in it during a year's lessons and then divide the cost by the number of hours. When viewed this way, an excellent chair isn't expensive at all!

Teacher's Side Desk

If the piano in the studio is a grand piano, its desk can serve as a writing surface. In addition, a nearby bookcase may serve as a storage area for reference material and other items necessary for the teaching process.

If one must work with an upright piano, the task of keeping lesson notes can be difficult. A low table on castors or wheels that can be kept adjacent to the keyboard can serve as an auxiliary writing surface as well as storage for other items. Such a table can be easily moved out of the way when the teacher must accompany the student. If this little auxiliary "desk" has a shelf, all the better. The one in use in the author's studio was made from the bottom of a broken secretary's chair mated with the top of a bedside table; it has served faithfully for years.

Student's Chair

This should be a comfortable chair in the teaching area for the student for use during long explanations, chatting, or if the student is not feeling well.

Bookcase for Reference Material

A small bookshelf for reference texts such as dictionaries, anatomy books, music texts, and so on, should be within arms reach of the voice teacher.

Bookcase for Recordings

Location

Since reference recordings are not usually an everyday need in voice sessions, bookshelves for recordings can be housed out of the immediate teaching area. If buying shelving for the first time, it is important to make sure there is plenty of room for expansion in the future.

Are the Shelves Sturdy Enough?

Also, consider the amount of weight that will go on the shelves. Books and recordings weigh a lot, and inexpensive shelving will warp with time. Discuss this with the salesperson. The author has constructed vertical panels that are wedged between each shelf at the midpoint (or, in the case of long shelves, at the "third" points). This helps carry the weight of the shelf contents to the floor so the shelving doesn't develop that "swayback" look.

Will Future Bookcases Match?

Practitioners should also buy bookcases from a manufacturer with a long track record. This way, they can reasonably expect to obtain matching shelving in the future.

Tissues

A box of tissues is an absolute must in the studio. Singers who arrive with upper-respiratory infections or who are emotionally upset will, more often as not, forget to bring their own tissues. Also make sure that there is a wastebasket with a plastic liner to receive the tissues discarded by those with upper-respiratory infections. The teacher shouldn't touch that refuse; it should be regarded as a biohazard!

ENVIRONMENTAL CONCERNS

Voice practitioners must learn to pay more attention to the environment in which they live, especially when it comes to the atmosphere that they breathe.

Air Temperature and Humidity

The air in the studio should *always* be at a comfortable level of temperature and humidity. Students should be able to walk in and sing and study in an exemplary atmosphere (one that, by example, they should try to recreate where they work and sleep). More important, the teacher is in need of a finely controlled atmospheric environment because of the number of hours he or she will spend in the room.

Warm Weather

In warm or hot weather, one may need:

- air conditioning
- humidifier

The humidifier may not be something that one thinks of during the summer except in areas that enjoy dry heat. Even in regions that suffer from a combination of heat and humidity, by the time an air conditioner drops the temperature to comfortable levels, the air can end up being too dry. One may need to *add* a little more humidity to keep the mucous membranes in the vocal system of both students and teacher at comfortable levels.

In Cold Weather

In cool or cold weather, one may need:

- thermostatic controls that allow very fine adjustment of the temperature.
- humidifier

When the *relative* humidity begins to drop below the comfort zone, it will be necessary to add humidity to the air. The best humidifiers for studio use are the small ones that hold approximately two gallons of water and create the humidity either by a heating coil (preferred) or an ultrasonic vaporizer. The heating coil type is preferred because there is some potential bactericidal effect when the mist is created. Another consideration is that the ultrasonic types tend to fail because of mineral buildup in areas with hard water.

Above all, one must keep all parts of the humidifier where water is stored or handled operating-room clean. This habit will protect everyone's health and lengthen the working life of the machine.

Lighting

The act of reading music from a distance requires a considerable amount of light. Local spot lighting (floor and piano lamps) should be available for the teacher, and overhead track lighting is a good solution for the area in which students stand during sessions. Overhead lighting (large panels on the ceiling), especially if it is of the fluorescent type, is usually unsatisfactory in the studio. Not only is it inferior light for reading music, but it also tends to make the atmosphere of the room a bit sterile.

BOOKKEEPING AND TAX CONSIDERATIONS

Run the Voice Studio as a Legal Business

Running a studio as a legitimate business enables one to declare all related expenses as *business tax* deductions:

- declare all the income on tax returns
- keep accurate and up-to-date records of all income and expenditures.

Does the Studio Business Need an Accountant?

Most voice studios are small, uncomplicated businesses. If one keeps careful records and remains familiar with tax code changes applicable to the type of business, one probably does not need an accountant. Federal, state, and local governments publish excellent guides that can help you.

Bookkeeping Software

Bookkeeping software for the computer can be extremely helpful. Today's software is easy to use (the same as using a checkbook) and inexpensive. Making sure that the records are entered promptly and accurately makes tax-filing time a breeze.

At Tax-Filing Time

Business owners should consult the current tax codes before declaring an item as deductible; tax codes change from year to year, especially those for small businesses. Those government publications referred to above are an invaluable source of guidance, and they are free. When dealing with the tax code, it is wise to remember the admonition, "Never argue with the government about facts, only interpretation."

SUMMARY

This book is about bringing more objectivity and professionalism into the craft of vocal pedagogy. While the inclusion of voice science and digital feedback are the text's major goals, it is easy to forget that the total image surrounding the craft is also important. This chapter opened by invoking memories of visits to the offices of other respected professions. Part of their aura is the care taken to *look* professional as well as to *be* professional. Voice teaching professionals should seek to impart the same level of professionalism in their studios.

AFTERWORD

By now, it is hoped that the reader has gained a sense of the potential embodied in the use of various forms of digital voice analysis and its applicability to the study of great singing. The technology and the equipment needed to employ the spectrogram and the power spectrum are easily available and affordable. The EGG, while still expensive, will add to any studio's capabilities and should be considered, especially for studios in schools with vocal pedagogy departments. With this triumvirate of feedback technology, we stand at the threshold of achieving gains in three principal areas.

SINGERS

Singers need every aid we can discover in their quest for greater and quicker access to vocal technique. The problems presented by the intervention of a singer's language habits coupled with lack of accuracy in his or her internal hearing are extensive and pervasive. Given these problems, this author has often wondered how we *do* manage to produce the numbers of glorious singers that populate the stage. The answer is, of course, the shear number of determined, talented singers co-joined with inventive, intuitive, and knowledgeable teachers who help those singers transcend the problems inherent in the development of the voice.

The use of the digital triumvirate has the potential of providing us with exciting tools to enhance already proven pedagogical techniques as well as potentially help develop new ones. Many students who are exposed to this technology will not only become fine stage artists, but will also carry on as the voice teachers of the next generation. Their proven comfort level with computers could facilitate the acceptance of this technology in the future of vocal pedagogy.

VOCAL PEDAGOGY

It is an old adage that teachers learn more while teaching their students than their students learn from them. The use of digital technology in the voice studio not only has the potential to improve the performance of singers but can also improve the understanding and technique of the teachers themselves. If the revelations observed on the monitor during lessons encourages teachers' curiosity, those teachers will be far more likely to stay current with the gains in voice science as a way of constantly improving their pedagogical craft. With that enhancement, there can be clearer, more objective communication between student and teacher on how to achieve agreed-upon technical norms. Finally, this increased knowledge will better prepare those students for the day when they will also teach. Each gain in the acquisition of true, objective understanding of the voice as a physics problem first, and an artistic problem second, has the potential of spawning greater understanding and with it, a concurrent improvement in the profession.

Developing and understanding the objective norms of fine singing has another benefit waiting in the wings. Armed with a more objective approach to technique, voice practitioners could be able to communicate with each other on more solid ground as they discuss and share pedagogical methods. No technical problem in the voice has a single solution, and the comparison of pedagogical methods among voice practitioners can only improve the craft. As more and more voice practitioners learn to use digital analysis in the studio and share their findings with others, exciting new prospects are possible; prospects that we can only dimly perceive at this point in the development of the field.

Finally, as vocal practitioners learn more about voice science and gain the ability to discuss singing in objective terms, we may find that the partnership which has already begun between enlightened voice practitioners and voice science may deepen and broaden. This shift from a subjective to an objective approach has the possibility of placing the dialogue between researchers and the practitioners on a more equal footing, permitting the voice practitioner to become a respected partner in voice research. Experienced voice practitioners may ask practical questions that may trigger research by voice scientists. This type of research could be crucial as to the future growth of our knowledge of the voice.

ELEVATING THE PROFESSION

The exciting prospect of having a means to measure and quantify what constitutes fine singing, as well as the means of testing the efficacy of corrective methods, may move our pedagogical work to a point where professional standards and certification can become a reality. With that achievement, vocal pedagogy will finally be able to take its place along with the sister professions of vocal pathology and voice therapy.

LET US OPEN OUR EYES, OUR EARS, AND OUR MINDS

Examples of great singing have always been abundantly available to us in the form of live performance and recordings. Voice practitioners need only open their ears and eyes to partake of the gifts that the great singers offer. As voice professionals, we must apportion the time we spend listening to those singers between being:

- consumers—enjoying the performance being both viscerally and emotionally thrilled, and

- professional listeners—carefully analyzing the means by which those singers produce the thrills.

By carrying the sounds of those singers into the studio/lab and experimenting with our own voices while utilizing digital analytical technology, more and more answers to the persistent question of *how* the great singers accomplish what they do will become available to us to possess and use.

CONCLUSION: TECHNIQUE IN THE SERVICE OF ART

This text began with a suggestion that the voice practitioner divide the training of singers into two subtasks: the teaching of technique and the coaching of artistic values. Without the technique, all the coaching in the world cannot produce a great singer. To walk on stage and plumb the depths of the human heart and the spirit, a singer needs a technical armada at his or her command.

No matter how useful the triumvirate of the spectrogram, the power spectrum, and the EGG may become, one fact stands paramount: The enlightened voice pedagogue will always be the most important factor in the training of great singers. It is the communication of spirit to spirit between the voice practitioner and the singer that enables that final leap from technique to art.

So let us join in a partnership and embrace the rich possibilities of both the use of the available technology and the utilization of the impressive gains in knowledge produced by recent voice research. In so doing, we just might raise the status of our profession, and with it, the level of service to our students and, ultimately, to the art itself.

APPENDIX

A

SINGER'S IPA TABLE

Garyth Nair

VOWELS

Front vowels

Type	IPA	ASCII	English	Italian	German	French	Remarks
	i[j]	105	keen	Si	Liebe	gui	See Chapter 8 for [j]
	y	121	–	–	müde	une	
	ɪ	73	pin,	–	bitte	–	See Chapter 8 for [j]
	ʏ	89	–	–	Glück	–	
	e	101	chaotic	stella	Leben	été	
	ɛ	69	bet	eccetto	Bett	tête	
	ɛ̃	69 +41	–	–	–	infame	
	æ	81	sat	–	–	–	

Central vowels

Type	IPA	ASCII	English	Italian	German	French	Remarks
	a	97	father	Maria	Mann	patte	Needed for unstressed "a" Maria.
	ʌ	195	cup	–	–	–	In American English, /ʌ/ is very prone to spreading.
	ɜ	206	–	–	Öffnen	–	No /r/ color.

Back vowels

Type	IPA	ASCII	English	Italian	German	French	Remarks
	u [w]	117	soon	subito	Uhr	genou	See Chapter 8 for [w].
	ʊ	85	put	–	Mutter	–	
	o	111	pope	non	Tot	mot	
	ɔ	141	soft	occhio	Morgen	ombrage	
	ɔ̃	141 +41	–	–	–	bon	
	œ	191	heard	–	zwölf	heure	

Diphthongs

Type	IPA	ASCII	English	Italian	German	French	Remarks
	œ̃	191 +41	—	—	—	un	
	ø	79	—	—	schön	peu	
	a	65	law	caro	Wagen	pas	
	ɑ̃	65 +41	—	—	—	sans, vent	
	oᵁ	111 +117	no	—	—	—	
	eⁱ	101 +105	day	dovei	—	—	
	ʌⁱ	195 +105	lie	—	Mai	—	In American English, /ʌ/ is very prone to spreading. See footnote.
	ɔⁱ	141 +105	boy	vuoi	Kreuz	—	
	ʌᵁ	195 +85	now	aura	Haus	—	In American English, /ʌ/ is very prone to spreading. Note that the secondary is /ᵁ/ not /u/.

English /r/ diphthongs

Type	IPA	ASCII	English	Italian	German	French	Remarks
	eə	—	air	—	—	—	Take care that these do not become triphthongs as in /eʷə/, or /ɔʷə/, or /moʷə/.
	iə	—	ear	—	—	—	
	ɔə	—	oar, or	—	—	—	
	uə	—	sewer	—	—	—	
	oə	—	mower	—	—	—	

(continued)

Type	IPA	ASCII	English	Italian	German	French	Remarks
English triphthongs ending in /r/							
	ʌiˑɚ	—	higher	—	—	—	As with the /r/ diphthongs, watch that the superscripted sound does not cause an unwanted accent on the ɚ secondary. It should be a gentle glide. In those combinations containing /ʌ/, beware of spreading.
	ɑuˑɚ	—	our	—	—	—	
	ɔˑɚ	—	foyer	—	—	—	
	ʌuˑɚ	—	flower	—	—	—	
CONSONANTS WITH PITCH							
Class I pitch consonants —least restriction in the oral cavity							Because this class of phoneme is performed at fairly transitory places in words, care must be taken to keep these on proper pitch.
English /r/ central vowels							Note: These two phonemes can be listed in either the vowel or pitch consonant classes. They are included in here, instead of in the vowels, to make them easier to find when readers are using this chart as a reference.
	ɚ	171 + 213	fathe<u>r</u>	—	—	—	Slight /r/ color. See Chapter 8.
	ɝ	206 + 213	su<u>rge</u>	—	—	—	More intense than ɚ. See Chapter 8.
Glides							
	j	72 or 74	yes	<u>i</u>osa	<u>j</u>a	b<u>i</u>en	Begins as /i/, glides to next vowel
	w	87	<u>w</u>ind	<u>u</u>omo	—	m<u>oi</u>	Begins as /ʊ/, glides to next vowel
Class II pitch consonants —moderate restriction in the oral cavity							
Liquid /l/							
	l	108	<u>l</u>ight	<u>l</u>argo	<u>l</u>achen	<u>l</u>ent	See Chapter 8.
Liquid glide							
	ʎ	180	—	g<u>li</u>	—	—	Actually ʎi. See Chapter 8.

Type	IPA	ASCII	English	Italian	German	French	Remarks
Other forms of /r/							
	ř	114 +224		rapporto			All must have definite pitch and care must be taken not to improperly scoop.
	ɹ	168	Hard	–	–	–	Retroflex (midwest, hard /r/)
	ʁ	210	–	–	rot	rouge	Parisian /r/ at the velum, also used in German.
	ɾ	82	(Brit.)—very	–	–	–	British; flipped at the front of the oral cavity /ʳ/ (once).
Class III pitch consonants —most restrictive in the oral cavity							
Nasals							
	m	109	mom	mamma	mit	moi	
	n	110	nun	nozze	nun	nez	
	ŋ	78	bong	–	singen	–	
Nasal glide							
	ɲ	248	onion	gnocco	–	agneau	
Fricatives, voiced							
	ð	68	that	–	–	–	With phonation (on definite pitch).
	v	118	vote	viva	was	vert	Care must be taken to make sure the pitch is definite and correct. A significant "scooping" class of phonemes.
	z	122	zebra	cosa	Seele	zéle	
CONSONANTS WITHOUT PITCH							
Fricatives, unvoiced							
	θ	84	think	–	–	–	Without phonation (pitch).
	f	103	face	forte	fahren	faux	

(continued)

Type	IPA	ASCii	English	Italian	German	French	Remarks
	s	115	saw	senza	Haus	ses	Used in French, front alveolar.
	ʃ	83	shine	scena	schön	creche	Alveolar, more frontal than the ç needed for German. When used in English, it is followed by a glide /j/.
	ɥ	231	—	—	—	lui	
	ç	254	hue	—	—	—	
	ʝ	67	—	—	noch	—	Palatal, needed for soft German ch.
	x	120	Ugh!	—	Ach!	—	Bernuoli trill at the velum, also needed in Hebrew.
	h	104	had	—	hoch	—	In English and German, the phoneme is made by creating turbulence at the glottis. There are other placements as well. In French, a glottal stoke, ʔ, is substituted for the ʰ. In Italian, it is silent.
Fricative "Glide"	ʍ	227	which	—	—	—	Almost archaic, but still elegantly useful. Begins with fricative, then ʷ on the way to the primary vowel.
Prevoiced plosives	b	98	bible	bambino	Bett	bien	Even though there is a pitch sounded in the prevoicing, it is not sustainable. Also, note that prevoicings can be a significant "scooping" site.
	d	100	dog	dolore	der	domire	
	g	103	go	gamba ghianda	Geist	galant	

Type	IPA	ASCII	English	Italian	German	French	Remarks
Pure plosives							
	p	112	pop	portare	Prinz	penser	
	t	116	top	tempo	Tag	timbre	
	k	107	kind	ecco, chi	Kaiser	que	
	ʔ	63	uh-uh	–	–	–	Glottal stop.
	ʔ	63 super- scripted	I'm on	–	–	–	Glottal stroke. Often needed to differentiate vowel joins between words. Used in English and German (indicated by superscripting the glottal symbol ʔ).
Affricates							
	tʃ	116 +83	church	lanciare	Klatsch	–	
Prevoiced affricate							
	dʒ	100 +90	judge	gioco	–	–	The prevoicing can be a significant source of "scooping."

Footnote: Most texts on speech and singing transliterate the diphthong in the word lie *as /aɪ/ or /aɪ/. The author prefers /ʌɪ/because, when well sung, /ʌ/ seems to join more easily with other phoenemes, resulting in richer and better defined diphthongs. The /ʌ/ vowel has a ɔad reputation because it is so often performed poorly. It is worth the studio time to learn to sing this phoneme with the richness it deserves.*

© Copyright 1999 by Garyth Nair.

APPENDIX

B

WARMUP TABLE:
CVC JOINS

Garyth Nair

Do each warm up singing on the consonant, then vowel, then returning to the consonant without pause. Work all possible CVC joins across each vowel row before moving down to the next consonant.

	Vowels		Front					Central		Back				
	IPA	ɪ	ɛ	e	i	æ	ʌ	ə	ʊ	ɑ	o	u	IPA
Consonants with pitch													
Class III: *most oral restriction*													
Nasals	m	ɪ	ɛ	e	i	æ	ʌ	ə	ʊ	ɑ	o	u	m
	n	ɪ	ɛ	e	i	æ	ʌ	ə	ʊ	ɑ	o	u	n
	ŋ	ɪ	ɛ	e	i	æ	ʌ	ə	ʊ	ɑ	o	u	ŋ
Voiced Fricatives	ð	ɪ	ɛ	e	i	æ	ʌ	ə	ʊ	ɑ	o	u	ð
	v	ɪ	ɛ	e	i	æ	ʌ	ə	ʊ	ɑ	o	u	v
	z	ɪ	ɛ	e	i	æ	ʌ	ə	ʊ	ɑ	o	u	z
	ʒ	ɪ	ɛ	e	i	æ	ʌ	ə	ʊ	ɑ	o	u	ʒ

Vowels		Front					Central		Back				
Class II: *moderate oral restriction*													
Liquid	l	ɪ	ɛ	e	i	æ	ʌ	ə	ʊ	ɑ	o	u	l
Rolled	ř	ɪ	ɛ	e	i	æ	ʌ	ə	ʊ	ɑ	o	u	ř
Class I: *least oral restriction*													
initial /r/	r	ɪ	ɛ	e	i	æ	ʌ	ə	ʊ	ɑ	o	u	r
interior /r/	ɝ	ɪ	ɛ	e	i	æ	ʌ	ə	ʊ	ɑ	o	u	ɝ
final /r/	ɚ	ɪ	ɛ	e	i	æ	ʌ	ə	ʊ	ɑ	o	u	ɚ
Consonants with a prevoiced pitch element													
Prevoiced plosives	b	ɪ	ɛ	e	i	æ	ʌ	ə	ʊ	ɑ	o	u	b
	d	ɪ	ɛ	e	i	æ	ʌ	ə	ʊ	ɑ	o	u	d
	g	ɪ	ɛ	e	i	æ	ʌ	ə	ʊ	ɑ	o	u	g
Prevoiced affricate	dʒ	ɪ	ɛ	e	i	æ	ʌ	ə	ʊ	ɑ	o	u	dʒ
Consonants without pitch													
Class III: *most oral restriction*													
Pure Fricatives	θ	ɪ	ɛ	e	i	æ	ʌ	ə	ʊ	ɑ	o	u	θ
	f	ɪ	ɛ	e	i	æ	ʌ	ə	ʊ	ɑ	o	u	f
	s	ɪ	ɛ	e	i	æ	ʌ	ə	ʊ	ɑ	o	u	s
	ʃ	ɪ	ɛ	e	i	æ	ʌ	ə	ʊ	ɑ	o	u	ʃ
	ç	ɪ	ɛ	e	i	æ	ʌ	ə	ʊ	ɑ	o	u	ç
	x	ɪ	ɛ	e	i	æ	ʌ	ə	ʊ	ɑ	o	u	x
Stops	p	ɪ	ɛ	e	i	æ	ʌ	ə	ʊ	ɑ	o	u	p
	t	ɪ	ɛ	e	i	æ	ʌ	ə	ʊ	ɑ	o	u	t
	k	ɪ	ɛ	e	i	æ	ʌ	ə	ʊ	ɑ	o	u	k
Affricate	tʃ	ɪ	ɛ	e	i	æ	ʌ	ə	ʊ	ɑ	o	u	tʃ
Class I: *least oral restriction*													
	h	ɪ	ɛ	e	i	æ	ʌ	ə	ʊ	ɑ	o	u	h

Note: this table does not contain all possible VCV joins, only the primary joins for English.

Other phonemes, both vowels and consonants, should be added to aid in the habitualization of excellent joins in non-English languages as well.

APPENDIX

C

DETAILED EXPLANATION OF GRAM CONTROLS AND SETTINGS

Richard Horne, Author of GRAM

PRINCIPLES OF OPERATION

A spectrogram is a plot of the frequency components of an audio signal as a function of time. In the Spectrogram program (GRAM.EXE), digital audio recordings (Windows *.wav files) or real-time audio (Windows sound card input) are analyzed to produce either a scrolling spectrogram display or a spectrum analyzer scope display revealing the hidden frequency structure of the sound.

DISPLAY MODES

Two display modes are provided, a scrolling spectrogram display and a spectrum analyzer scope display.

Spectrogram Display

The scrolling spectrogram display depicts the audio signal as a frequency versus time plot with signal amplitude at each frequency represented by intensity (or color). The display can be configured for either dual channel or single channel audio with a wide selection of frequency resolutions and either linear or logarithmic frequency scales. In dual channel operation, the spectrogram window is split into left and right halves with separate scrolling spectrograms for the left and right audio channels.

A continuous readout of time (milliseconds), frequency (Hz), and signal level (dB) at the position of the mouse pointer (cursor) is displayed at the bottom left of the display. A coordinate grid can also be added or removed by clicking the "Toggle Grid" button at the bottom right of the display.

Spectrogram can play back the audio sample through the sound card when the user clicks the "Play" or "PlayWdw" buttons at the bottom right of the display. "PlayWdw" replays only the segment of the spectrogram visible in the display window, whereas Play replays the entire width of the spectrogram.

Spectrum Analyzer Scope Display

A spectrum analyzer scope display is also available for viewing the sound spectrum. The scope display can be configured for either dual-channel or single-channel audio with a wide selection of frequency resolutions and either linear or logarithmic frequency scales. In dual-channel operation, the left channel data are plotted in blue, and the right channel data are plotted in yellow. This allows for an evaluation of the spectral differences between the two channels.

The scope display can be configured as either a histogram bar display (BScope) where component amplitude is represented at each frequency by a vertical bar or as a continuous line plot of component amplitude at each frequency (LScope).

A continuous readout of time (milliseconds), frequency (Hz), and signal level (dB) at the position of the mouse pointer (cursor) is shown at the bottom left of the display. A coordinate grid can also be added or removed by clicking the "Toggle Grid" button at the bottom right of the display.

The scope display can be calibrated using the vertical scroll bar at the right side of the display window. The scope display shows a fixed 90 dB signal range. However, many interacting factors will affect the absolute level of frequency components shown on the display. While the relative levels of frequency components to each other will always be correct, the gain of the sound card and the combination of frequency analysis parameters selected will affect absolute measurement. Use the vertical scroll bar to adjust the amplitude of a known frequency component to its exact value. Then absolute measurement of all other components will also be correct.

MODES OF OPERATION

The Spectrogram program provides two modes of operation, Analyze and Scan.

Analyze Modes

The Analyze File and Analyze Input modes are used to produce a permanent spectrogram plot from either recorded wave files or real-time audio data from the sound card. The Analyze Modes allow repeated manipulation of the analysis parameters to obtain the best possible spectrogram plot. Choose "File—Analyze File" from the main menu to analyze an existing wave file. Choose "File—Analyze Input" to analyze incoming audio from the sound card.

Scan Modes

The Scan File and Scan Input modes are used to produce a real-time spectrogram or scope display from either a recorded wave file or real-time audio data from the sound card. The Scan Modes do not allow further manipulation of the analysis parameters. However, scanning of either a wave file or audio input will provide a real-time high resolution display of audio data of unlimited length. Choose "File—Scan File" from the main menu to scan an existing wave file. Choose "File—Scan Input" to scan incoming audio from the sound card.

ANALYSIS PARAMETERS

Before analyzing or scanning files or audio, the user will be presented with a dialog box for selection of the analysis parameters for the spectrogram. Each of these parameters is described below.

Sample Characteristics

Sample Rate (Hz)

The digital sampling rate is the frequency at which an audio signal is sampled by the Windows sound card. The spectrogram plot will cover a frequency band from zero to half the sampling rate. For Analyze Input or Scan Input, these buttons offer a choice of sampling rates of 5.5K, 11K, 22K, and 44K samples per second. Use the lowest sampling rates possible, taking into account that the sampling rate should be at least twice the frequency of the highest frequency component in the audio sample. Lower sampling rates can be used for Spectrograms with linear frequency scales. Logarithmic frequency scales will require higher sampling rates.

Resolution (Bits)

Resolution is the size of the sample data word in bits. Windows sound cards provide a resolution of either 8 bits or 16 bits. Generally, 16-bit data resolution should be used for all high-resolution spectrograms.

Type

A digital audio signal can be sampled as either a monaural or stereo type. Monaural recording is recommended when memory is limited.

Length (Sec)

The Analyze File and Analyze Input modes use this parameter to designate the length of a recorded wave file. In the Analyze File mode, the length of the previously recorded file is indicated. In the Analyze Input mode, the user can choose a sample length of 10, 20, 30, or "Any" seconds for a recorded file of unlimited length.

Display Characteristics

Channels

In analyzing or scanning a stereo type file or signal, the user has a choice of displaying either the left, the right, or both (dual) channels for either the scrolling spectrogram display or the spectrum analyzer scope display.

Display Type

For Analyze Input, Scan Input, and Scan File modes, the display type may be chosen as either the scrolling spectrogram display or the spectrum analyzer scope display. The spectrogram display consists of a scrolling 256 point frequency versus time spectrum plot for either single or dual channels. The scope display consists of real-time amplitude versus frequency display in typical scope format for either single or dual channels with 256 frequency points. The scrolling spectrogram display is automatically selected in the Analyze File mode.

Latency

For Analyze Input, Scan Input, and Scan File modes, latency is the length of time (in milliseconds) that it takes for the sound card to process a data sample and record it in memory. A spectrogram display that shows a series of closely spaced vertical spikes, or that fades in and out over time, probably has the latency value set too low. Choose the lowest value of latency that produces an undistorted spectrogram display. Once set for the sound card, this control will not need to be adjusted again.

Attenuation

The user is given a choice of display attenuation in order to reduce clutter in noisy digital recordings. Attenuation can be selected at any value between 0 and 18 dB. Use a threshold of 0 dB regularly, and select greater attenuation only if necessary to reduce clutter.

Palette

The user also has a choice of four color palettes; color on a black background (CB), color on a gray background (CG), black on a white background (BW), and white on a black background (WB). For a CB or CG display, red represents the strongest frequency component and dark blue the lowest. For a BW display, darker black represents the strongest component; for a WB display, brighter white represents the strongest component.

Frequency Analysis

Freq Scale

The user has a choice of either a linear or logarithmic frequency scale for computing a spectrogram. A linear scale spaces frequency components equally across the entire spectrum, while a logarithmic scale expands the low-frequency region of the spectrogram and compresses the high-frequency region.

FFT Size

The user can compute a spectrogram using 512, 1024, 2048, 4096, 8192, or 16384 point Fast Fourier Transforms (FFTs). The number of points used determines the frequency resolution of the spectrogram display. The highest possible frequency resolution of the spectrogram will be the

digital sampling rate divided by the number of FFT points. Use the larger FFTs only for high-resolution analysis or with the logarithmic frequency scale. The higher resolution FFTs require more time to compute the spectrogram. For this reason, it is sometimes preferable to decrease sampling rate when recording audio data if increased frequency resolution is needed, rather than to use a higher resolution FFT.

Freq Resolution

Frequency resolution determines the closest frequency components that can be visually separated on the display. For usual narrow-band frequency analysis, use the lowest value of frequency resolution. Where broadband analysis is required (such as for observation of speech formants), use a larger value of frequency resolution.

Freq Band

If the user has chosen a linear frequency scale, the highest resolution spectrograms may not fit entirely in the display window, which has a maximum height of 256 points. In this case, the Freq Band defines which portion of the spectrum bandwidth to display.

Spectrum Average

Spectrum average is the number of sequential spectrum measurements that are averaged together before display on either the scrolling spectrogram display or the scope display. Averaging is particularly useful in recovering weak periodic signals from a noisy background, but is probably not of much interest in analysis of speech or other rapidly varying signals. The user can choose averaging from 1 (no averaging) to 128 spectrum measurements. In general, the Spectrum Analyzer Scope display needs averaging of at least four spectrum measurements to produce a stable display.

RECORDING

Recording can be accomplished using either the Analyze Input Mode or the Scan Input Mode.

Recording Using Analyze Input

The Analyze Input mode allows the user to record fixed-length wave files or to record a continuous wave file of any length (limited only by the hard drive). Choose "File-Analyze Input" from the main menu. The user will first be prompted for a file name and then will see the Analyze Input dialog box for selection of analysis parameters as described in the Analysis Parameters section. If the user chooses a sample length of 10, 20, or 30 seconds, the sample will be both stored on disk and stored in RAM for immediate spectrum analysis. The user can also choose "Any" sample length, which is limited only by the size of the hard drive. In this case, the sample will be stored on the hard drive, but not in RAM, for immediate spectrum analysis. To analyze this sample, the user must process it separately using the Analyze Audio mode.

Recording Using Scan Input

The Scan Input mode allows the user to scan an incoming audio signal and turn recording on and off at times of interest. Choose "File—Scan Input" from the main menu and note the Scan Input dialog box for selection of analysis parameters as described previously. The dialog box also gives the user a **"Quick Save"** option which allows recording to be turned on and off while scanning audio input. After selecting "Quick Save On," the user will be prompted for a file name. Then, clicking the "Save" and "Stop Save" buttons will turn recording on and off while scanning. Note that it may take a few seconds before recording can be started again after turning recording off. Each time the user restarts recording, however, the new data segment is added to the end of the wave file specified. This feature allows recording of interesting events without having to record continuously for long periods.

Please note that use of the Quick Save feature requires that the hard drive be continuously powered. Some computers can operate in power-saving mode, in which the hard-drive power is turned off if the drive is not accessed for a fixed amount of time (usually 10 to 20 minutes). If Quick Save is attempted after the hard-drive power has been turned off, the time delay required to turn the drive on and bring it up to operating speed will disrupt the timing of the Spectrogram program and introduce this delay into data display and recording. If the user intends to run Quick Save after an extended period of scanning, then the computer's power saving mode must be disabled so that the hard drive will remain continuously powered.

MODIFYING, PLAYING, PRINTING, AND SAVING SPECTROGRAMS

Display Markers

In the real-time scanning modes (Analyze Input, Scan Input, and Scan File), the user has the option of adding a fixed reference cross mark to either the scrolling spectrogram display or the scope display. This marker can be useful for identification of amplitude or frequency peaks in the audio signal. Click the left mouse button to set this cross mark at the cursor position on the display.

In addition, the user has the option of adding one or two fixed frequency markers to the either the scrolling spectrogram display or the scope display. These markers can be useful when using Spectrogram to tune an audio source to a particular frequency. To activate the frequency markers, choose "Cursors—Freq Mark" from the main menu. Enter the frequency values

(Hz) for each marker, and they will then appear on the screen as fixed lines at the chosen frequencies.

Modifying Spectrograms

Once the user has computed a spectrogram, it is possible to make changes to its length, vertical or horizontal scale, threshold, or color to improve the frequency analysis. Choose "Parameters—Change" from the File Menu to bring up a dialog box to "Modify Analysis Parameters." The parameters that can be changed here are identical to those used to define the original spectrogram.

The user can select a section of the spectrogram for modification, rather than the entire length, by drag-selecting this section from the spectrogram display. This is accomplished by positioning the mouse pointer at the desired starting point, pressing the left mouse button, and dragging the mouse to the desired ending point. The dialog box will appear with the starting and ending locations filled according to the user's selection.

One can return to the initial spectrogram prior to any modification by choosing "Parameters—Restore" from the File menu. The starting spectrogram display is established the first time "Parameters—Change" is selected. The user can return to the starting spectrogram again and again until analyzing a new data file or recording a new sample. Note that this function is not available if the computer has only 8MB of RAM memory.

Playing Spectrograms

With a Windows-compatible sound card installed, the user will also be able to play back the spectrogram by clicking the "Play" or "Play Wdw" buttons. The Play button plays back the entire length of the .wav file, while the Play Wdw button plays back only that portion of the spectrogram that is visible in the Spectrogram Window.

Printing

With a graphics-capable printer attached to the computer, the user can print the spectrogram display from the Analyze File and Analyze Input modes by choosing "File—Print Window" from the main menu. The user will be presented with the "Print" dialog box for selection of a printer and printer properties. Click "Properties" to change paper orientation or other print characteristics. When printing a spectrogram to a black-and-white printer, it may be best to choose the black-on-white color palette (BW) for the spectrogram. Otherwise, the printer will use a very large amount of black ink filling in the black background on the printed image.

The user can also print the scope display from the Scan File, Scan Input, and Analyze Input modes with a graphics-capable printer. Stop the display at the desired point and then choose "File—Print Window" from the main menu. The scope display will always be printed with a white background rather than a black background in order to conserve printer ink.

Saving Audio and Bitmap Files

One can save a .wav file of the digital audio of the spectrogram by choosing "Save Wave" from the File Menu. The user can also save a bitmap of the Spectrogram Window by choosing "Save Bitmap" from the File Menu. One can choose to save either the visible section of the display bitmap by choosing "Window Bitmap" or the entire display bitmap, including area outside the display window, by choosing "Entire Bitmap." The bitmap save feature is available only for single-channel spectrograms.

Data Logging

The Spectrogram program provides an automatic data logging capability for researchers who wish to record the time, frequency, and harmonic level of events in an audio file. To save the amplitude and phase of every frequency point in a single channel spectrogram, choose "Log Data—Full Spectrum" from the File menu after computing a spectrogram. Data are saved in a text file that records each FFT output point, frequency, amplitude (16 bit), and phase. The amplitude levels in the full-spectrum log are calculated without any averaging of sequential spectrum measurements. The log file for the entire spectrogram can be very large, so it is best to drag select a smaller segment of interest on the spectrogram before saving a full-spectrum log.

To save the amplitude and phase of every frequency component at a single point in time, choose "Log Data—Spectrum" from the File menu after computing a single-channel spectrogram. After a file name is selected, a dialog box for recording of events will be presented. Data are saved in a text file that records each FFT output point, frequency, amplitude (16 bit), and phase. The amplitude levels in the single-spectrum log are calculated without any averaging of sequential spectrum measurements. Click the left mouse button on the event of interest on the spectrogram display, and the spectrum will be displayed in the dialog box. Choose "Save/Exit" to close and save the data-log file.

To save the dB signal level and time of individual points, choose "Log Data—Points" from the File menu after computing a single channel spectrogram. After a file name is selected, a dialog box for recording events will be presented. Data are saved in a text file that records an event identifier (usually a letter of the alphabet), the frequency, the time, and the harmonic level in dB (20 log amplitude) at the selected event on the spectrogram. Events to be recorded are defined by the researcher and could be such things as signal start, signal stop, highest pitch, lowest pitch, highest level, or lowest level, and so forth. Click the left mouse button on the event of interest on the spectrogram display, and the corresponding data-log values will be computed and entered. Enter an event identifier by clicking one of the buttons marked "a" through "h" or by typing an entry in the text box provided. Click "Enter Data" to record the event to the data-log file, and then move on to the next event and repeat the process. Enter as many events as needed, and then choose "Save/Exit" to close and save the data-log file. Opening an existing data-log file will allow the user to append data without starting a new file.

APPENDIX

D

COMPUTERIZED FEEDBACK SYSTEMS

Robert A. Volin

Gram is just one of a number of computer-based systems available for speech feedback and analysis. Here is a short list of commercially available systems that are in current use in speech-language pathology practices across the nation.

VoceVista

A new program that combines the power spectrum with waveform and EGG. It was developed by the Voice Research Lab at the University of Groningen, Netherlands, in conjunction with Richard S. Horne (the author of Gram). See Chapters 12 and 13 for more information on the workings of VV. *Contact:* Donald Miller by e-mail at d.g.miller@med.rug.nl.

Visi-Pitch II, Model 3300

The current version of the Visi-Pitch is comprised of six modules, three of which are likely to be of interest to the reader of this text. The *Pitch and Intensity Module* provides real-time displays of F_0 and intensity, either separately or combined in a single display. A split-screen option allows the clinician/teacher to provide a visual model for the learner to emulate. The system is highly adjustable with respect to duration and speed of display and is consequently very useful for work on glottal onset timing. The *Vowel and Sibilant Module* permit the modeling—again, in real-time—of continuants across a wide frequency band, as does Gram. There is a spectrum display which is much like Gram's BScope display, in which the clinician/teacher is ableto display a target for real-time emulation. Visually, the Visi-Pitch target is more satisfying than the Frequency Markers in Gram, but is probably no more effective. The Vowel and Sibilant Module also features a powerful display that captures vocalic F_1 and F_2 and displays these two frequencies as a single point on a two-dimensional vowel chart. This permits learners to attempt to match their vowel production to a specific target point on the screen. The Visi-Pitch has a *Voice Analysis Module* that provides a detailed analysis of several voice production parameters. This model does not provide real-time feedback, however. Another module contains a clever and visually striking set of games, in which the screen is controlled by the speaker's manipulation of various parameters of voice production. These displays are entertaining but are probably not precise enough to meet the demands of the readers of this text.

Contact: Kay Elemetrics Corporation, 2 Bridgewater Lane, Lincoln Park, NJ 07035-1488, 1-800-289-5297. Internet: http://www.kayelemetrics.com/.

IBM SpeechViewer III

The SpeechViewer was designed principally for use with young speakers. Most of its displays are entertaining graphic representations of simple parameters of voice or articulation. The modules that are likely to be most useful for readers of this text are the *Pitch and Loudness* and *Spectra* displays. The Pitch and Loudness module provides up to eight seconds of continuous display of intensity and F_0. The pitch and intensity ranges of the display can be adjusted to suit speaker and task. The Spectra display provides a real-time spectrum suitable for modeling vowel formants. The display allows a clinician/teacher to set a target outline for immediate, real-time emulation by the student.

Contact: Edmark Corporation, Attn: Customer Service, P.O. Box 97021, Redmond,

WA, 98073-9721. (800) 691-2986, E-mail: edmarkteam@edmark.com, Internet: http://www.Edmark.com/. Or contact IBM through the Internet at http://www.austin.ibm.com/sns/snsspv3.html.

Video Voice

The makers of Video Voice created a voice and speech feedback system designed to help deaf and hard of hearing children to speak. They were the first to combine a pitch/intensity display with an F_1/F_2 formant display and a set of speech-controlled games, complete with graphic rewards, in a single system. The Formant display provides a continuous trace of the F_1/F_2 coordinates throughout an utterance. This enables therapy applications, including vowel training (accuracy, onset/offset, and drift), voiced/voiceless phoneme discrimination, gross sibilant production, and correction of phonemic errors.

Contact: Micro Video, 210 Collingwood, Suite 100, P.O. Box 7357, Ann Arbor, MI 48107. Internet: http://www.videovoice.com/.

Dr. Speech

This system takes advantage of the sound card that is installed in most new PCs and does not require the user to install additional and expensive hardware. Earlier incarnations of this program did not run in real time and so were not effective for therapeutic applications. This has changed, according to a representative of Tiger Electronics, who wrote the following in a recent e-mail response: "Everything, I mean everything, is in real-time, audio, F_0, Intensity, Formants, Spectrograms, F_1-F_2, video, Nasal, Spectrums . . . on one screen you can see Audio, EGG F_0 and formants in real-time together" (Robert O'Brien, e-mail personal communication, December 14, 1998). If these claims are accurate, then Dr. Speech represents a formidable array of feedback and analysis modules at a comparatively reasonable cost (which, of course, is substantially greater than the cost of Gram).

Contact: Tiger DRS, Inc. P.O. Box 75063, Seattle, WA 98125. E-mail: tiger-electronics@worldnet.att.net. Internet: http://www.drspeech.com/.

Cafet

Cafet is a program, supported by proprietary hardware that must be installed in the computer, designed by a speech-language pathologist for the clinical treatment of stuttering in adults and adolescents. The system receives input about chest wall movement through a chest bellows and gathers acoustic input with a clip-on microphone. It provides continuous real-time visual feedback that simultaneously integrates respiratory movement characteristics with voice timing, continuity, and amplitude. While this system is originally specialized for the treatment of stuttering, it has been adapted for voice. One can readily imagine applications designed to develop breath support and other techniques for singing.

Contact: Cafet, Inc., 4208 Evergreen Lane, Suite 213, Annandale, VA 22003, (703) 941-8903.

Gram in Comparison

In some respects, Gram may be less versatile than other systems. Its data output may be less precise and less comprehensive, and its control features may be less adaptable for various tasks and conditions. If, however, the reader has used the program while following this text, it is apparent that Gram offers virtually real-time visual feedback with wide applicability for the training of singers and speakers. Beyond the program's evident utility, its primary advantage is its availability and cost. Gram is available to anyone with an Internet connection, and it is completely free of charge! Moreover, upgrades of the program are made available without charge by the author as soon as they are completed. As this chapter was begun, the latest version of Gram was v. 4.2.7. As the chapter was completed, version 4.2.10 was current. Which version are you using today?

APPENDIX

E

DIGITAL ANALYSIS OF SUNG PHONEMES AND SAGITTAL VIEWS OF SINGING PRODUCTION

Italic type = table and Roman type = Figure

Vowels	Spectrograms	Power Spectra	Sagittal Views
ɑ	4-11, 5-3, 8-1, 9-7, 9-8, 11-6	5-2, 12-1, 12-3, 12-6, 12-7, 12-8 12-9 12-10, 13-2, 13-5,	4-10, 8-1
æ	8-1, 10-4	–	8-1
ə	8-29	8-30	8-1
e	7-9, 8-1, 8-28	–	8-1
ɛ	8-1, 9-10	12-4, 12-5, 12-12, 13-3	8-1
i	4-8, 7-11, 7-12, 8-1, 8-3, 8-14, 8-22, 9-8, 9-10	8-6, 8-7, 13-4	4-9, 7-13, 7-15, 7-16, 8-1, 8-2

(continued)

Vowels	Spectrograms	Power Spectra	Sagittal Views
ɪ	8-1, 8-3, 8-4, 8-5, 9-10	8-6	8-1
o	8-1, 8-16, 8-17, 9-7	–	8-1
ɔ	7-12, 8-1, 10-5	13-3	7-13, 8-1
u	8-1, 8-16	–	7-16, 8-1
ʊ	8-1	–	8-1
ʌ	8-1, 8-29, 9-8	5-2, 8-30	8-1
Pitch consonants			
l	9-2, 9-7	–	9-13
m	9-5, 9-8	–	9-17
n	9-8	–	9-17
ŋ	9-8	–	9-17
r	9-7	–	9-12
ɚ	9-6	–	–
ř	9-14	–	–
ð	–	–	9-18
v	–	–	9-18
z	–	–	9-18
ʒ	–	–	9-18
Non-pitch consonants			
f	–	–	9-18
s	–	–	9-18
ʃ	–	–	9-18
θ	–	–	9-18
b	10-9	–	–
d	10-9	–	–
g	10-3, 10-4, 10-9	–	–
t	10-2, 10-3, 10-4, 10-5, 10-6	–	–
p	10-2, 10-5, 10-6	–	–
k	10-2, 10-6	–	–
dʒ	–	–	–
tʃ	10-3	–	–

GLOSSARY

Entries that are new terms or terms redefined in this text by the author are shown in bold italics. Nonbolded, italicized words within the definitions indicate a word that is defined elsewhere in this glossary.

Affricate: a compound *consonant* that begins as a stop and is released as a *fricative*, that is, /dʒ/.

Alveolar ridge: the ridge of the gum behind the upper teeth.

Amplitude: the degree of displacement of a sound wave. The greater the displacement, the greater the amplitude. Our perception of loudness is derived from amplitude.

Anterior: toward the front of a structure (opposite of *posterior*).

Aperiodic: vibrations that occur at irregular periods.

ARTF: closed-loop aural feedback used in *real-time*.

Articulators: structures in the vocal tract that can be used interactively to create speech or singing language sounds, that is, tongue, lips, teeth, *soft palate,* and hard palate.

Arytenoid: one of a pair of movable *cartilages* in the *larynx* that serve as attachment points for the vocal folds. These cartilages help shape and determine the *glottal* aperture.

Back vowel: a vowel produced by pulling the tongue back from its at-rest (neutral) position.

Bernoulli effect (principle): named after Daniel Bernoulli (pronounced /bə-nuli/), an 18th-century Swiss mathematician and physician who developed the kinetic theory of fluids (in physics, gas is considered a fluid). The principle states that, at a point of constriction, a stream of fluid (air in the case of the voice) must simultaneously undergo a decrease in pressure and an increase in particle velocity.

Benchmark: a standard by which other like things are judged.

Bilabial covering: using both lips to constrict the opening of the mouth and thus "cover" the sound, that is, attenuate the upper harmonics of the radiated sound.

Blooming: beginning a vowel with an incomplete *set* of the articulators. As the vowel progresses, the articulators continue to move until they are in the proper position for the phoneme. This effect can be heard, as well as seen on the spectrogram. Blooming can occur on vowel onsets as well as word-interior vowels.

Break: a transition point between vocal *registers*. Also see, *lift* and *passaggio*.

Cartilage: connecting tissue that is more flexible than bone.

Central vowel: a vowel produced with the tongue at or near the rest or neutral position.

Chest voice: heavy registration with particular emphasis on the formants of the lower spectrum.

Coarticulation: a state where the production of one *phoneme* influences the production of the *phonemes* on either side of it; this can result in a disturbance in the clarity and/or *timbre* of the surrounding sounds.

Complex periodic vibration: a sound that regularly repeats a pattern of simultaneously sounding *partials*.

Compression: an increase in the density of molecules.

Consonants: a class of language sounds that are not *vowels* and are executed with a partial or complete constriction of the vocal tract.

Consonant resonance: the concept of maintaining a vowel-like *resonance* behind the point of constriction or occlusion that is needed in the production of *consonants*.

Also referred to in this text by its acronym, *CR*.

Consonant shadow: a term used in the author's studio for any form of *coarticulation* caused by the presence of a consonant. In a vowel preceding a consonant, the timbre shadow can be heard when a singer "presets" some of the articulator configuration needed for the following consonant into the vowel. When vowels follow consonants, the shadow falls when a singer has failed to release the articulator set of the consonant, resulting in an improperly formed vowel.

Continuants: vocal sounds that can be sustained because the airflow in the vocal tract is not blocked. The sound can be sustained for as long as *subglottal pressure* can be maintained on one breath.

Cricothyroid: the ring-like cartilage that forms the base for the complex of laryngeal cartilages.

CR: See *consonant resonance*.

Cough: a reflex action consisting of a build-up of pressure beneath a closed *glottis* followed by a precipitous release of the pressure in an attempt to free foreign matter from the *larynx*. The action can be performed at will or subconsciously by singers who are attempting to clear *phlegm* from the vocal folds. This action is contraindicated as it can lead to *vocal fold* injury.

CV: A syllable consisting of a *consonant-to-vowel join*. Example: the syllable "me" of the word "memory."

Cycle: the interval of time comprising one complete set of regularly recurring actions.

Damped oscillation: *oscillation* in which energy is gradually lost during each *cycle* until vibratory movement ceases.

dB: abbreviation for *decibel*.

Decibel: unit of sound pressure named to honor Alexander Graham Bell's pioneering work with vocal acoustics.

Dialect: a variety of spoken language produced by geographical, political, social, or economic isolation.

Diaphragm: a large dome-shaped muscle separating the lungs from the *viscera* of the abdomen. When this muscle flexes, it moves downward, compressing the viscera. It is an important component of inspiration. It also functions as the antagonistic muscle working against the abdominal wall during *support* in singing.

Diphthong: two consecutive *vowels* occurring in the same syllable. During a spoken diphthong, the *articulators* move smoothly from the position of one vowel to the other. In singing, the shift between vowels is not gradual throughout the performance of diphthongs, as they are often sung for longer periods of time than those in speech. When this occurs, this text refers to the two sounds as *primary* and *secondary* vowels.

Dysphonia: impairment of voicing (*phonation*).

Edema: a swelling of tissue brought about by excessive fluid concentration.

EGG: abbreviation for *electroglottograph*.

Electroglottogram: the printed or recorded signal produced by an electroglottograph. See *EGG* and *electroglotograph*.

Electroglottograph: an electrical instrument used to monitor and display the behavior of the contact area between the *vocal folds*. Information is obtained by reading electrical conductance through the *larynx* in the *glottal* region. See *electroglottogram* and *EGG*.

Epiglottal tube: see *epilarynx*.

Epiglottis: the *cartilage* flap that seals the top of the *larynx* during swallowing.

Epilarynx: a small resonating region bound by the rim of the *epiglottis* and the *glottis*. This is the area where the *singer's formant* is thought to originate. The term epiglottal tube is synonymous.

Exit: the act of ceasing *phonation*.

Extent: term applied to vibrato indicating the degree of F_0 *pitch* variation from the median during a *vibrato cycle*. Also see *VExtent*.

F_0: see *fundamental*.

Falsetto: the usual term used for the voice above the *middle voice* (also called *loft* voice). This term is used in voice science but may cause confusion in the voice studio, as falsetto is also a term used for the extreme upper *register* of the male voice.

Feedback: modification of control of a process or system by its results or effects. This is different from *biofeedback*, where an external stimulus is used to acquire voluntary control of a process or system.

Formant: a vocal-tract *resonance* seen on *spectrograms* as a concentrated band of high energy.

Formant tuning: tuning the vocal resonance so the *fundamental* (F_0) or one of its *harmonics* coincides exactly with a *formant frequency* thus increasing the intensity.

F-pattern: literally, *formant* pattern, the relative placement of the formants on the sound spectrum.

Frequency: the rate of repetition of a *periodic* event. In sound, it is the number of vibrational *cycles* per second and is expressed in hertz (*Hz*). This word is not equivalent to the word *pitch*, which is a human perception of frequency.

Fricative: a *consonant* produced by constricting the vocal tract to produce *turbulence* (i.e., /f/, /v/, /s/, etc.).

Front vowel: a vowel that requires the tongue to shift forward of its at-rest (neutral) position.

Fundamental: the lowest *frequency* of a *periodic waveform*. Written as F_0.

Genioglossus: two fan-shaped muscles that radiate from the chin and insert in the tongue, attach to the sides of the *pharynx*, and insert on the *hyoid bone*.

Geniohyoid: two slender muscles that insert into the *hyoid bone* and connect to the *mandible.*

Glide: a written consonant that is actually a vowel sound, produced in transition to a following vowel (e.g., /w/ or /j/).

Glottal: pertaining to the *glottis.*

Glottis: the space between the *vocal folds.*

Glottal focus: the aperture of the *glottis* at any given point in time.

Glottal stop: the precipitous release of air pressure built behind an *occlusion* of the vocal folds. If performed chronically and with sufficient force, the use of *glottal* stops can contribute to vocal fold injury.

Glottal stroke: a transient *glottal* event where the air pressure is increased behind the occluded glottis and then released. It is a much gentler event than the glottal stop and is commonly used in language to separate *phonemes* where meaning of words might be misconstrued, for example, "some ice" being heard as "some mice" if there is not glottal stroke between the /m/ of "some" and the /ʌⁱ/ of "ice."

Harmonics: components of the sound spectrum that are an integer multiple of the *fundamental* (F_0).

Hertz: one complete cycle of a periodic vibration. Named for the physicist, Heinrich Hertz. See *Frequency* and *Hz.*

Hyoid bone: U-shaped bone at the base of the tongue that connects both the tongue and the *larynx* by means of *ligaments.*

Hz: abbreviation for *hertz.*

Inferior: below.

Insertion: the part of the muscle that attaches to a bone that it can move.

Intercostal: external and internal muscles between the ribs that are involved in the process of inhalation/exhalation.

IPA: International Phonetic Alphabet; also can refer to the International Phonetic Association.

Italianization: the utilization of the production norms of well-sung Italian to enrich and open the sounds of other languages.

Jaw elevation: the position of the jaw on the vertical plane. Jaw elevation is the major determinant of the degree of aperture of the mouth as well as *laryngeal elevation.*

Jitter: short-term (*cycle*-to-cycle) variability in the F_0.

Join: a point of change between two language sounds.

Klang: abbreviated form of the German word, "Klangfarbe" (tone color). The term is often shortened to "klang" and synonymous with the word *timbre.*

Labiodental: a *consonant* produced with the lower lip contacting the upper front teeth.

Laminar flow: airflow that moves in smooth layers over a surface. Opposite of *turbulent* air flow.

Laryngeal elevation: the relative vertical position of the larynx.

Larynx: the vocal organ, situated in the neck, which houses the vocal folds. Pronounced /lærɪŋks/ not /lærnɪks/.

Lateral: away from the center, toward the outside.

Lift: a transition point between vocal *registers.* Also see, *break, passaggio.*

Ligament: tissue that connects the articular extremities of bones.

Lingua: referring to the tongue.

Linguadental: a *consonant* produced with tongue-teeth contact.

Linguapalatal: a *consonant* produced with tongue-hard palate contact. Also called *palatal.*

Lip covering: the use of either the upper lip, lower lip, or both lips to attenuate the upper harmonics of a vocal sound (making the sound less "bright"). Also see *bilabial covering* and *lip drop.*

Lip drop: the involuntary lowering of the upper lip that produces unwanted attenuation of the upper *harmonics* of the vocal sound.

LPC: acronym for linear predictive coding; a method by which a spectrum is derived.

LTAS: acronym for long term average spectrum. This form of spectrographic analysis calculates the mean of all spectra of sounds during a relatively long sample.

Loft voice: another term for the vocal *register* above the *middle voice*. Sometimes also called *falsetto*.

Longitudinal movement: movement of the tongue on its *anterior/posterior* axis. In speech, this movement is called tongue advancement.

Mandible: the jaw.

Medial: meaning toward the center (mid-plane or midline). Mesial is a synonym for medial.

Melisma: two or more notes sung on a single syllable.

Middle voice: the voice between the chest voice and the *loft register*.

Millisecond: one-thousandth of a second. Abbreviated, ms or msec.

Model/imitation: a traditional behavior-modification technique employed in voice studios in which the voice teacher sings a passage to model proper technique for the student. The student then attempts to imitate the teacher's model. Further modifications are often needed until the desired technique has been established.

Monophthong: a single vowel that has no change of *resonance* affecting its *timbre* during the time it is produced.

Mucosal: referring to the mucous producing membranes lining the vocal tract.

Muscle memory: the ability to move a muscle system to a relatively specific point in space. The memory is acquired after many successful repetitions of the movement.

Myoelasticity: muscle elasticity; the tendency of a muscle to return to its place of rest after being moved, stretched, or tightened.

Neutral vowel: a vowel made in the center of the oral cavity. The two types of schwa, /ə/ and /ʌ/ as well as the *rhotacized schwas* are made in that region. Also see, *front* and *back vowels*.

Nodules: benign growths on the vocal folds caused by chronic voice abuse.

Occlusion: complete closure.

Offglide: the transition from a speech vowel of longer duration to one of shorter duration (e.g., /ʌⁱ/, as in the word "eye"). See *Primary/Secondary vowel*.

Onglide: the transition from a speech sound to a vowel of longer duration (e.g., /ʲɛ/, as in the word "yes"). See *Primary/Secondary vowel* and *glide*.

Onset: the act of beginning *phonation*.

Oscillation: a back-and-forth movement that is repeated.

Overtone: a component of the sound spectrum that is an integer multiple of the *fundamental* (F_0). They are numbered beginning with the first component above the fundamental (hence the word "over-"). Not to be confused with the term *partial* which includes the fundamental in the series.

Palatal: a *consonant* produced with tongue-hard palate contact. Also called *linguapalatal*.

Palatogram: a graphic representation of the degree of tongue-molar contact as viewed from below the jaw.

Partial: a component of the sound spectrum that is an integer multiple of the *fundamental* (F_0). Unlike the related term overtone, the numbering of the partials includes the fundamental in the series. See, *overtone, harmonic*.

Passaggio (plural, passaggi): two definitions occur for this word,

- The point of shift between two vocal *registers*. This is the preferred definition in the voice science literature.
- The area (usually four notes) surrounding the shift point between registers where the singer must gradually move the mode of vocal production from one register to the other. This definition is usually employed by teachers and teachers of singing. Technically, this area should be called the *zona di passaggio*.

Patter song: a type of song requiring the singer to execute long passages of notes, one to a syllable, at considerable speed. Examples include Gilbert and Sullivan's, *I am the very model of a modern major general*, and the second central section of the aria, "La vendetta" from Mozart's *Nozzi di Figaro*.

Periodic: a regularly recurring action or set of actions.

Perturbation: minor changes from expected behavior.

Pharynx: the airway in the vocal tract from the *velum* down to the top of the *larynx*.

Phlegm: a thick, semi-fluid, viscous secretion produced by the mucous membranes of the respiratory passages. Pronounced /flɛm/.

Phonation: vibration of the vocal folds during the production of vowels or *pitch consonants* (there is also a brief moment of *phonation* during the *prevoicing* of the *prevoiced* pitch *consonants* such as /b/ or /d/).

Phoneme: a unit of sound within a specific language, or a family of sounds that can signal differences in meaning within a language.

Physioacoustics: the union of the study of the anatomy and physiology of the singing voice with computer-aided analysis of vocal acoustics.

Pitch: a listener's perception of the highness or lowness of a tone, based on *frequency*.

Plosive: a synonym for stop *consonants*; sometimes called stop-plosives.

Posterior: toward the back of a structure.

Power spectrum: a type of sound analysis that produces a two-dimensional graphic. The x-axis shows *frequency* and the y-axis shows *amplitude*.

Pressed voice: *phonation* produced by a tight *glottal focus* and high *subglottal* pressure. It is a mode of *phonation* that is considered voice abuse and can lead to vocal fold injury.

Prevoiced stop: a stop *consonant* that is preceded by a prevoicing. Also see *simple stop*.

Prevoicing: momentary *phonation* that occurs prior to the release of pressure in a *prevoiced* stop. The prevoicing is performed with the vocal instrument occluded so the time that *phonation* can occur is as brief as the time required to equalize the sub- and *supraglottal* pressure. At that point in time, the built-up pressure is released as a stop *consonant*. Because the prevoicing is sung on a pitch, the *pitch* carries through the release of the pressure component.

Primary and **Secondary vowels:** the two *monophthongs* of a diphthong as executed while singing. In singing, the primary vowel is sustained for a longer period of time than its corollary in a spoken diphthong. The secondary vowel is the monophthong that takes minimal execution time in a sung diphthong. These terms, suggested by the author, are meant to replace the speech terms, *onglide, offglide*, and nucleus, when discussing sung diphthongs. In this text, the secondary vowel of the diphthong is indicated by superscripting (i.e., /ʌⁱ/ as in the word "my").

Ramus: the vertical, *posterior* part of the jaw that articulates with the skull.

Rarefaction: a decrease in the density of molecules.

Rate: term applied to vibrato indicating the number of vibrato *cycles* per second. Also see *Vrate*.

Real-time: a result that appears virtually simultaneously with its cause. A *spectrogram* is said to running in real-time when the lag between the sound produced by the subject and its appearance on the monitor is short enough that the subject does not sense the lag.

Register: a scalar area of the voice that has equal (or similar) *timbre*.

Resonance: the vibratory response to an applied force.

Resonator: a physical entity that is set into vibration by the proximity of another vibration. In the human voice, the resonator consists of all the empty, air-filled *supraglottal* spaces.

Rhotic; rhoticized: a vowel sound produced with r-coloring.

Rhoticized schwa: a schwa /ə/ produced with a slight /r/ color /ɚ/ .

Risorius: a narrow band of muscle fibers inserted into the tissue at the corners of the mouth.

RTF: real-time feedback. Also see, *ARTF* and *VRTF*.

Sagittal: an imaginary slice down the center of the anatomy as viewed from the side.

Schwa: the neutral, unstressed vowel, /ə/. Also see, *unstressed* and *rhoticized schwa*.

Scrolling: the ribbon-like display of a *real-time spectrogram*.

Secondary vowel: see *Primary/Secondary vowels*.

Semivowel: a *consonant* that has vowel-like *resonance*.

Set: The placement of *articulators* in the vocal instrument during the singing of a *phoneme* at a given point in time.

Shimmer: short-term variability of *amplitude* (*cycle*-to-cycle).

Simple harmonic motion: smoothest possible back-and-forth motion.

Simple stop: *Stop* consonants that have no pitch element (i.e., /t/, /k/, and /p/). Also see *prevoiced stop*.

Singer's formant: an area of vocal *resonance* in the area between 2.3 and 3.5 kHz that singers call "ring" or "point." It is a brilliance in the voice that is principally associated with Western concert and operatic singing styles.

Skill accelerando: the author's pedagogical technique in which a sung phrase is slowed down far from the actual tempo of the piece in order to give the singer time to think about and habitualize phonemic joins. As the singer is able to sing the entire line, the tempo is increased gradually until it can be sung at speed with all of the technical norms in place.

Soft palate: the velum, *posterior* roof of the mouth made up of soft tissue.

Sound: the movement of a specific type of energy in waves through a medium such as air.

Spectrogram: a three-dimensional graphic representation of the analysis of sound showing time on the horizontal axis, *frequency* on the vertical axis, and *amplitude* as intensity of color or grayscale. If the spectrogram is running in *real-time*, it is said to be scrolling.

Spectrograph: the apparatus or computer software that produces a *spectrogram*.

Spike: the thin vertical component of the spectrographic display that results from the performance of a *transient* (such as the *consonant* /t/).

Spreading: the use of oral structures on the horizontal plane instead of the vertical plane.

Stop or **Stop consonant:** a *consonant* produced by building air pressure behind an *occlusion* of the vocal cavity and then suddenly releasing that pressure. See *simple stop* and *prevoiced stop*.

Stop gap: term used in conjunction with either stop or affricate *consonants* corresponding to the closure of the *articulators* and the consequent accumulation of pressure before the release of the consonant.

Structured building: the author's pedagogical technique in which a sung phrase is reduced to only the vowels, then pitch consonants are added, and finally all phonemes are sung. The technique gives the singer a chance to build the production norms slowly and carefully.

Subglottal: airway structures below the *glottis.*

Subglottal pressure: pressure of the air stream below the *glottis.*

Superior: above.

Support: the abdominal muscles exerting inward and upward pressure on the abdominal *viscera,* simultaneously opposed by the *diaphragm* (the muscle of antagonism). Support provides much of the *subglottal* air pressure needed in singing.

Supraglottal: areas above the *glottis.*

Target undershoot: in a change of *phoneme,* falling short of the ideal formant pattern for the second phoneme because of phonetic context. In cases of *target undershoot,* the *F-pattern* is close enough to the ideal model that the listener can still understand the sound and place it into context.

Timbre: the unique quality of sound as determined by the relative *amplitude* of its *harmonics.*

Toggle exercise: an exercise where a subject alternates between two modes of production to discover the differences between the two. An example would be to alternate between an /a/ produced too far forward in the oral cavity with one produced at an optimal point.

Tone generator: a vibratory sound source. In the human voice, the tone generator is the *larynx,* in particular, the paired system of the vocal folds found within that organ.

Transient: not lasting, a very brief vocal event such as the production of /t/.

Transliterate: to represent the sounds of a language by a system of symbols different from those employed in the everyday written language. *IPA* is the preferred method of transliterating language sounds in the speech and voice science literature. Example: the English word "noise" is transliterated in *IPA* as, /nɔiz/. Transliteration can also be called phonetic transcription.

Triphthong: three consecutive vowels that constitute the same syllable.

Turbulence: the opposite of *laminar* when speaking of airflow. Airflow that is turbulent contains eddies or vortices, whirlpools or rotating particles of air.

Turbulent: the state of *turbulence.*

Unstressed schwa: the *neutral vowel* /ə/. See *schwa.*

Unvoiced: a language sound made without *phonation* (possessing no *pitch*). Synonymous with *voiceless.*

Uvula: the cone-shaped lobe of the lower *medial* border of the *velum.*

VC: A syllable consisting of a vowel changing to a *consonant.* Example: the syllable "em" of the word "memory."

Velum: the region of the *soft palate* and adjacent nasopharynx. In language, the *posterior* velum closes the *velo-pharyngeal port* during swallowing and language production. This closure is necessary for the production of most *vowels* and *consonants.* Also see *pharynx.*

VExtent: shorthand for vibrato extent, the amount of F_0 *pitch* variation above and below the mean *frequency* line.

Velo-pharyngeal port: the region of the nasopharynx that forms a passageway from the nasal cavities to the *pharynx.* This area can be closed by the *posterior velum.*

Vibration: the oscillating motion of a fluid or elastic solid in which the equilibrium has been disturbed. The disturbance of the equilibrium of the material radiates sound energy. In humans, the vocal folds vibrate to create the sound source used in the creation of language sounds as well as the pitched tones needed for singing.

Vibrato: a 4–6 *Hz* undulation of the singing voice occurring in both *pitch* and *frequency*.

Viscera: the stomach and the intestines (soft compressible tissues) in the abdomen.

Vocal cords: common usage synonym for *vocal folds*; vocal fold is the preferred usage.

Vocal folds: a paired system of structures in the *larynx* consisting of muscle and mucous membranes. The vocal folds are the source of *phonation* for the voice.

Vocal fry: The extreme low end of the singing range; an oscillation of the vocal folds that produces periodic disturbances in the air stream with perceived temporal gaps. This type of vocalization is not considered as one of the norms of good singing but can be used by a skilled practitioner to simulate extreme low notes (especially when employed by Slavic basses). Also called "pulse voice" or "Strohbass."

Vocal tract: all of the anatomical structures needed for speech/song production. These structures include the trachea, *larynx*, *pharynx*, oral cavity, and nasal cavity.

Vocalize: a pedagogical or warmup exercise involving sung sounds. Most singers utilize a *vowel vocalize*, an exercise that is sung exclusively on vowels.

Voice box: common usage for word *larynx*.

Voice onset time (VOT): the interval between the release of a *stop consonant* and the beginning of *phonation* for the following vowel.

Voiced: a language sound made with *phonation* of the *vocal folds* (has *pitch*). Also see *unvoiced and voiceless*.

Voiceless: synonym for *unvoiced*, that is, a language sound made without *phonation* of the vocal folds.

Voice practitioner: anyone who has a higher level involvement with the singing voice. The term is an all-purpose inclusive that applies to singers, voice teachers, coaches, teachers of vocal pedagogy, vocal pathologists working with singers, and so forth.

VOT: see *voice onset time*.

Vowel-color: Another term for the vowel *timbre* or *klang*.

VRate: the *frequency* of the *oscillation* of the *vibrato* given in *Hz*.

VRTF: Visual real-time feedback. See *RTF* and *ARTF*.

Waveform: graphic representations of vibration that plot *amplitude* versus time.

Wobble: normally defined as a *vibrato rate* in the 2- to 4-*Hz* range, coupled with an *extent* greater than ±3%. At these parameters, the brain of the listener can no longer average the extent into one tone and begins to perceive the vibrato as an *oscillation* of two notes (±3% = ± .5 semitone).

REFERENCES

Alexander, F. M. (1974). *The Alexander Technique: The essential writings of F. Matthias Alexander.* London: Thames and Hudson.

Appelman, D. R. (1967). *The science of vocal pedagogy, theory and application.* Bloomington, IN: Indiana University Press.

Bartholomew, W. T. (1934). A physical definition of "good voice quality." *Journal of the Acoustical Society of America, 6,* 25–33.

Basmajian, J. V. (1982). Clinical use of biofeedback in rehabilitation. *Psychosomatics, 23*(1), 67–69.

Benade, A. (1976/1990). *Fundamentals of musical acoustics.* New York: Dover Publications.

Bernac, P. (1970). *The interpretation of French song* (W. Radford, trans.). New York: W. W. Norton & Company.

Bilodeau, E. A., Bilodeau, I. M., & Schumsky, D. A. (1959). Some effects of introducing and withdrawing knowledge of results early and late in practice. *Journal of Experimental Psychology, 58,* 142–144.

Borden, G. J., Harris, K. S. & Raphael, L. J. (1994). *Speech science primer: Physiology, acoustics and perception of speech* (3rd ed). Baltimore, MD: Williams & Wilkins.

Carter, M. C., & Shapiro, D. C. (1984). Control of sequential movements: Evidence for generalized motor programs. *Journal of Neurophysiology, 52,* 787–796.

Chiba, R., & Kajiyama, M. (1946). *The vowel: Its nature and structure.* Tokyo: Phonetic Society of Japan.

Curry, F. (1967). A comparison of left-handed and right-handed subjects on verbal and non-verbal listening tasks. *Cortex, 8,* 343–352.

Damasio, A. R. (1989). Time-locked multiregional retroactivation: A systems-level proposal for the neural substrates of recall and recognition. *Cognition, 33,* 25–62.

Dewey, G. (1971). *English spelling: Roadblock to reading.* New York: Teachers College Press.

Dmitriev, L., & Kiselev, A. (1979). Relationship between the formant structure of different types of singing voices and the dimension of supraglottal cavities. *Folia Phoniatrica, 31,* 238–241.

Doscher, B. (1994). *The functional unity of the singing voice* (2nd ed.). Lanham, MD: The Scarecrow Press, Inc.

Edwards, H. T. (1997). *Applied phonetics* (2nd ed.). San Diego: Singular Publishing Group.

Epstein, S. (1994). Integration of the cognitive and psychodynamic unconscious. *American Psychologist, 49,* 709–724.

Estill, J. (1995). *Voice craft: A user's guide to voice quality.* Copyright Estill Voice Training Systems.

Estill, J., Baer, T., Honda, J., & Harris, C. (1983). Supralaryngeal activity in a study of six voice qualities. In *Proceedings of the Stockholm Music Acoustics Conference, Sweden 1,* pp. 157–174.

Fant, G. (1960). *Acoustic theory of speech production.* The Hague: Mouton.

Fitts, P. M., & Posner, M. I. (1967). *Human performance.* Belmont, CA: Brooks/Cole.

Garcia, M. (1984). *Hints on singing* (B. Garcia, trans.). New York: Edward Schuberth Co.

Hakes, J., Doherty, T., & Shipp, T. (1990). Trillo rates exhibited by professional early music singers. *Journal of Voice, 4,* 148–156.

Henderson, C., with Palmer, C. (1940). *How to sing for money.* New York: Harcourt, Brace and Company.

Hirano, M. (1995). Physiological aspects of vibrato. In P. H. Dejonckere, M. Hirano, & J. Sundberg (Eds.), *Vibrato.* San Diego, CA: Singular Publishing Group.

Jacoby, L. L., & Dallas, M. (1981). On the relationship between autobiographical memory and perceptual learning. *Journal of Experimental Psychology: General, 110,* 306–340.

Kandel, E. R., Schwartz, J. H., & Jessell, T. M. (1991). *Principles of neural science* (3rd ed.). Norwalk, CT: Appleton & Lange.

Kantner, C. E., & West, R. W. (1960). *Phonetics, an introduction to the principles of phonetic science from the point of view of English speech.* New York: Harper.

Keefe, M., & Dalton, R. (1989). An analysis of velopharyngeal timing in normal adult speakers using a microcomputer based photodetector system. *Journal of Speech Hearing Research, 32,* 39–48.

Kent, R. D. (1997) *The speech sciences.* San Diego, CA: Singular Publishing Group.

Kent R. D., & Read, C. (1992). *The acoustic analysis of speech.* San Diego, CA: Singular Publishing Group.

Kimura, D. (1964). Left-right differences in the perception of melodies. *Journal of Experimental Psychology, 16,* 355–358.

Krebs, D. E., & Behr, D. W. (1994). Biofeedback. In S. B. O'Sullivan & T. J. Schmitz (Eds.), *Physical rehabilitation: Assessment and treatment procedures.* New York: F. A. Davis.

Kreiman, J., Gerratt, B. R., Kempster, G. B., Erman, A., & Berke, G. S. (1993). Perceptual evaluation of voice quality: Review, tutorial, and a framework for future research. *Journal of Speech and Hearing Research, 36,* 21–40.

Kuehn. D. (1976). A cineradiographic investigation of velar movement variables in two normals. *Cleft Palate Journal, 13,* 88–103.

Lehmann, L. (1903). *How to sing.* New York: Macmillan. As cited in R. Miller (1997).

Marchesi, M. (1970). *Bel canto: A theoretical and practical vocal method* (P. L. Miller, Ed.). New York: Dover Publications.

Marshall, M. (1953). *The singer's manual of English diction.* New York: Schirmer Books.

McKinney, J. C. (1982). *The diagnosis and correction of vocal faults.* Nashville, TN: Grenevox.

Miller, D., & Doing, J. (1998). Male passaggio and the upper extension in the light of visual feedback. *Journal of Singing, 54*(1), 3–14.

Miller, D. G., & Schutte, H. K. (1986). The effect of F_0/F_1 coincidence in soprano high notes on pressure at the glottis. *Journal of Phonetics, 14,* 385–392.

Miller, D. G., & Schutte, H. K. (1990). Feedback from spectrum analysis applied to the singing voice. *Journal of Voice, 4,* 329–334.

Miller, D. G., & Schutte, H. K. (1993). Physical definition of the "flageolet register." *Journal of Voice, 7*(3), 206–212.

Miller, D. G., & Schutte, H. K. (1994). Toward a definition of male "head" register, passaggio, and "cover" in Western operatic singing. *Folia Phoniatrica Logopaedica, 46,* 157–170.

Miller, D. G., Sulter, A. M., Schutte, H. K., & Wolf, R. F. (1997). Comparison of vocal tract formants in singing and nonperiodic phonation. *Journal of Voice, 11*(1), 1–11.

Miller, R. (1977). *English, French, German and Italian techniques of singing: A study in national tonal preferences and how they relate to functional efficiency.* Metuchen, NJ: The Scarecrow Press.

Miller, R. (1986). *The structure of singing: System and art in vocal techique.* New York: Schirmer Books.

Miller, R. (1998). The singing teacher in the age of voice science. In R. T. Sataloff (Ed.), *Vocal health and pedagogy.* San Diego, CA: Singular Publishing Group.

Milner, B. (1962). Les troubles de la memoire accompagnant des lesions hippocampique bilaterales [Memory problems accompanying bilateral hippocampal lesions]. In P. Passouant (Ed.), *Physiologie de l'hippocampique.* Paris: Centre National de la Recherche Scientifique.

Moriarty, J. (1975). *Diction*. Boston: E. C. Schirmer Music Company.

Neely, J. H. (1977). Semantic priming and retrieval from lexical memory: Roles of inhibitionless spreading activation and limited-capacity attention. *Journal of Experimental Psychology: General, 106*, 226–254.

Oxendine, J. P. (1984). *Psychology of motor learning* (2nd ed.). Englewood Cliffs, NJ: Prentice-Hall.

Peterson, G. E., & Lehiste, I. (1961).Transitions, glides, and diphthongs. *Journal of the Acoustical Society of America, 33*, 268–277.

Posner, M. I., & Snyder, C. R. R. (1975). Facilitation and inhibition in the processing of signals. In P. M. A. Rabbitt & S. Dornie (Eds.), *Attention and performance V*. New York: Academic Press.

Raibert, M. H. (1977). *Motor control and learning by the state-space model* (*Technical Report, Artificial Intelligence Laboratory*, AI - TR-439). Boston, MA: Massachusetts Institute of Technology.

Ramig, L., & Shipp, T. (1987). Cinoaratuve measures of vocal tremor and vocal vibrato. *Journal of Voice, 1*(2), 162–167.

Reid, C. (n.d.). *A dictionary of vocal terminology: An analysis*. New York: Joseph Patelson Music House.

Salmon, D. P., & Butters, N. (1995). Neurobiology of skill and habit learning. *Current Opinion in Neurobiology, 5*, 184–190.

Sataloff, R. T. (1997). *Professional voice, the science and art of clinical care* (2nd ed.). San Diego, CA: Singular Publishing Group.

Sataloff, R. T. (1998). *Vocal health and pedagogy*. San Diego, CA: Singular Publishing Group.

Sataloff, R. T., Spiegel, J. R., & Rosen, D. C. (1998). The effects of age on the voice. In R. T. Sataloff (Ed.), V*ocal health and pedagogy*. San Diego, CA: Singular Publishing Group.

Schmidt, R. A. (1987). The acquisition of skill: Some modifications to the perception-action relationship through practice. In H. Heuer & A. Sanders (Eds.), *Perspectives on perception and action*. Hillsdale, NJ: Lawrence Erlbaum Associates.

Schmidt, R. A. (1988). *Motor control and learning*. Champaign, IL: Human Kinetics Publishers.

Schmidt, R. A., Lange, C., & Young, D. E. (1990). Optimizing summary knowledge of results for skill learning. *Human Movement Science, 9*, 325–348.

Schutte, H. K., & Miller, D. G. (1986). The effect of F_0/F_1 coincidence in soprano high notes on pressure at the glottis. *Journal of Phonetics, 14*, 385–392.

Schutte, H. K., Miller, D. G., & Svec, J. G. (1995). Measurement of formant frequencies and bandwidths in singing. *Journal of Voice, 9*(3), 290–296.

Scoville, W. B., & Milner, B. (1957). Loss of recent memory after bilateral hippocampal lesions. *Journal of Neurology, Neurosurgery, and Psychiatry, 20*, 11–21.

Shaffer, L. H. (1980). Analyzing piano performance. A study of concert pianists. In G. E. Stelmach & J. Requin (Eds.), *Tutorials in motor behavior*. Amsterdam: North Holland.

Shaffer, L. H. (1984). Timing in solo and duet piano performances. *Quarterly Journal of Experimental Psychology, 16A*, 577–595.

Shuster, L., Ruscello, D. M., & Smith, K. D. (1992). Evoking [r] using visual feedback. *American Journal of Speech-Language Pathology, 1*(3), 29–34.

Squire, L. R., & Moore, R. Y. (1979). Dorsal thalamic lesions in a noted case of chronic memory dysfunction. *Annals of Neurology, 6*, 503–506.

Strange, W., & Jenkins, J. J. (1978). The role of linguistic experience in the perception of speech. In R. D. Walk and H. L. Pick (Eds.), *Perception and experience* (pp. 125–169). New York: Plenum Press.

Sundberg, J. (1972). *An articulatory interpretation of the "singing formant."* (Quarterly Progress Status Report, Vol. 1, 45–53). Stockholm: Speech Transmission Laboratory.

Sundberg, J. (1972). Production and function of the singing formant. *Report of the 11th Congress of the International Musicological Society*, Copenhagen, *2*, 679–88.

Sundberg, J. (1974). Articulatory interpretation of the "singing formant." *Journal of the Acoustical Society of America, 55*, 838–84.

Sundberg, J. (1977, March). The acoustics of the singing voice. *Scientific American*, 82–91.

Sundberg, J. (1978). Synthesis of singing. *Swedish Journal of Musicology, 60*, 107.

Sundberg, J. (1987). *The science of the singing voice*. DeKalb, IL: Northern Illinois University Press.

Teager, H. M., & Teager, S. M. (1992). Evidence for nonlinear sound production mechanisms in the vocal tract. In W. J. Hardcastle & A. Marchal (Eds.), *Speech production and speech modelling* (pp. 241–261). Dordrecht, Netherlands: Kluwer.

Terzuolo, C. A., & Viviani, P. (1979). The central representation of learning motor programs. In R. E. Talbot & D. R. Humphrey (Eds.), *Posture and movement.* New York: Raven Press.

The concise Oxford dictionary of current English (6th ed.). (1976). Oxford: Oxford at the Clarendon Press.

Titze, I. R. (1994). *Principles of voice production.* Englewood Cliffs, NJ: Prentice Hall.

Titze, I. R. (1998). The wide pharynx. *Journal of Singing, 55*(1), 27–28.

Vennard, W. (1967). *Singing, the mechanism and the technic.* New York: Carl Fischer.

Verdolini, K. (1997). Principles of skill acquisition applied to voice training. In M. Hampton & B. Acker (Eds.), *The vocal vision: Views on voice.* New York: Applause.

Victor, M., Adams, R. D., & Collins, G. H. (1971). *The Wernicke-Korsakoff syndrome.* Philadelphia: F. A. Davis.

Wall, J., & Caldwell, R. (1996). *The singer's voice: The vocal tract* (videotape). Available from PST...Inc.

Wulf, G., Schmidt, R. A., & Duebel, H. (1993). Reduced feedback frequency enhances generalized motor program learning but not parameterization learning. *Journal of Experimental Psychology: Learning, Memory, and Cognition, 19*(5), 1134–1150.

Yanagisawa, E., Estill, J., Kmucha, S. T., & Leder, S. B. (1989). The contribution of aryteplglottic constriction to "ringing" voice quality: A videolaryngoscopic study with acoustic analysis. *Journal of Voice, 3,* 342–350.

Young, D. E., & Schmidt, R. A. (1992). Augmented kinematic feedback for motor learning. *Journal of Motor Behavior, 24*(3), 261–273.

Zemlin, W. R. (1998). *Speech and hearing science: Anatomy and physiology* (4th ed.). Boston: Allyn & Bacon.

Zola-Morgan, S., Squire, L. R., & Mishkin, M. (1982). The neuroanatomy of amnesia: Amygdala-hippocampus versus temporal stem. *Science, 218,* 1337–1339.

SUGGESTED READING

For those readers unfamiliar with voice science, the following reading list may help in their quest for greater knowledge. Of course, this field changes month-to-month and the vocal practitioner must update the knowledge by reading the journals applicable to both speech and voice. But, this list is a good starting point.

Books, Based on Voice Science, Written by Voice Teachers

Appelman, D. R. (1967). *The science of vocal pedagogy, theory and application.* Bloomington, IN: Indiana University Press.

There is much to be gleaned from this venerable work. The x-ray imagery at the end of the book is worth the purchase alone.

Doscher, B. (1994). *The functional unity of the singing voice* (2nd ed.). Lanham, MD: The Scarecrow Press, Inc.

An excellent, general look at vocal production by a voice teacher steeped in voice science.

Miller, R. (1986). *The structure of singing: System and art in vocal technique.* New York: Schirmer Books.

Miller's classic book, is mostly about his personal view of vocal pedagogy but it is a work that is thoroughly informed by voice science.

Vennard, W. (1967). *Singing, the mechanism and the technic.* New York: Carl Fischer.

This is the book that started the author's foray into voice science and also gave him the first idea that the spectrogram might be useful in the everyday voice studio. Considering when this book was written, it is filled with the science that existed up to that time and much of it still applies to our practice today.

Books About Vocal Health

Sataloff, R. T. (1997). *Professional voice, the science and art of clinical care* (2nd ed.). San Diego, CA: Singular Publishing Group.

This book, and its companion, *Vocal Health and Pedagogy,* are ground zero for any singer desiring to know about the healthy workings of the voice. It should be on the reference shelf of every voice teacher and singer.

Sataloff, R. T. (1998). *Vocal health and pedagogy.* San Diego, CA: Singular Publishing Group.

Books by Voice Scientists

Baken, R. J. (1996). *Clinical measurement of speech and voice.* San Diego, CA: Singular Publishing Group.

This work quickly became a classic. It is a thorough examination of instrumentation and methods for studying the voice. Voice practitioners who wish to know more about the instruments and techniques applied to them should own this book.

Sundberg, J. (1987). *The science of the singing voice.* DeKalb, IL: Northern Illinois University Press.

When one thinks of voice scientists, the names Sundberg and Titze loom as the giants of the field. This engaging book is packed with knowledge about the singing voice.

Titze, I. R. (1994). *Principles of voice production.* Englewood Cliffs, NJ: Prentice Hall.

This is a highly technical book, filled with mathematical equations. When read after Sundberg's book, it can take one a bit deeper into the physics of the voice. If the reader has no physics background, it can be slow reading. Since I have no physics background, I borrowed the talents of some of my math and physics major students, and came away both humbled and enlightened.

Books by Speech Scientists Particularly Helpful to the Singer

Borden, G. J., Harris, K. S., & Raphael, L. J. (1994). *Speech science primer: Physiology, acoustics and perception of speech* (3rd ed). Baltimore, MD: Williams & Wilkins.

Perhaps the best introduction to speech and speech science. This book is a classic textbook that is used in countless classes as the beginning point in the speech sciences.

The following three books should be on every vocal practitioner's shelf.

Edwards, H. T. (1997). *Applied phonetics* (2nd ed.). San Diego: Singular Publishing Group.

This book is a must for every singer who is interested in phonetics. Every entry is packed with information about its subject phoneme, and the education that it affords will bring many rewards to the reader.

Kent R. D., & Read, C. (1992). *The acoustic analysis of speech.* San Diego, CA: Singular Publishing Group.

A helpful adjunct to *Voice Tradition and Technology.* In some respects, some of the reasoning behind both books is the same; both attempt to teach about spectrography and show basic principles of vocal production.

Kent, R. D. (1997) *The speech sciences.* San Diego, CA: Singular Publishing Group.

There is no collection of illustrations currently on the market that can come close to the excellence of this book. The author passed this book up on many occasions thinking that it was primarily for the speech field. Everything in this book applies to the singing voice, and the illustrations will make fundamental principles of anatomy, physiology, physics, and phonetics clear to the reader. It belongs in the voice studio as a reference.

Journals

Journal of Singing (The Official Journal of the National Association of Teachers of Singing). James E. McKinney (Ed.). Published 5 times per year. San Diego: Singular Publishing Group.

Journal of Voice (The Official Journal of the Voice Foundation). Robert T. Sataloff (Ed.). Published quarterly. San Diego: Singular Publishing Group.

INDEX

of musical sound, 189–191
and spectrogram, 79–81
  playing displays, 80–81
as tool for vowel identity work, 99–101
PPAF. *See* Postperformance aural feedback
Prephonation airflow, 256
Pressed voice, 105–106
spectrographic evidence, 105
Pressure
subglottal, 38
supraglottal, 38
Prevoiced stops, 156, 160–162
nature of, 161–162
voice bars, 160–161
and VOT, 162
Primary vowel, 116
Primo passaggio, problems in, 173
Professionalism of voice studio, 262–263
Professionals, improved communication
      among, 17
Prosody and rate control of pitch, 253

Q

Quality of voice in speech and singing, 230

R

/r/-colored schwa, 121–122
Range, table of, 171
Rarefaction, definition of, 23
Real-time
computer-aided feedback in studio, 1–2
definition of, 15
digital feedback in, 16–17
software-produced acoustic analysis in,
      16–17
Real-time exercises in Gram. *See* Gram,
      learning
Real-time feedback, for speech. *See* Speech
Recordings
causing shifting standards of diction, 56–57
influence on standards of diction, 56
resonance strategies determined from,
      204–205
universalization of diction, 56
utilizing for research, 10
Registers, table of, 171
Reid, Cornelius, 11
Relative timing of consonants and vowels, 229
Release burst, 159–160
Release of simple stops, 158–160
Reliability, definition of, 236
Resonance
"ch" class consonants, 164

collapse, 112–113
creation checklist, 167
laryngeal elevation, low, 124
mandible, low, 122–123
pharynx open and relaxed, 123
set of lips, 123
tongue configuration, 123
velum raised, 123
definition, 35
interaction between and sound source, 31
resonator
definition of, 30
kinds of resonators, 30
reshaping, 42
singer's formant, 46–47
source-filter theory, 42–43
schematic of, 43
strategies
determined from commercial recording,
      204–205
effective adjustment of formant
      frequencies, 195–207
sympathetic vibration and resonance,
      30–31
TMJ syndrome and, 62
vocal tract, 35, 41–48, 191–193
articulators, 42
definition of resonator, 41
formants and vowels, 191–192
higher formants, 192–193
identifying formants in power spectrum,
      193
resonating space exercise, 42
source-filter theory, 42–44
Resonating space exercise, 42
Resonator. *See* Resonance
Respiration and voice, 249–251
Retroflex /ɹ/, 140–141
Rhoticized schwa. *See* Schwar

S

S/Z ratio, 250
SAS exercise, 51–53
Sagan, Carl, 7
Sagittal views of the vocal resonator
Appelman's X-ray images, 93
articulators, 61
general view showing regions and
      articulators, 41
/a/, 45, 96
/æ/, 95
/e/, 95
/ɛ/, 95
/i/, 45, 86, 88, 95, 97

bass-itis, 106
breathiness, 105
excessive lip rounding, 107–109
exits, 112–114
glottal stop and stroke, 183–186
high voice, problem of, 180–181
inhalation problems, 181–183
jaw elevation as major coarticulative
    problem, 101–102
lip covering, 106–107
lip rounding, excessive, 107–108
onsets, 109–112
other uses for, 186–187
passaggio issues, 169–175
schwa, mastering production of, 120–121
spreading, 60, 103–105
tight glottal aperture, 105–106
tongue massing, 106
vertical configuration, 89–90
    spread production, 89
vibrato, 175–180
word-interior vowel blooming, 102–103
X-axis, 29, 79
Y-axis, 79
Spectral analyzer, use of as possible solution
    for vocal problems, 235–236
Spectrograms of phonemes. *See* Appendix E
Spectrum analysis. *See* Power Spectrum
Speech
    learning from speech science, 53–54
    necessary translation for singing, 53–54
    pitch
        and loudness, duration of , 228–229
        prosody and rate control, 253
        range, 251–253
        targeting, 253
    real-time feedback.
        delay, 244
        display modes, 244
        parameters, 245–246
        signal acquisition, 244
        simple arithmetic, 245
    and singing terms, possible confusion
        between, 164
    and song science, new terminology for, 12
Speech and singing, similarity and differences
        between, 228–231
    differences, 51
    coarticulation, 229–230
    loudness and pitch, duration of, 228–229
    neural substrates, 230–231
    relative timing, 229
    summary, 238–239
    two template model, 50–51, 231–233, 235
    voice quality, 230

Speech habit interference, 241–242
Speech interference
    challenge, 235
    hypothesis, 231–233
    solution for, 233
Speech template, 50–51, 231–233, 235
Speech and voice therapy tasks adapted to
        Gram
    articulatory accuracy, 246–249
        fricatives, 249
        plosives, 246, 248–249
        targeting vowels and vocalic continuants,
            246
    configured, 257–258
    pitch, 251–253
        prosody and rate control, 253
        range, 251–253
    reduction of vocal hyperfunction, hard
            glottal attack, 256–257
        alternate voiced and unvoiced
            continuant cognate pairs, 256
        prephonation airflow, 256
        whispered onset, 256
        yawn-sign technique, 256
    vocal coordination and control, 253–255
        continuous phonation, 253–254
        effort closure exercises, 255
        vocal clarity, 254–255
    voice and respiration, 249–251
        duration, 249–251
        intensity, 251
Spreading, 59, 60, 103–105, 129, 132, 155
    correcting, 132
    definition, 129
    observing on spectrogram, 89, 106
    photo of mouth configuration, 129
Staccato ASAI onsets, 110
Standardized vocal terminology, 11
Standardization of vocal sounds
    shifts in, 56
Standing wave, singing and, 216, 218
State-of-the-art voice studio, creating. *See*
        Voice studio, creating state-of-the-art
Stop, glottal, 48, 185
Stops, 156, 157–160, 246, 248–249
    gap, 157–158
    glottal, 48, 185
    prevoiced, 160–162
        definition, 156
        nature of prevoicing, 161–162
        onset, 157–158
        prevoiced stops and VOT, 162
        voice bars, 160–161
    release of, 158–160
        release burst, 159–160